The Ultimate Lean and Green Cookbook 2021

500+ Lean & Green Meals and Fueling Snacks to enjoy Everyday. The Most Comprehensive Cookbook to Make Weight Loss and Fat Burning Easy for lifelong results

Rachel Kim

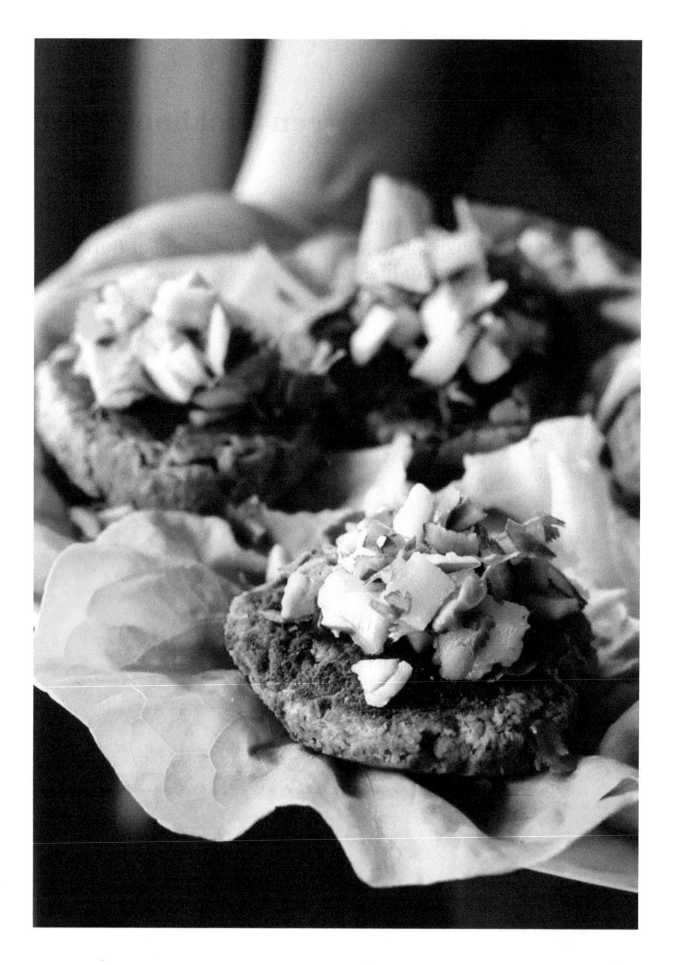

Table Of Contents

BREKFAST RECIPES

1. Avocado Toast with Eggs

Prep Time: 15 min | **Cook Time:** 4 min | **Serve:** 4
- 1 large avocado, peeled, pitted, and chopped roughly ¼ teaspoon fresh lemon juice
- Salt and ground pepper, as required 4 whole-wheat bread slices
- 4 boiled eggs, peeled and sliced

1. In a bowl, add the avocado and, with a fork, mash roughly.
2. Add the lemon juice, salt, and black pepper and stir to combine well. Set aside.
3. Heat a nonstick pan on meedium/high heat and toast 1 slice for about 2 minutes per side.
4. Repeat with the remaining slices.
5. Arrange the slices onto serving plates.
6. Spread the avocado mixture over each slice evenly.
7. Top each with egg slices and serve immediately.

Nutrition: Calories: 206, Fat: 13.9g, Carbohydrates: 14g, Fiber: 4.5g, Sugar: 1.4g, Protein: 9.6g

2. Toast with Egg & Asparagus

Prep Time: 10 min | **Cook Time:** 6 min | **Serve:** 2
- Olive oil cooking spray
- 10 asparagus spears
- 1 teaspoon olive oil
- 2 large eggs
- 2 large sourdough bread slices, toasted Salt and ground black pepper, as required 1 teaspoon fresh rosemary leaves

1. Heat a griddle pan with cooking spray and heat over high heat.
2. Place the asparagus and cook for about 2-3 minutes per side.
3. Transfer the asparagus onto a plate and drizzle with a little oil.
4. Meanwhile, in a large pan, add the water and a little salt and bring to a boil over high heat.
5. Adjust the heat to low.
6. Carefully crack the eggs in the simmering water and cook for about 3 minutes.
7. With a slotted spoon, transfer the eggs onto a paper towel-lined plate to drain.
8. Divide the bread slices onto serving plates.

9. Top each slice with asparagus spears, followed by 1 egg.
10. Sprinkle with salt and black pepper and serve with the garnishing of rosemary.

Nutrition: Calories: 157, Fat: 7.5g, Carbohydrates: 14g, Fiber: 1.9g, Sugar: 1.9g, Protein: 9.8g

3.Eggs in Bell Pepper Rings

Prep Time: 10 min | **Cook Time:** 6 min | **Serve:** 2

- Olive oil cooking spray
- 1 pepper, seeded and cut into 4 (¼-inch) rings
- 4 eggs
- Salt and ground black pepper, as required ¼ teaspoon dried parsley, crushed

1. Heat a nonstick pan with cooking spray and heat over medium heat.
2. Place 4 bell pepper rings in the pan and cook for about 2 minutes.
3. Carefully flip the rings.
4. Crack an egg of each bell pepper ring and sprinkle with salt and black pepper.
5. Cook for about 2-4 minutes or until the desired doneness of eggs.
6. Carefully transfer the bell pepper rings on serving plates and serve with the garnishing of parsley.

Nutrition: Calories: 139, Fat: 8.9g, Carbohydrates: 3.6g, Fiber: 1.1g, Sugar: 2.2g, Protein: 11.7g

4.Spinach Waffles

Prep Time: 10 min | **Cook Time:** 20 min | **Serve:** 4

- 1 large egg, beaten
- 1 cup ricotta cheese, crumbled
- ½ cup part-skim Mozzarella cheese, shredded ¼ cup low-fat Parmesan cheese, grated
- 4 ounces spinach, thawed and squeezed dry
- 1 garlic clove, minced
- Salt and ground black pepper, as required

1. Preheat and then grease the mini waffle iron.
2. Add cheeses, spinach, garlic, salt, and black pepper in a medium mixing bowl and mix until well blended.
3. Place ¼ of the mixture into preheated waffle iron and cook for about 4-5 minutes or until golden brown.
4. Repeat with the remaining mixture.

Nutrition: Calories: 138, Fat: 8.1g, Carbohydrates: 4.8g, Fiber: 0.6g, Sugar: 0.4g, Protein: 11.7g

5.Kale Scramble

Prep Time: 10 min | **Cook Time:** 6 min | **Serve:** 2

- 4 eggs
- 1/8 teaspoon ground turmeric
- 1/8 teaspoon red pepper flakes, crushed
- Salt and ground black pepper, as required
- 1 tablespoon water
- 2 teaspoons olive oil
- 1 cup fresh kale, tough ribs removed and chopped

1. In a bowl, add the eggs, turmeric, red pepper flakes, salt, black pepper, and water and beat until foamy.
2. In a pan, heat the oil over meedium heat.
3. Add the egg mixture and stir to combine.
4. Immediately adjust the heat to medium-low and cook for about 1-2 minutes, stirring frequently.
5. Stir the kale in and cook for about 3-4 minutes, stirring frequently.
6. Remove from the heat and serve immediately.

Nutrition: Calories: 183, Fat: 13.4g, Carbohydrates: 4.3g, Fiber: 0.5g, Sugar: 0.7g, Protein: 12.1g

6.Tomato Scramble

Prep Time: 10 min | **Cook Time:** 5 min | **Serve:** 2

- 4 eggs
- ¼ spoon red pepper flakes, crushed Salt and ground black pepper, as required ¼ cup fresh basil, chopped ½ cup tomatoes, chopped
- 1 tablespoon olive oil

1. Add the eggs, red pepper flakes, salt, and black pepper in a large bowl and beat well.
2. Add the basil and tomatoes and stir to combine.
3. In a non-stick pan, heat the oil over medium-high heat.
4. Add the egg mixture and cook for about 3-5 minutes, stirring continuously.

Nutrition: Calories: 195, Fat: 15.9g, Carbohydrates: 2.6g, Fiber: 0.7g, Sugar: 1.9g, Protein: 11.6g

7.Salmon & Arugula Scramble

Prep Time: 10 min | **Cook Time:** 6 min | **Serve:** 4

- 6 eggs
- 2 tablespoons unsweetened almond milk Salt and ground black pepper, as required 2 tablespoons olive oil
- 4 ounces smoked salmon, cut into bite-sized chunks
- 2 cups fresh arugula, chopped finely
- 4 scallions, chopped finely

1. In a bowl, place the eggs, almond milk, salt, and black pepper and beat well. Set aside.
2. In a non-stick paan, heat the oil over medium heat.
3. Place the egg mixture evenly and cook for about 30 seconds without stirring.
4. Place the salmon, arugula, and scallions on top of the egg mixture evenly.
5. Adjust the heat to low and cok for about 3-5 minutes, stirring continuously.

Nutrition: Calories: 196, Fat: 15g, Carbohydrates: 2g, Fiber: 0.6g, Sugar: 1.1g, Protein: 14g

8.Apple Omelet

Prep Time: 10 min | **Cook Time:** 9 min | **Serve:** 1

- 2 teaspoons olive oil, divided
- ½ of large green apple, cored and sliced thinly ¼ teaspoon ground cinnamon 1/8 teaspoon ground nutmeg
- 2 large eggs
- 1/8 teaspoon vanilla extract
- Pinch of salt

1. In a non-stick frying pan, heat 1 spoon of oil over medium-low heat.
2. Add the apple slices and sprinkle with nutmeg and cinnamon.
3. Cook for about 4-5 minutes, turning once halfway through.
4. Meanwhile, in a bowl, add eggs, vanilla extract, and salt and beat until fluffy.
5. Add the reemaining oil to the pan and let it heat completely.
6. Place the egg mixture over apple slices evenly and cook for about 3-4 minutes or until desired doneness.
7. Carefully turn the pan over a serving plate and immediately fold the omelet.

Nutrition: Calories: 258, Fat: 19.5g, Carbohydrates: 9g, Fiber: 1.2g, Sugar: 7g, Protein: 12.8g

9. Veggie Omelet

Prep Time: 15 min | **Cook Time:** 15 min | **Serve:** 4

- 1 teaspoon olive oil
- 2 cups fresh fennel bulb, sliced thinly
- ¼ cup canned artichoke hearts, rinsed, drained, and chopped ¼ cup green olives, pitted and chopped 1 Roma tomato, chopped
- 6 eggs
- Salt and ground black pepper, as required ½ cup goat cheese, crumbled

1. Preheat your oven to 325 degrees F.
2. Heat olive oil in a large ovenprof pan over medium-high heat and sauté the chopped fennel bulb for about 5 minutes.
3. Stir in the artichoke, olives, and tomato and cook for about 3 minutes.
4. Meanwhile, in a bowl, add eggs, salt, and black pepper and beat until well blended.
5. Place the egg mixture over the veggie mixture and stir to combine.
6. Cook for about 2 minutes.
7. Sprinkle with the goat cheese evenly and immediately transfer the pan into the oven.
8. Bake for approximately 5 minutes or until eggs are set completely.
9. Remove the paan from the oven and carefully transfer the omelet onto a cutting board.
10. Cut into desired sized wedges and serve.

Nutrition: Calories: 185, Fat: 12.7g, Carbohydrates: 6.3g, Fiber: 2.3g, Sugar: 1.9g, Protein: 12g

10. Mushroom & Bell Pepper Quiche

Prep Time: 25 min | **Cook Time:** 15 min | **Serve:** 4

- 6 large eggs
- ½ cup unsweetened almond milk
- Salt and ground black pepper, as required ½ of onion, chopped
- ¼ cup bell pepper, seeded and chopped ¼ cup fresh mushrooms, sliced
- 1 tablespoon fresh chives, minced

1. Preheat your oven to 350 degrees F.
2. Lightly grease a pie dish.
3. In a bowl, add eggs, almond milk, salt, and black pepper and beat until well blended.
4. In a separate bowl, add the onion, bell pepper, and mushrooms and mix.
5. Place the egg mixture into the prepared pie dish evenly and top with vegetable mixture.
6. Sprinkle with chives evenly.
7. Bake for approximately 20-25 minutes.
8. Remove the pie-dish from the oven and set aside for about 5 minutes.
9. Cut into 4 portions and serve immediately.

Nutrition: Calories: 121, Fat: 0g, Carbohydrates: 8g, Fiber: 0.6g, Sugar: 0.1g, Protein: 10g

11. Green Veggies Quiche

Prep Time: 15 min | **Cook Time:** 20 min | **Serve:** 4

- 6 eggs
- ½ cup unsweetened almond milk

- Salt and ground pepper, as required 2 cups fresh baby kale, chopped
- ½ cup bell pepper, seeded and chopped 1 scallion, chopped
- ¼ cup fresh parsley, chopped
- 1 tablespoon fresh chives, minced

1. Preheat your oven to 400 degrees F.
2. Lightly grease a pie dish.
3. In a bowl, add eggs, almond milk, salt, and black pepper and beat until well blended. Set aside.
4. In another bowl, add the vegetables and herbs and mix well.
5. In the bottom of the prepared pie dish, place the veggie mixture evenly and top with the egg mixture.
6. Bake for approximately 20 minutes.
7. Remove the pie-dish from the oven and set aside for about 5 minutes before slicing.
8. Cut into desired sized wedges and serve warm.

Nutrition: Calories: 123, Fat: 7.1g, Carbohydrates: 5.9g, Fiber: 1.1g, Sugar: 1.4g, Protein: 9.8g

12. Zucchini & Carrot Quiche

Prep Time: 10 min | **Cook Time:** 40 min | **Serve:** 3

- 5 eggs
- Salt and ground black-pepper, as required 1 carrot, peeled and grated 1 small zucchini, shredded

1. Preheat your oven to 350 degrees F.
2. Lightly grease a small baking dish.
3. In a large bowl, add eggs, salt, and black pepper and beat well.
4. Add the carrot and zucchini and stir to combine.
5. Transfer the mixture into the prepared baking-dish evenly.
6. Bake for approximately 40 minutes.
7. Remove the baking-dish from the oven and set aside for about 5 minutes.
8. Cut into equal-sized wedges and serve.

Nutrition: Calories: 119, Fat: 7.4g, Carbohydrates: 3.9g, Fiber: 0.9g, Sugar: 2.2g, Protein: 9.9g

13. Pineapple Sorbet

Prep Time: 5 min | **Cook Time:** None | **Serve:** 4

- cup mint, fresh
- can pineapple-chunks (1 can = 20oz. in juice, or ½ real pineapple)

1. Wipe the tin or cut the real pineapple and drop it in a freezer bowl (this should freeze for around 2 hours). Keep a few chunks or a loop for garnish.
2. Using a hand blender or food mixer to mix with mint when frozen (keep a few mint leaves aside as well).
3. This seems to work better if you're using fresh pineapple, then we suggest blending first and freezing afterward.
4. When nicely combined, put in bowls and garnish each with the leftover chunks and leaves.

14. Bell Pepper Frittata

Prep Time: 15 min | **Cook Time:** 10 min | **Serve:** 6

- 8 eggs
- 1 tablespoon fresh cilantro, chopped
- 1 tablespoon fresh basil, chopped
- ¼ spoon red pepper flakes, crushed Salt, and ground black pepper, as required 2 tablespoons olive oil
- 1 bunch scallions, chopped

- 1 cup bell pepper, seeded and sliced thinly ½ cup goat cheese, crumbled

1. Preheat the broiler of the oven.
2. Arrange a rack in the upper third portion of the oven.
3. In a bowl, add the eggs, fresh herbs, red pepper flakes, salt, and black pepper and beat well.
4. In an ovenproof pan, melt the butter over medium heat and sauté the scallion and bell pepper for about 1 minute.
5. Add the egg mixture over the bell pepper mixture evenly and lift the edges to let the egg mixture flow underneath and cook for about 2-3 minutes.
6. Place the cheese on top in the form of dots.
7. Now, transfer the pan under the broiler and broil for about 2-3 minutes.
8. Removee the pan from the oven and set aside for about 5 minutes before serving.
9. Cut the frittata into desired size slices and serve.

Nutrition: Calories: 167, Fat: 13g, Carbohydrates: 3.3g, Fiber: 0.6g, Sugar: 2.2g, Protein: 9.6g

15. Zucchini Frittata

Prep Time: 15 min | **Cook Time:** 19 min | **Serve:** 6
- 2 tablespoons unsweetened almond milk
- 8 eggs
- Salt and ground-black pepper, as required 1 tablespoon olive oil 1 garlic clove, minced
- 2 medium zucchinis, cut into ¼-inch thick round slices ½ cup feta cheese, crumbled

1. Preheat your oven to 350 degrees F.
2. In a bowl, add the almond milk, eggs, salt, and black pepper and beat well. Set aside.
3. In an ovenproof-pan, heat oil over medium heat and sauté the garlic for about 1 minute.
4. Stir in the zucchini and cook for about 5 minutes.
5. Add the egg mixture and stir for about 1 minute.
6. Sprinkle the cheese on top evenly.
7. Immediately transfer the pan into the oven and bake for approximately 10-12 minutes or until eggs become set.
8. Remove the pan from the oveen and set aside to cool for about 3-5 minutes.
9. Cut into desired sized wedges and serve.

Nutrition: Calories: 149, Fat: 11g, Carbohydrates: 3.4g, Fiber: 0.8g, Sugar: 2.1g, Protein: 10g

16. Chicken & Asparagus Frittata

Prep Time: 15 min | **Cook Time:** 12 min | **Serve:** 4
- ½ cup cooked chicken, chopped
- ½ cup low-fat Parmesan cheese, grated and divided 6 eggs, beaten lightly
- Salt and ground black-pepper, as required 1/3 cup boiled asparagus, chopped ¼ cup cherry tomatoes, halved

1. Preheat the broiler of the oven.
2. In a bowl, add ¼ cup of the Parmesan cheese, eggs, salt, and black pepper and beat until well blended.
3. In a large oven-proof pan, melt the butter over medium-high heat and cook the chicken and asparagus for about 2-3 minutes.
4. Add the egg mixture and tomatoes and stir to combine.
5. Cook for about 4-5 minutes.
6. Remove from the heeat and sprinkle with the remaining Parmesan cheese.
7. Now, transfer the pan under the broiler and broil for about 3-4 minutes or until slightly puffed.

8. Cut into desired sized wedges and serve immediately.

Nutrition: Calories: 158, Fat: 9.6g, Carbohydrates: 1.6g, Fiber: 0.4g, Sugar: 1g, Protein: 16.2g

17. Eggs with Spinach

Prep Time: 10 min | **Cook Time:** 22 min | **Serve:** 2
- 6 cups fresh baby spinach
- 2-3 tablespoons water
- 4 eggs
- Salt and ground black pepper, as required 2-3 tablespoons feta cheese, crumbled

1. Preheat your oven to 400 degrees F.
2. Lightly grease 2 small baking dishes.
3. In a large frying-pan, add spinach and water over medium heat and cook for about 3-4 minutes.
4. Remove the frying pan from heat and drain the excess water completely.
5. Divide the spinach into prepared baking dishes evenly.
6. Carefully crack 2 eggs in each baking dish over spinach.
7. Sprinkle with salt and peppeer and top with feta cheese evenly.
8. Arrange the baking dishes onto a large cookie sheet.
9. Bake for approximately 15-18 minutes.

Nutrition: Calories: 171, Fat: 11.1g, Carbohydrates: 4.3g, Fiber: 2g, Sugar: 1.4g, Protein: 15g

18. Eggs with Spinach & Tomatoes

Prep Time: 15 min | **Cook Time:** 25 min | **Serve:** 4
- 2 tablespoons olive oil
- 1 yellow onion, chopped
- 2 garlic cloves, minced
- 1 cup tomatoes, chopped
- ½ pound fresh spinach, chopped
- 1 teaspoon ground cumin
- ¼ spoon red pepper flakes, crushed Salt, and ground black pepper, as required 4 eggs
- 2 tablespoons fresh parsley, chopped

1. In a non-stick pan, heeat the olive oil over medium heat and sauté the onion for about 4-5 minutes.
2. Add the garlic and sauté for approximately 1 minute.
3. Add the tomatoes, spices, salt, and black pepper and cook for about 2-3 minutes, stirring frequently.
4. Add in the spinach and cook for about 4-5 minutes.
5. Carefully crack eggs on top of spinach mixture.
6. With the lid, cover the pan and cook for about 10 minutes.
7. Serve hot with the garnishing of parsley.

Nutrition: Calories: 160, Fat: 11.9g, Carbohydrates: 7.6g, Fiber: 2.6g, Sugar: 3g, Protein: 8.1g

19. Chicken & Zucchini Muffins

Prep Time: 15 min | **Cook Time:** 15 min | **Serve:** 4
- 4 eggs
- ¼ cup olive oil
- ¼ cup of water
- 1/3 cup coconut flour
- ½ teaspoon baking powder
- ¼ teaspoon salt
- ¾ cup cooked chicken, shredded
- ¾ cup zucchini, grated
- ½ cup low-fat Parmesan cheese, shredded 1 tablespoon fresh oregano, minced 1 tablespoon fresh thyme, minced
- ¼ cup low-fat cheddar cheese, grated

1. Preheat your oven to 400 degrees F.
2. Lightly greease 8 cups of a muffin tin.
3. In a bowl, add the eggs, oil, and water and beat until well blended.
4. Add the flooura, baking powder, and salt, and mix well.
5. Add the remaining ingredients and mix until just blended.
6. Place the muffin mixture into the prepared muffin cup evenly.
7. Bake for approximately 13-15 minutes or until tops become golden brown.
8. Remove muffin tin from oven and place onto a wire rack to cool for about 10 minutes.
9. Invert the muffins onto a platter and serve warm.

Nutrition: Calories: 270, Fat: 20g, Carbohydrates: 3.5g, Fiber: 1.4g, Sugar: 0.9g, Protein: 18g

20. Turkey & Bell Pepper Muffins

Prep Time: 15 min | **Cook Time:** 20 min | **Serve:** 4

- 8 eggs
- Salt and ground pepper, as required 2 tablespoons water
- 8 ounces cooked turkey meat, chopped finely
- 1 cup bell pepper, seeded and chopped
- 1 cup onion, finely chopped

1. Preheat your oven to 350 degrees F.
2. Grease 8 cups of a muffin tin.
3. In a bowl, add the eggs, salt, black pepper, and water and beat until well blended.
4. Add the meat, bell pepper, and onion and stir to combine.
5. Place the mixture into the prepared muffin cups evenly.
6. Bake for approximately 17,30-20,30 minutes or until golden brown.
7. Remove the muuffin tin from the oven and place onto a wire rack to cool for about 10 minutes.
8. Carefully invert the muffins onto a platter and serve warm.

Nutrition: Calories: 238, Fat: 11.7g, Carbohydrates: 4.4g, Fiber: 1g, Sugar: 2.5g, Protein: 28.2g

21. Tofu & Mushroom Muffins

Prep Time: 15 min | **Cook Time:** 30 min | **Serve:** 6

- 2 teaspoons olive oil, divided
- 1½ cups fresh mushrooms, chopped
- 1 scallion, chopped
- 1 teaspoon garlic, minced
- 1 teaspoon fresh rosemary, minced Freshly ground black pepper, as required
- 1 (12.3-ounce) package lite firm silken tofu, drained ¼ cup unsweetened almond milk
- 2 tablespoons nutritional yeast
- 1 tablespoon arrowroot starch
- ¼ teaspoon ground turmeric

1. Preheat your oven to 375 degrees F.
2. Grease a 12 cups muffin tin.
3. In a non-stick pan, heat 1 spoon of oil over medium heat and sauté scallion and garlic for about 1 minute.
4. Add the mushrooms and sauté for about 5-7 minutes.
5. Stir in the rosemary and black pepper and remove from the heat.
6. Set aside to cool slightly.
7. In a food processor, add the tofu, remaining oil, almond milk, nutritional yeast, arrowroot starch, turmeric, and pulse until smooth.
8. Transfer the tofu mixture into a large bowl.
9. Add the mushroom mixture and gently stir to combine.

10. Move the mixture uniformly into the muffin cups that have been prepared.
11. Bake for 20-22 minutes or until it comes out clean with a toothpick inserted in the center.
12. Remove the mufin tin from the oven and place onto a wire rack to cool for about 10 minutes.
13. Invert the muffins onto the wire rack carefully.

Nutrition: Calories: 70, Fat: 3.6g, Carbohydrates: 4.3g, Fiber: 1.3g, Sugar: 1.1g, Protein: 55.7g

22. Alkaline Blueberry Spelt Pancakes

Prep Time: 6 min | **Cook Time:** 20 min | **Serve:** 3

- 2 cups Spelt Flour
- 1 cup Coconut Milk
- 1/2 cup Alkaline Water
- 2 tbsps. Grapeseed Oil
- 1/2 cup Agave
- 1/2 cup Blueberries
- 1/4 tsp. Sea Moss

1. Mix the spelled flour, agave, grapeseed oil, hemp seeds, and sea moss in a bowl.
2. Add in 1 cup of hemp milk and alkaline water to the mixture until you get the consistency mixture you like.
3. Crimp the blueberries into the batter.
4. Heat the skillet to moderate heat, then lightly coat it with the grapeseed oil.
5. Pour the batter into the skillet, then let them cook for approximately 5 minutes on every side.

Nutrition: Calories: 203 kcal Fat: 1.4g Carbs: 41.6g Proteins: 4.8g

23. Alkaline Blueberry Muffins

Prep Time: 5 min | **Cook Time:** 20 min | **Serve:** 3

- 1 cup Coconut Milk
- 3/4 cup Spelt Flour
- 3/4 Teff Flour
- 1/2 cup Blueberries
- 1/3 cup Agave
- 1/4 cup Sea Moss Gel
- 1/2 tsp. Sea Salt
- Grapeseed Oil

1. Adjust the temperature of the oven to 365 degrees.
2. Grease 6 regular-size muffin cups with muffin liners.
3. In a bowl, mix sea salt, sea moss, agave, coconut milk, and flour gel until they are properly blended.
4. You then crimp in blueberries.
5. Coat the muffin pan lightly with the grapeseed oil.
6. Pour in the muffin batter.
7. Bake for at least 30 minutes until it turns golden brown.

Nutrition: Calories: 160 kcal Fat: 5g Carbs: 25g Proteins: 2g

24. Crunchy Quinoa Meal

Prep Time: 5 min | **Cook Time:** 25 min | **Serve:** 2

- 3 cups of coconut milk
- 1 cup rinsed quinoa
- 1/8 tsp. ground cinnamon
- 1 cup raspberry
- 1/2 cup chopped coconuts

1. In a saucepan, pour milk and bring to a boil over moderate heat.
2. Add the quinoa to the milk and then bring it to a boil once more.

3. You then let it simmer for at least 15 minutes on medium heat until the milk is reduced.
4. Stir in the cinnamon, then mix properly.
5. Cover it, then cook for 8 minutes until the milk is completely absorbed.
6. Add the raspberry and cook the meal for 30 seconds.
Nutrition: Calories: 271 kcal Fat: 3.7g Carbs: 54g Proteins: 6.5g

25.Coconut Pancakes
Prep Time: 5 min | **Cook Time:** 15 min | **Serve:** 4
- 1 cup coconut flour
- 2 tbsps. arrowroot powder
- 1 tsp. baking powder
- 1 cup of coconut milk
- 3 tbsps. coconut oil

1. In a medium container, mix in all the dry ingredients.
2. Add the coconut milk and 2 tbsps. Of the coconut oil, then mix properly.
3. Drop a spoon of flour into the skillet and then swirl the pan into a smooth pancake to distribute the batter uniformly.
4. Cook it for like 3 minutes on medium heat until it becomes firm.
5. Turn the pancake to the other side, then cook it for another 2 minutes until it turns golden brown.
6. Cook the remaining pancakes in the same process.
Nutrition: Calories: 377 kcal Fat: 14.9g Carbs: 60.7g Protein: 6.4g

26.Quinoa Porridge
Prep Time: 5 min | **Cook Time:** 25 min | **Serve:** 2
- 2 cups of coconut milk
- 1 cup rinsed quinoa
- 1/8 tsp. ground cinnamon
- 1 cup fresh blueberries

1. In a saucepan, boil the coconut milk over high heat.
2. Add the quinoa to the milk, then bring the mixture to a boil.
3. You then let it simmer for 15 minutes on medium heat until the milk is reduced.
4. Add the cinnamon, then mix it properly in the saucepan.
5. Cover the saucepan and cook for at least 8 minutes until the milk is completely absorbed.
6. Add in the blueberries, then cook for 30 more seconds.
Nutrition: Calories: 271 kcal Fat: 3.7g Carbs: 54g Protein:6.5g

27.Amaranth Porridge
Prep Time: 5 min | **Cook Time:** 30 min | **Serve:** 2.
- 2 cups of coconut milk
- 2 cups alkaline water
- 1 cup amaranth
- 2 tbsps. coconut oil
- 1 tbsp. ground cinnamon

1. In a saucepan, mix the milk with water, then boil the mixture.
2. You stir in the amaranth, then reduce the heat to medium.
3. Cook on medium heat and then simmer for at least 30 minutes as you occasionally stir it.
4. Turn off the heat.
5. Add in cinnamon and coconut oil, then stir.
Nutrition: Calories: 434 kcal Fat: 35g Carbs: 27g Protein: 6.7g

28.Banana Barley Porridge
Prep Time: 15 min | **Cook Time:** 5 min | **Serve:** 2
- 1 cup divided unsweetened coconut milk 1 small peeled and sliced banana 1/2 cup barley
- 3 drops liquid stevia
- 1/4 cup chopped coconuts

1. In a bowl, properly mix barley with half of the coconut milk and stevia.
2. Cover the mixing bowl, then refrigerate for about 6 hours.
3. In a saucepan, mix the barley mixture with coconut milk.
4. Cook for about 5 minutes on moderate heat.
5. Then top it with the chopped coconuts and the banana slices.
Nutrition: Calories: 159kcal Fat: 8.4g Carbs: 19.8g Proteins: 4.6g

29.Zucchini Muffins
Prep Time: 10 min | **Cook Time:** 25 min | **Serve:** 16
- 1 tbsp. ground flaxseed
- 3 tbsps. alkaline water
- 1/4 cup walnut butter
- 3 medium over-ripe bananas
- 2 small grated
- zucchinis
- 1/2 cup coconut milk
- 1 tsp. vanilla extract
- 2 cups coconut flour
- 1 tbsp. baking powder
- 1 tsp. cinnamon
- 1/4 tsp. sea salt

1. Tune the temperature of your oven to 375°F.
2. Grease the muffin tray with the cooking spray.
3. In a bowl, mix the flaxseed with water.
4. In a glass bowl, mash the bananas, then stir in the remaining ingredients.
5. Properly mix and then divide the mixture into the muffin tray.
6. Bake it for 25 minutes.
Nutrition: Calories: 127 kcal Fat: 6.6g Carbs: 13g Protein: 0.7g

30.Millet Porridge
Prep Time: 10 min | **Cook Time:** 20 min | **Serve:** 2
- Sea salt
- 1 tbsp. finely chopped coconuts
- 1/2 cup unsweetened coconut milk
- 1/2 cup rinsed and drained millet
- 1-1/2 cups alkaline water
- 3 drops liquid stevia

1. Sauté the millet in a non-stick skillet for about 3 minutes.
2. Add salt and water, then stir.
3. Let the meal boil, then reduce the amount of heat.
4. Cook for 15 minutes, then add the remaining ingredients. Stir.
5. Cook the meal for 4 extra minutes.
6. Serve the meal with toping of the chopped nuts.
Nutrition: Calories: 219 kcal Fat: 4.5g Carbs: 38.2g Protein: 6.4g

31.Jackfruit Vegetable Fry
Prep Time: 5 min | **Cook Time:** 5 min | **Serve:** 6
- 2 finely chopped small onions

- 2 cups finely chopped cherry tomatoes
- 1/8 tsp. ground turmeric
- 1 tbsp. olive oil
- 2 seeded and chopped red bell peppers
- 3 cups seeded and chopped firm jackfruit
- 1/8 tsp. cayenne pepper
- 2 tbsps. chopped fresh basil leaves
- Salt

1. In a greased skillet, sauté the onions and bell peppers for about 5 minutes.
2. Add the tomatoes, then stir.
3. Cook for 2 minutes.
4. Then add the jackfruit, cayenne pepper, salt, and turmeric.
5. Cook for about 8 minutes.
6. Garnish the meal with basil leaves.

Nutrition: Calories: 236 kcal Fat: 1.8g Carbs: 48.3g Protein: 7g

32. Zucchini Pancakes

Prep Time: 15 min | **Cook Time:** 8 min | **Serve:** 8
- 12 tbsps. alkaline water
- 6 large grated zucchinis
- Sea salt
- 4 tbsps. ground Flax Seeds
- 2 tips. olive oil
- 2 finely chopped jalapeño peppers
- 1/2 cup finely chopped scallions

1. In a bowl, mix water and the flax seeds, then set it aside.
2. Pour oil into a large non-stick skillet, then heat it on medium heat.
3. The add the black pepper, salt, and zucchini.
4. Cook for 3 minutes, then transfer the zucchini into a large bowl.
5. Add the flaxseed and the scallion mixture, then properly mix it.
6. Preheat a griddle, then grease it lightly with the cooking spray.
7. Pour 1/4 of the zucchini mixture into the griddle, then cook for 3 minutes.
8. Flip the side carefully, then cook for 2 more minutes.
9. Repeat the procedure with the remaining mixture in batches.

Nutrition: Calories: 71 kcal Fat: 2.8g Carbs: 9.8g Protein: 3.7g

33. Squash Hash

Prep Time: 2 min | **Cook Time:** 10 min | **Serve:** 2
- 1 tsp. onion powder
- 1/2 cup finely chopped onion
- 2 cups spaghetti squash
- 1/2 tsp. sea salt

1. Using paper towels, squeeze extra moisture from spaghetti squash.
2. Place the squash into a bowl, then add the salt, onion, and onion powder.
3. Stir properly to mix them.
4. Spray a non-stick cooking skillet with cooking spray, then place it over moderate heat.
5. Add the spaghetti squash to the pan.
6. Cook the squash for about 5 minutes.
7. Flip the hash browns using a spatula.
8. Cook for 5 minutes until the desired crispness is reached.

Nutrition: Calories: 44 kcal Fat: 0.6g Carbs: 9.7g Protein: 0.9

34. Hemp Seed Porridge

Prep Time: 5 min | **Cook Time:** 5 min | **Serve:** 6
- 3 cups cooked hemp seed
- 1 packet Stevia
- 1 cup of coconut milk

1. In a saucepan, mix the rice and the coconut milk over moderate heat for about 5 minutes as you stir it constantly.
2. Take the pan out of the burner, then add it to the Stevia. Stir.
3. Serve in 6 bowls.

Nutrition: Calories: 236 kcal Fat: 1.8g Carbs: 48.3g Protein: 7g

35. Pumpkin Spice Quinoa

Prep Time: 10 min | **Cook Time:** 0 min | **Serve:** 2
- 1 cup cooked quinoa
- 1 cup unsweetened coconut milk
- 1 large mashed banana
- 1/4 cup pumpkin puree
- 1 tsp. pumpkin spice
- 2 tips. chia seeds

1. In a container, mix all the ingredients.
2. Seal the lid, then shake the container properly to mix.
3. Refrigerate overnight.

Nutrition: Calories: 212 kcal Fat: 11.9g Carbs: 31.7g Protein: 7.3g

36. Easy, healthy Greek Salmon Salad

Prep Time: 10 min | **Cook Time:** 8 min | **Serve:** 4
- ¼ cup olive oil
- 3 tablespoons red wine vinegar
- 2 tablespoons freshly crush lemon juice (from 1 lemon)
- 1 clove of garlic, chopped
- ¾ teaspoon dried oregano
- 1/2 teaspoon Kosar salt
- ¼ teaspoon fresh black pepper
- One finely chopped red onion
- A cup of cold water
- 4 (6 oz) salmon fillets, peeled
- 2 medium-sized Korean salads, such as Boston or Bibb (about 1 kilogram), broken into bite-size pieces
- 2 medium-sized tomatoes, cut into 1-inch pieces
- 1 medium English cucumber, quadrilateral and then cut into 1/2-inch pieces
- ½ cup of half-length Kalamata olives 4 oz Feta Cheese, minced (about 1 cup)

1. In the middle of the oven, arrange a shelf and heat to 425 degrees Fahrenheit. While the oven is warming, marinate the salmon and soften the onion (instructions below).
2. Put the olive oil, vinegar, lemon juice, garlic, oregano, salt and pepper in a large bowl, then transfer three tablespoons of vinegar large enough into a baking dish to keep all the salmon chunks in one layer. Add the salmon, lightly rotate a few times to wrap evenly in the wings. Cover the fridge. Pour the onion and water into a small bowl and set aside 10 minutes to make the onion stronger. Drain and release the liquid.
3. Discover the salmon and grill for 8 to 12 minutes until they are cooked and lightly fried. Thermometer instant-read in

the middle of the thickest tab should record 120 degrees Fahrenheit to 130 degrees Fahrenheit for the rare medium or 135 degrees Fahrenheit to 145 degrees Fahrenheit. The cooking depends on the thickness of the salmon, depending on the thickest portion of the fillet. It Al depends on the salad.

4. Add the salad, tomatoes, cucumbers, olives, and red onion to the Gina Vine bowl and salt to combine. Divide into four plates or shallow bowl. When the salmon is ready, place one fillet over each salad. Sprinkle with feta and serve quickly.

Nutrition: Calories: 351 Total fat: 4g Cholesterol: 94mg Fiber: 2g Protein: 12g Sodium: 327mg

37.*Mediterranean Pepper*

Prep Time: 5 min | **Cook Time:** 20 min | **Serve:** 4
- 1/2 teaspoon restrained oil 1/2 cup sun-dried tomatoes
- 2 cups of spinach (fresh or frozen)
- 1/2 spoon drops of zaatar spices
- 10 eggs, screaming
- 1/2 cup Feta cheese
- 1-2 tablespoons
- salt and pepper

1. At 350 degrees Fahrenheit, firstly preheat the oven
2. Heat a cast-iron boiler over medium heat. Add the olive oil and peas, slowly and slowly cooking until you want to release the liquid and start to brown and brown. Then, sauté the sun-dried tomatoes with a little reserved oil, spinach and zucchini, and cook for 2-3 minutes until the spinach is crushed.
3. When the spinach has faded, pour the vegetable mixture evenly into the cast iron fish and then add the boiled eggs, turning the pan so that the eggs cover the vegetables evenly. Bake on medium heat until the eggs start about halfway through. Pour the eggs and vegetables with the spatula into the pan, leave the eggs to cook until the frittata is placed.
4. When the eggs are almost half cooked, add the Feta cheese and spoon the horseradish sauce on top and dust with salt and pepper. Remove the cast iron from the oven and place it in the middle rack in the oven. Bake until cooked on the ferrite; it will take about five minutes.
5. Bring out from the oven and let it cool slightly. For cedar, cut or square the pie and pour with a pan.

Nutrition: Calories: 311 Total fat: 4g Cholesterol: 84mg Fiber: 2g Protein: 12g Sodium: 357mg

38.*Black Beans and Sweet Potato Tacos*

Prep Time: 10 min | **Cook Time:** 30 min | **Serve:** 6
- 1 lb. sweet potato (about 2 medium teaspoons), skin cut and cut
- into 1/2-inch pieces
- Divide into 2 tablespoons of olive oil
- 1 tablespoon Kosar salt, divided
- ¼ teaspoon fresh black pepper on large white or yellow onion, finely chopped
- 2 teaspoons of red pepper
- 1 cumin with a teaspoon
- 1 (15 oz.) can be black beans, drained and drained Cup of water
- ¼ cup freshly chopped garlic
- 12 pcs. Corn
- To serving guacamole
- Sliced cheese or feta cheese (optional)
- Wood Wedge

1. In the oven, set out a shelf in the middle and place to 425 degrees Fahrenheit. Set a big sheet of aluminum foil on the work surface. Collect the tortillas from the top and wrap them completely in foil. Put it aside
2. Put sweet potatoes on a small baking sheet. Mix with one tablespoon oil and sprinkle with 1/2 teaspoon salt and 1/4 teaspoon black pepper. Discard to mix and play in one layer. Fry for 20 minutes. Sprinkle the potatoes with a flat lid and set aside until a corner of the oven is clear.
3. Put the foil wrapping in the space and continue to cook for about 10 minutes until the sweet potatoes are browned and stained and the seasonings are heated. Also, cook the beans.
4. You then heat one tablespoon remaining in a large skillet over low heat. Put the onion and cook, occasionally stirring, until translucent, about 3 minutes. Mix the pepper powder, cumin, and 1/2 teaspoon salt. Add the beans and water.
5. Shield the pan and reduce the heat to low heat. Cook for 5 minutes, then slice and use the fork's back to chop the beans a little, about half of the total. If water still remains in the vessel, stir the exposed mixture for about 30 seconds until evaporated.
6. Peel the sweet potatoes and add the cantaloupe to the black beans, and mix. If used, fill the yolk with a mixture of black beans and top with guacamole and cheese. Serve with lime wedges.

Nutrition: Calories: 251 Total fat: 4g Cholesterol: 94mg Fiber: 2g Protein: 15g Sodium: 329mg

39.*Seafood Cooked from Beer*

Prep Time: 30 min | **Cook Time:** 1 h | **Serve:** 8
Seafood:
- Canola oil for roasting
- 1/2 Cup Coarse cornmeal
- 1/2 tablespoon red pepper
- 1/4 baking soda
- 1 1/2 Cup Flour for all purposes is divided
- Kosher salt and freshly ground black pepper
- 1 12 oz can drink beer in style
- 1 code and skin without skin, cut into 8 strips
- 1 large cup (number 25/25) of peeled and spread shrimp (remaining tail)
- 16 percentiles, shake
- 1 lemon sliced with cedar wedge
- Tartar sauce, mignon, chimichurri, hot sauce, and malt vinegar, for cedar.

Sos tartar:
- 1/2 Cup Mayonnaise
- 2 teaspoons, pickled, chopped or pureed
- 1 tablespoon fresh lemon juice
- 1 tablespoon three-quarter pants
- 1 tablespoon mustard
- Kosher salt and freshly ground black pepper
- 1/2 cup Red wine vinegar
- 1 small rest, finely chopped

Kosher salt and chimichurri of freshly ground black pepper:
- 1/2 Cup Fresh parsley on a flat-leaf
- 1/4 Cup White wine vinegar
- 2 tablespoons olive oil
- 2 cloves of minced garlic
- 1 stem, seeds and mincemeat
- 1 tablespoon fresh oregano, chopped
- Sare Kosar

1. Heat 1 1/2-inch oil in a large Dutch oven over medium heat at 375 degrees F (deep-fried temperature with a thermometer).

2. Meanwhile, chop corn, bell pepper, baking soda, 1 cup of flour, 1/2 teaspoon salt, and 1/2 teaspoon pepper in a bowl. Add the broth and the phloem to mix.

3. Put 1/2 cup of the remaining flour in a bowl. Add salt, pepper and the fish, shrimps, shells, and lemon slices, and serve little.

4. Work several pieces at once, remove the seafood and the lemons from the flour, shake too much, drain the dough and allow the excess drops to return to the container. Carefully add the hot oil, being careful not to overload the pot. Roast golden brown and cook for 1 to 2 minutes. Transfer to a sheet of paper towel — season with salt.

5. Make the tartar sauce: mayonnaise, pickled or mixed the cloves, and pour the lemon juice, pepper, and mustard whole in a bowl. Season with Kosar salt and freshly ground pepper; feel free to add more lemon juice. Face 2/3 glass.

6. To Make a Mignonette: add red wine vinegar and finely minced mustard in a bowl. Season with Kosar salt and freshly ground pepper; allow standing for at least 30 minutes or up to 24 hours. Make 1/2 cup.

7. Make Chimichurri: Combine parsley, white wine vinegar, olive oil, garlic, jalapeño, and fresh oregano in a bowl. It is seasoned with Kosar salt. Face 2/3 glass.

8. It is served with lemon wedges, tartar sauce, mignon, chemicals, hot sauce, and malt vinegar.

Nutrition: Calories: 221 Total fat: 4g Cholesterol: 94mg Fiber: 2g Protein: 12g Sodium: 327mg

40. Crab Chicken

Prep Time: 20 min | **Cook Time:** 40 min | **Serve:** 8
- Canola oil for roasting
- 1c coarse cornflour
- 1/2 Cup Flour, spoon, and surface used
- 3/4 Cup Baking powder
- 1/2 spoon
- 1/4 tablespoon
- Sare Kosar
- 2 graphic, finely chopped
- 1 tablespoon crushed peas
- Eat 8 ounces of claw crab meat (2.11 c)
- 4 oz. of Gruyère cheese, chilled (about 1 cup)
- 1 c Dough water
- 1 you tie

1. Heat 1 1/2-inch oil in a large Dutch oven over medium heat up to 350 degrees F (deep-fry).

2. Meanwhile, mix the cornmeal, flour, baking powder, cayenne, baking soda, and 3/4 teaspoon salt in a bowl. Add onion and onion and mix to combine. Add the crab meat and cheese and mix with a fork to combine. In the center of a well, add the butter and egg and mix to combine.

3. Spoon soup into the hot oil and be careful not to spill the pan and fry, occasionally turning until browned, 3 to 5 minutes. Transfer toa sheet of paper towel — season with salt repeat with the remaining dough.

Nutrition: Calories: 351 Total fat: 4g Cholesterol: 94mg Fiber: 2g Protein: 12g Sodium: 319mg

41. Slow Lentil Soup

Prep Time: 10 min | **Cook Time:** 20 min | **Serve:** 6
- 4 cups (1 quart) of low sodium vegetable juice
- 1 (14 oz.) tomatoes can (no leak)
- 1 small, fried yellow onion
- 1 medium carrot, sliced
- 1 medium-sized celery stalk, one-piece
- 1 cup green lentils
- 1 teaspoon of olive oil, plus more for cedar
- 2 cloves of garlic, turn
- 1 teaspoon Kosar salt
- 1 teaspoon tomato paste
- 1 leaf
- 1/2 teaspoon below ground
- 1/2 teaspoon of ground coriander
- 1/4 teaspoon of smoked peppers
- 2 tablespoons red wine vinegar
- Serving options: plain yogurt, olive oil, freshly chopped parsley or coriander leaves

1. Put all ingredients, except vinegar, in a slow cooker for 1/3 to 2-4 quarts and mix to combine. Cover and cook in the LOW settings for about 8 hours until the lentil is tender.

2. Remove bay leaf and mix in red wine vinegar. If desired, place a pot, a drop of olive oil and fresh parsley or crushed liquid in a bowl.

Nutrition: Calories: 231 Total fat: 4g Cholesterol: 64mg Fiber: 2g Protein: 12g Sodium: 368mg

42. Light Bang Shrimp Paste

Prep Time: 10 min | **Cook Time:** 20 min | **Serve:** 4
For crunchy crumbs:
- 1 tablespoon oil without butter
- Fresh cups or pancakes
- 1/8 teaspoon Kosar salt
- 1/8 teaspoon fresh black pepper
- Pepper racks
- Spend garlic powder

For shrimp pasta:
- Cooking spray
- ½ cup of Greek yogurt whole milk
- 2 tablespoons of Asian sweet pepper sauce, such as the iconic eel
- 1 teaspoon of honey
- ¼ teaspoon of garlic powder
- The juice is divided into 2 medium lemons (about 1/4 glass)
- 12 ounces of dried spaghetti
- 1 cup shrimp without skin and peeled
- 1 teaspoon Kosar salt, plus for pasta juice
- ¼ teaspoon fresh black pepper
- 1/8 teaspoon cayenne pepper
- 2 Moderated onions, sliced, sliced

1. Make crisp crumbs:

2. Over low heat, defrost the butter in a skillet. Add crumbs, salt, black pepper, cayenne pepper, and garlic powder. Cook while constantly stirring, until golden, crispy and fragrant. It will take 4 - 5 minutes, then put it aside.

3. Make shrimps:

4. Place a shelf in the middle of the oven and heat to 400 degrees Fahrenheit. Cover with a lightly cooked baking sheet with cooking spray. Put it aside

5. Boil salt water in a big pot. Meanwhile, chop yogurt, pepper sauce, honey, garlic powder and half of the lemon juice in a small bowl. Put it aside

6. Add the pasta when the water boils and boil the pasta for up to 10 minutes, or as directed. Dry the shrimps and place

them on a sheet of ready-made cooking. Season with salt, black pepper and coffee and mix to cook. It stretches in a uniform layer. Roast once, until the shrimps are matte and pink, 6 to 8 minutes. Pour the remaining lemon juice over the shrimps, pour over it and pour the flavored pieces onto the baking sheet.

7. Evacuate the pasta and return it to the pot. Pour into the yogurt sauce and serve until well cooked. Put shrimp and juice on a baking sheet with half of the onion and lightly add it again. Generously sprinkle each portion with a crunchy crumb and remaining onion. Serve immediately.

Nutrition: Calories: 351 Total fat: 4g Cholesterol: 94mg Fiber: 2g Protein: 12g Sodium: 327mg

43. *Sweet and Smoked Salmon*

Prep Time: 35 min | **Cook Time:** 1 h | **Serve:** 8
- 2 tablespoons light brown sugar
- 2 tablespoons smoked peppers
- 1 tablespoon shaved lemon peel
- Sare Kosar
- Freshly chopped black pepper
- Salmon fillets on the skin 1/2 kilogram

1. Soak a large plate (about 15 cm by 7 inches) in water for 1 to 2 hours.
2. It is heated over medium heat. Combine sugar, pepper, lemon zest, and 1/2 teaspoon of salt and pepper in a bowl. Mix the salmon with the salt and rub the mixture of spices in all parts of the meat.
3. Put the salmon on the wet plate, skin down — oven, covered, in the desired color, 25 to 28 minutes for medium.

Nutrition: Calories: 321 Total fat: 4g Cholesterol: 54mg Fiber: 2g Protein: 12g Sodium: 337mg

44. *Chocolate Cherry Crunch Granola*

Prep Time: 10 min | **Cook Time:** 20 min | **Serve:** 6
- 3 cups rolled oats
- 2 cups assorted seeds, such as sesame, chia, sunflower, and pepitas (hulled pumpkin seeds)
- 1 cup sliced almonds
- 1 cup unsweetened coconut flakes
- 2 teaspoons vanilla extract
- 2 teaspoons ground cinnamon
- 1 teaspoon fine sea salt
- ½ cup of cocoa powder
- ½ cup pure maple syrup
- ¼ cup coconut oil or canola oil
- 1 cup dried cherries (unsweetened, if possible)
- 1 cup of chocolate chips

1. Preheat the oven to 350°F. Spread 2 large baking sheets with parchment paper.
2. In a large bowl, stir together the oats, seeds, almonds, and coconut. Add the vanilla, cinnamon, salt, and cocoa powder. Stir to combine.
3. Heat the maple syrup and coconut-oil in a low-heat frying pan. Pour the warm syrup and oil over the oat mixture and stir to coat. On the prepared baking sheets, spread the granola in even layers.
4. Bake for 15 to 18 minutes, scraping and mixing occasionally, then remove from the oven.
5. Put in the dried cherries and chocolate chips, then return to the oven, now turned off but still warm, and let the granola cool and dry completely.

Nutrition: Calories: 570 Total fat: 31g Cholesterol: 94mg Fiber: 2g Protein: 12g Sodium: 204mg

45. *Creamy Raspberry Pomegranate Smoothie*

Prep Time: 5 min | **Cook Time:** 5 min | **Serve:** 1
- 1½ cups pomegranate juice
- ½ cup unsweetened coconut milk
- 1 scoop vanilla protein powder (plant-based if you need it to be dairy-free)
- 2 packed cups fresh baby spinach
- 1 cup frozen raspberries
- 1 frozen banana (see Tip)
- 1 to 2 tablespoons freshly compressed lemon juice

1. In a blender, combine the pomegranate juice and coconut milk. Add the protein powder and spinach. Give these a whirl to break down the spinach.
2. Add the raspberries, banana, and lemon juice, then top it off with ice. Blend until smooth and frothy.

Nutrition: Calories: 303 Total fat: 3g Cholesterol: 0mg Fiber: 2g Protein: 15g Sodium: 165mg

46. *Mango Coconut Oatmeal*

Prep Time: 5 min | **Cook Time:** 5 min | **Serve:** 2
- 1½ cups water
- ½ cup 5-minute steel cut oats
- ¼ cup unsweetened canned coconut milk, plus more for serving (optional)
- 1 tablespoon pure maple syrup
- 1 teaspoon sesame seeds
- Dash ground cinnamon
- 1 mango, stripped, pitted, and divide into slices
- 1 tablespoon unsweetened coconut flakes

1. In a frying pan over high heat, boil water. Put the oats and lower the heat. Cook, occasionally stirring, for 5 minutes.
2. Put in the coconut milk, maple syrup, and salt to combine.
3. Get two bowls and sprinkle with the sesame seeds and cinnamon. Top with sliced mango and coconut flakes.

Nutrition: Calories: 373 Total fat: 11g Cholesterol: 0mg Fiber: 2g Protein: 12g Sodium: 167mg

47. *Spiced Sweet Potato Hash with Cilantro-Lime Cream*

Prep Time: 20 min | **Cook Time:** 30 min | **Serve:** 2
- For the cilantro-lime cream
- 1 avocado, halved and pitted
- ¼ cup packed fresh cilantro leaves and stems
- 2 tablespoons freshly squeezed lime juice
- 1 garlic clove, peeled
- 1 teaspoon kosher salt
- ½ teaspoon ground cumin
- 2 tablespoons extra-virgin olive oil
- For the hash
- ½ teaspoon kosher salt
- 1 large sweet potato, cut into ¾-inch pieces
- 2 tablespoons extra-virgin olive oil
- 1 onion, thinly sliced
- 2 garlic cloves, crushed
- 1 red bell pepper, thinly sliced
- 1 teaspoon ground cumin
- ¼ teaspoon ground turmeric
- Pinch freshly ground black pepper
- 2 tablespoons fresh cilantro leaves, chopped
- ½ jalapeño pepper, seeded and chopped (optional)

- Hot sauce, for serving (optional)

1. To make the cilantro-lime cream
2. Add the avocado flesh in a food compressor. Add the cilantro, lime juice, garlic, salt, and cumin. Whirl until smooth when the processor is running slowly, softly. Taste and adjust seasonings, as needed. If there is no food processor or blender for you,, simply mash the avocado well with a fork; the results will have more texture but will still work. Cover and refrigerate until ready to serve.
3. To make the hash
4. Boil saltwater in a medium pot over high heat. Add the sweet potato and cook for about 20 minutes until tender. Drain thoroughly.
5. Over low heat, heat the olive oil. In a large skillet until it shimmers. Add the onion and sauté for about 4 minutes until translucent. Put the garlic and cook, turning, for about 30 seconds. Add the cooked sweet potato and red bell pepper. Season the hash with cumin, salt, turmeric, and pepper. For 5 to 7 minutes, Saute until the sweet potatoes are golden and the red bell pepper is soft.
6. Divide the sweet potatoes between 2 bowls and spoon the sauce over them. Scatter the cilantro and jalapeño (if using) over each and serve with hot sauce (if using).

Nutrition: Calories: 520 Total fat: 43g Cholesterol: 0mg Fiber: 2g Protein: 12g Sodium: 1719mg

48. Open-Face Egg Sandwiches with Cilantro-Jalapeño spread

Prep Time: 20 min | **Cook Time:** 10 min | **Serve:** 2

For the cilantro and jalapeño spread
- 1 cup filled up fresh cilantro leaves and stems (about 1 bunch)
- 1 jalapeño pepper, seeded and roughly chopped
- ½ cup extra-virgin olive oil
- ¼ cup pepitas (hulled pumpkin seeds), raw or roasted
- 2 garlic cloves, thinly sliced
- 1 tablespoon freshly squeezed lime juice
- 1 teaspoon kosher salt

For the eggs
- 4 large eggs
- ¼ cup milk
- ¼ to ½ teaspoon kosher salt
- 2 tablespoons butter

For the sandwich
- 2 slices bread
- 1 tablespoon butter
- 1 avocado, halved, pitted and divided into slices Microgreens or sprouts, for garnish

1. To make the cilantro and jalapeño spread
2. In a food processor, combine the cilantro, jalapeño, oil, pepitas, garlic, lime juice, and salt. Whirl until smooth. Refrigerate if making in advance; otherwise, set aside.
3. To make the eggs
4. In a medium bowl, whisk the eggs, milk, and salt.
5. Dissolve the butter in a skillet over low heat, swirling to coat the pan's bottom. Pour in the whisked eggs. Cook until they begin to set then, using a heatproof spatula, push them to the sides, allowing the uncooked portions to run into the bottom of the skillet. Continue until the eggs are set.
6. To assemble the sandwiches
7. Toast the bed and spread it with butter.
8. Spread a spoonful of the cilantro-jalapeño spread on each piece of toast. Top each with scrambled eggs.

9. Arrange avocado over each sandwich and garnish with microgreens.

Nutrition: Calories: 711 Total fat: 4g Cholesterol: 54mg Fiber: 12g Protein: 12g Sodium: 327mg

49. Scrambled Eggs with Soy Sauce and Broccoli Slaw

Prep Time: 5 min | **Cook Time:** 10 min | **Serve:** 2
- 1 tablespoon peanut oil, divided
- 4 large eggs
- ½ to 1 tablespoon soy sauce, tamari, or Bragg's liquid aminos
- 1 tablespoon water
- 1 cup shredded broccoli slaw or another shredded vegetable
- Kosher salt
- Chopped fresh cilantro for serving
- Hot sauce, for serving.

1. In a medium nonstick skillet or cast-iron skillet over medium heat, heat 2 teaspoons of peanut oil, swirling to coat the skillet.
2. In a small bowl, whip the eggs, soy sauce, and water until smooth. Pour the eggs into the pan and let the bottom set. Using a wooden spoon, spread the eggs from one side to the other a couple of times so the uncooked portions on top pool into the bottom. Cook until the eggs are set.
3. In a medium container, stir together the broccoli slaw, the remaining 1 teaspoon of peanut oil, and a salt touch. Divide the slaw between 2 plates.
4. Top with the eggs and scatter cilantro on each serving. Serve with hot sauce.

Nutrition: Calories: 222 Total fat: 4g Cholesterol: 374mg Fiber: 2g Protein: 12g Sodium: 737mg

50. Tasty Breakfast Donuts

Prep Time: 5 min | **Cook Time:** 5 min | **Serve:** 4
- 43 grams' cream cheese
- 2 eggs
- 2 tablespoons almond flour
- 2 tablespoons erythritol
- 1 ½ tablespoons coconut flour
- ½ teaspoon baking powder
- ½ teaspoon vanilla extract
- 5 drops Stevia (liquid form)
- 2 strips bacon, fried until crispy

1. Rub coconut oil over the donut maker and turn it on.
2. Pulse all ingredients except bacon in a blender or food processor until smooth (should take around 1 minute).
3. pour batter into the donut maker, leaving 1/10 in each round for rising.
4. Leave for 3 minutes before flipping each donut. When you pierce them, leave for another 2 minutes or until the fork comes out clean.
5. Take donuts out and let cool.
6. Repeat steps 1-5 until all batter is used.
7. Crumble bacon into bits and use to top donuts.

Nutrition: Calories: 60 Fat: 5g Carbs: 1g Fiber: 0g Protein: 3g

51. Cheesy Spicy Bacon Bowls

Prep Time: 10 min | **Cook Time:** 22 min | **Serve:** 12
- 6 strips Bacon, pan-fried until cooked but still malleable

- 4 eggs
- 60 grams' cheddar cheese
- 40 grams' cream cheese, grated
- 2 Jalapenos, sliced and seeds removed
- 2 tablespoons coconut oil
- ¼ teaspoon onion powder
- ¼ teaspoon garlic powder
- Dash of salt and pepper

1. Preheat oven to 375 degrees Fahrenheit
2. In a bowl, beat together eggs, cream cheese, jalapenos (minus 6 slices), coconut oil, onion powder, garlic powder, and salt and pepper.
3. Using leftover bacon grease on a muffin tray, rubbing it into each insert. Place bacon-wrapped inside the parameters of each insert.
4. Pour the beaten mixture halfway up each bacon bowl.
5. Garnish each bacon bowl with cheese and leftover jalapeno slices (placing one on top of each).
6. Leave in the oven for about 22 minutes, or until the egg is thoroughly cooked and cheese is bubbly.
7. Remove from oven and let cool until edible.
Nutrition: Calories: 259 Fat: 24g Carbs: 1g Fiber: 0g Protein: 10g

52.Goat Cheese Zucchini Kale Quiche
Prep Time: 35 min | **Cook Time:** 1 h 10 min | **Serve:** 4
- 4 large eggs
- 8 ounces' fresh zucchini, sliced
- 10 ounces' kale
- 3 garlic cloves (minced)
- 1 cup of soy milk
- 1 ounce's goat cheese
- 1cup grated parmesan
- 1cup shredded cheddar cheese
- 2 teaspoons olive oil
- Salt & pepper, to taste

1. Preheat oven to 350°F.
2. Heat 1 TSP of olive-oil in a casserole dish over medium-high heat.
6. Slightly grease a baking dish with cooking spray and spread the kale leaves across the bottom. Add the zucchini and top with goat cheese.
7. Pour the egg, milk and parmesan mixture evenly over the other ingredients. Top with cheddar cheese.
8. Bake for 50–60 minutes until golden brown. Check the center of the quiche; it should have a solid consistency.
9. Let chill for a few minutes before serving.
Nutrition: Total Carbohydrates: 15g Dietary Fiber: 2g Net Carbs: 13g Protein: 19g Total Fat: 18g Calories: 290

53.Cream Cheese Egg Breakfast
Prep Time: 5 min | **Cook Time:** 5 min | **Serve:** 4
- 2 eggs, beaten
- 1 tablespoon butter
- 2 tablespoons soft cream cheese with chives

1. Melt the butter in a small skillet. Add the eggs and cream cheese. Stir and cook to desired doneness.
Nutrition: Calories: 341 Fat: 31g Protein: 15g Carbohydrate: 0g Dietary Fiber: 3g

54.Avocado Red Peppers Roasted Scrambled Eggs
Prep Time: 10 min | **Cook Time:** 12 min | **Serve:** 3
- 1/2 tablespoon butter
- Eggs, 2
- 1/2 roasted red pepper, about 1 1/2 ounces
- 1/2 small avocado, coarsely chopped, about 2 1/4 ounces Salt, to taste

1. Heat the butter over heat in a nonstick skillet. Break the eggs into the pan and break the yolks with a spoon. Sprinkle with a little salt.
2. Stir to stir and continue stirring until the eggs start to come out. Quickly add the bell peppers and avocado.
3. Cook and stir until the eggs suit your taste. Adjust the seasoning, if necessary.
Nutrition: Calories: 317 Fat: 26g Protein: 14g Dietary Fiber: 5g Net Carbs: 4g

55.Mushroom Quickie Scramble
Prep Time: 10 min | **Cook Time:** 10 min | **Serve:** 4
- 3 small-sized eggs, whisked
- 4 pcs. bella mushrooms
- ½ cup of spinach
- ¼ cup of red bell peppers
- 2 deli ham slices
- 1 tablespoon of ghee or coconut oil
- Salt & pepper to taste

1. Chop the ham and veggies.
2. Put half a tbsp of butter in a frying pan and heat until melted.
3. Sauté the ham and vegetables in a frying pan, then set aside.
4. Get a new frying pan and heat the remaining butter.
5. Add the whisked eggs into the second pan while stirring continuously to avoid overcooking.
6. When the eggs are done, sprinkle with salt & pepper to taste.
7. Add the ham and veggies to the pan with the eggs.
8. Mix well.
9. Remove it from the burner and transfer it to a tray.
Nutrition: Calories: 350 Total Fat: 29 g Protein: 21 g Total Carbs: 5 g

56.Coconut Coffee and Ghee
Prep Time: 10 min | **Cook Time:** 10 min | **Serve:** 5
- ½ Tbsp. of coconut oil
- ½ Tbsp. of ghee
- 1 to 2 cups of preferred coffee (or rooibos or black tea, if preferred)
- 1 Tbsp. of coconut or almond milk

1. Place the almond (or coconut) milk, coconut oil, ghee and coffee in a blender (or milk frother).
2. mix for around 10 seconds or until the coffee turns creamy and foamy.
3. Pour contents into a coffee cup.
Nutrition: Calories: 150 Total Fat: 15 g Protein: 0 g Total Carbs: 0 g Net Carbs: 0 g

57.Yummy Veggie Waffles
Prep Time: 10 min | **Cook Time:** 9 min | **Serve:** 3
- 3 cups raw cauliflower, grated
- 1 cup cheddar cheese
- 1 cup mozzarella cheese
- ½ cup parmesan
- 1/3 cup chives, finely sliced

- 6 eggs
- 1 teaspoon garlic powder
- 1 teaspoon onion powder
- ½ teaspoon chili flakes
- Dash of salt and pepper

1. Turn the waffle maker on.
2. Mix all the ingredients in a bowl.
3. Once the waffle maker is hot, distribute the waffle mixture into the insert.
4. Let cook for about 9 minutes, flipping at 6 minutes.
5. Remove from waffle maker and set aside.
6. Repeat the steps with the batter until it's gone (4 waffles should come out)

Nutrition: Calories: 390 Fat: 28g Carbs: 6g Fiber: 2g Protein: 30g

58. Omega 3 Breakfast Shake

Prep Time: 5 min | **Cook Time:** 5 min | **Serve:** 2
- 1 cup vanilla almond milk (unsweetened)
- 2 tablespoons blueberries
- 1 ½ tablespoons flaxseed meal
- 1 tablespoon MCT Oil
- ¾ tablespoon banana extract
- ½ tablespoon chia seeds
- 5 drops Stevia (liquid form)
- 1/8 tablespoon Xanthan gum

1. In a blender, pulse vanilla almond milk, banana extract, Stevia, and 3 ice cubes.
2. When smooth, add blueberries and pulse.
3. Once blueberries are thoroughly incorporated, add flaxseed meal and chia seeds.
4. Let sit for 5 minutes.
5. After 5 minutes, pulse again until all ingredients are nicely distributed.

Nutrition: Calories: 264 Fats: 25g Carbs: 7g Protein: 4g

59. Bacon Spaghetti Squash Carbonara

Prep Time: 20 min | **Cook Time:** 40 min | **Serve:** 4
- 1 small spaghetti squash
- 6 ounces' bacon (roughly chopped)
- 1 large tomato (sliced)
- 2 chives (chopped)
- 1 garlic clove (minced)
- 6 ounces' low-fat cottage cheese
- 1 cup Gouda cheese (grated)
- 2 tablespoons olive oil
- Salt and pepper, to taste

1. Preheat the oven to 350°F.
2. Cut the squash spaghetti in half, brush with some olive oil and bake for 20–30 minutes, skin side up. Remove from the oven and remove the core with a fork, creating the spaghetti.
3. In a pan, heat one tablespoon of olive oil. Cook the bacon for about 1 minute until crispy.
4. Quickly wipe out the pan with paper towels.
5. Heat another tablespoon of oil and sauté the garlic, tomato and chives for 2–3 minutes. Add the spaghetti and sauté for another 5 minutes, occasionally stirring to keep from burning.
6. Begin to add the cottage cheese, about 2 tablespoons at a time. If the sauce becomes thick, add about a cup of water. It should be smooth with the sauce but not too runny or thick. Allow cooking for another 3 minutes.

Nutrition: Calories: 305 Total Fat: 21g Net Carbs: 8g Protein: 18g

60. Lime Bacon Thyme Muffins

Prep Time: 10 min | **Cook Time:** 20 min | **Serve:** 3
- 3 cups of almond flour
- 4 medium-sized eggs
- 1 cup of bacon bits
- 2 tsp. of lemon thyme
- ½ cup of melted ghee
- 1 tsp. of baking soda
- ½ tsp. of salt, to taste

1. Pre-heat oven to 350° F.
2. Put ghee in the mixing bowl and melt.
3. Add baking soda and almond flour.
4. Put the eggs in.
5. Add the lemon thyme (if preferred, other herbs or spices may be used).
6. Drizzle with salt.
7. Mix all ingredients well.
8. Sprinkle with bacon bits.
9. Line the muffin pan with liners.
10. Spoon mixture into the pan, filling the pan to about ¾ full.
11. Bake for about 20 minutes. Test by inserting a toothpick into a muffin. If it comes out clean, then the muffins are done.

Nutrition: Calories: 300 Total Fat: 28 g Protein: 11 g Total Carbs: 6 g Fiber: 3 g

61. Gluten -Free Pancakes

Prep Time: 5 min | **Cook Time:** 2 min | **Serve:** 2
- 6 eggs
- 1 cup low-fat cream cheese
- 1 1/12; teaspoons baking powder
- 1 scoop protein powder
- 1/4; cup almond meal
- ¼ teaspoon salt

1. Combine dry ingredients in a food processor. Add the eggs one after another and then the cream cheese. Edit until you have a blast.
2. Lightly grease a skillet with spray and place over medium-high heat.
3. Pour the batter into the pan. Turn the pan gently to create round pancakes.
4. Cook for about 120 seconds on each side.
5. Serve pancakes with your favorite topping.

Nutrition: Dietary Fiber: 1g Net Carbs: 5g Protein: 25g Total Fat: 14g Calories: 288

62. Mushroom & Spinach Omelet

Prep Time: 20 min | **Cook Time:** 20 min | **Serve:** 3
- 2 tablespoons butter, divided
- 6-8 fresh mushrooms, sliced, 5 ounces
- Chives, chopped, optional
- Salt and pepper, to taste
- 1 handful baby spinach, about 1/2 ounce
- Pinch garlic powder
- 4 eggs, beaten
- 1-ounce shredded Swiss cheese,

1. In a very large saucepan, sauté the mushrooms in 1 tablespoon of butter until soft. Season with salt, pepper and garlic.

2. Remove the pan from the mushrooms and keep warm. Once the egg is almost out, place the cheese over the middle of the tortilla.

4. Fill the cheese with spinach leaves and hot mushrooms. Let cook for about a minute for the spinach to start to wilt. Fold the tortilla's empty side carefully over the filling and slide it onto a plate and sprinkle with chives, if desired.

5. Alternatively, you can make two tortillas using half the mushroom, spinach, and cheese filling in each.

Nutrition: Calories: 321 Fat: 26g Protein: 19g Carbohydrate: 4g Dietary Fiber: 1g

63.Gluten-Free Pancakes

Prep Time: 5 min | **Cook Time:** 2 minutes **Serve:** 2

- 6 eggs
- 1 cup low-fat cream cheese
- 1 1/12; teaspoons baking powder
- 1 scoop protein powder
- 1/4; cup almond meal
- ¼ teaspoon salt

1. Combine dry ingredients in a food processor. Add the eggs one after another and then the cream cheese. Edit until you have a blast.
2. Lightly grease a cooking spray skillet and position it over medium-high heat.
3. Pour the batter into the pan. Turn the pan gently to create round pancakes.
4. Cook on each side for about 2,5 minutes.
5. Serve pancakes with your favorite topping.

Nutrition: Dietary Fiber: 1g Net Carbs: 5g Protein: 25g Total Fat: 14g Calories: 288

64.Sweey and Smoked Salmon

Prep Time: 35 min | **Cook Time:** 1 h | **Serve:** 8

- 2 tablespoons light brown sugar
- 2 tablespoons smoked peppers
- 1 tablespoon shaved lemon peel
- Sare Kosar
- Freshly chopped black pepper Salmon fillets on the skin 1/2 kilogram

1. Soak a large plate (about 15 cm by 7 inches) in water for 1 to 2 hours.
2. It is heated over medium heat. Combine sugar, pepper, lemon zest, and 1/2 teaspoon of salt and pepper in a bowl. Mix the salmon with the salt and rub the mixture of spices in all parts of the meat.
3. Put the salmon on the wet plate, skin down — oven, covered, in the desired color, 25 to 28 minutes for medium.

Nutrition: Calories: 321 Total fat: 4g Cholesterol: 54mg Fiber: 2g Protein: 12g Sodium: 337mg

65.Vitamina C Smoothie Cubes

Prep Time: 5 min | **Cook Time:** 8 h to chill | **Serve:** 1

- 1/8 large papaya
- 1/8 mango
- 1/4 cups chopped pineapple, fresh or frozen
- 1/8 cup raw cauliflower florets, fresh or frozen
- 1/4 large navel oranges, peeled and halved
- 1/4 large orange bell pepper stemmed, seeded, and coarsely chopped

1. Halve the papaya and mango, remove the pits, and scoop their soft flesh into a high-speed blender.

2. Add the pineapple, cauliflower, oranges, and bell pepper. Blend until smooth.
3. Evenly divide the puree between 2 (16-compartment) ice cube trays and place them on a level surface in your freezer. Freeze for at least 8 hours.
4. The cubes can be left in the ice cube trays until use or transferred to a freezer bag. The frozen cubes are good for about three weeks in a standard freezer or up to 6 months in a chest freezer.

Nutrition: Calories: 96, Fat: 1 g, Protein: 2 g, Carbohydrates: 24 g, Fiber: 4 g

66.Polenta with Seared Pears

Prep Time: 10 min | **Cook Time:** 50 min | **Serve:** 1

- One cup water, divided, plus more as needed
- 1/2 cups coarse cornmeal
- One tablespoon pure maple syrup
- 1/4 tablespoon molasses
- 1/4 teaspoon ground cinnamon
- 1/2 ripe pears, cored and diced
- 1/4 cup fresh cranberries
- 1/4 teaspoon chopped fresh rosemary leaves

1. In a pan, cook 5 cups of water to a simmer.
2. While whisking continuously to avoid clumping, slowly pour in the cornmeal. Cook, often stirring with a heavy spoon, for 30 minutes. The polenta should be thick and creamy.
3. While the polenta cooks, in a saucepan over medium heat, stir together the maple syrup, molasses, Whit the remaining 1/4 cup of water and when paired, the cinnamon. Bring it to a simmer. Add the pears and cranberries. Cook for 10 minutes, occasionally stirring, until the pears are tender and start to brown.
4. Remove from the heat. Stir in the rosemary and let the mixture sit for 5 minutes. If it is too thick, add another 1/4 cup of water and return to the heat.
5. Top with the cranberry-pear mixture.

Nutrition: Calories: 282, Fat: 2 g, Protein: 4 g

67.Bell-Pepper Corn Wrapped in Tortilla

Prep Time: 5 min | **Cook Time:** 15 min | **Serve:** 1

- 1/4 small red bell pepper, chopped
- 1/4 small yellow onion, diced
- 1/4 tablespoon water
- 1/2 cobs grilled corn kernels
- One large tortilla
- One-piece commercial vegan nuggets, chopped
- Mixed greens for garnish

1. Preheat the Instant Crisp Air Fryer to 400°F.
2. In a skillet heated over medium heat, sauté the vegan nuggets and the onions, bell peppers, and corn kernels. Set aside.
3. Place filling inside the corn tortillas.
4. Lock the air fryer lid. Fold the tortillas and place inside the Instant Crisp Air Fryer, cook for 15 minutes until the tortilla wraps are crispy.
5. Serve with mixed greens on top.

Nutrition: Calories: 548, Fat: 20.7g, Protein: 46g

68.Eggplant Curry

Prep Time: 5 min | **Cook Time:** 30 min | **Serve:** 2

- ½ tbsp. pepper
- ½ cups coconut milk (1 cup = 250ml)

- tin tomatoes (chopped) (roughly 14oz./400g)
- tbsp. Ground coriander
- tbsp. turmeric
- 1 tbsp. gram masala powder or curry powder
- clove garlic
- 1 red onion
- tbsp. Olive oil
- ½ tbsp. salt
- 1 aborigine (medium)
- Optional:
- tbsp. sugar (or 1-2 tbsp. mango chutney)

1. Cook as per packet directions when using rice.
2. Break your aubergine into tiny cubes. Fry with olive oil in a wide pan over high heat for 3-4 minutes. Mix well enough that it won't smoke.
3. Meanwhile, chop-the onion, and put it in as well. Put it back to medium heat and cook for 5-6 minutes.
4. Crush the garlic or dice it.
5. Garlic, curry powder, turmeric, and ground cilantro should be mixed in. Cook, stirring well, for the next 3-4 minutes.
6. Add in the sliced tomatoes and coconut milk. Add salt.
7. Boil for 15 minutes, roughly.
8. The coconut milk gets thicker, so when it is at the right consistency for you, stop cooking.
9. If you like it a little-sweeter, stir in the honey or mango chutney.
10. Serve according to taste, with salt and pepper.

69. Authentic Vegan Banana Pancakes

Prep Time: 5 min | **Cook Time:** 15 min | **Serve:** 4
- 2 tbsp. Chia seeds
- ripe, med-sized banana
- tbsp. baking powder
- ⅓ cup wholemeal flour
- pinch salt
- cup soy milk (or your fave None-dairy)
- tbsp. olive oil (or coconut oil work great)
- cup rolled oats

1. Put all the products into a large bowl and use a hand blender to mix them.
2. In a None-stick pan, spray or drizzle with oil and scatter around with a paper towel. Heat (do not go higher!) at low-medium heat.
3. Place about a tiny volume of the batter. The pancakes should be tiny and fluffy.
4. Put a lid-on-it and let it softly steam the pancake. The other hand is through until the side facing you starts bubbling. Time for tossing! The smallest is a spatula.
5. Let the other side cook when turned, too. After a minute or two, take a look at the underside with the spatula. It is ready when it is good and brown (but not burnt!). Woo! Only repeat.
6. If you have a big pan, it's easy to simultaneously cook two or three small pancakes. Alternatively, if you experience a single flash, you should cook at the same time with two pans. Serve directly, or stack the pancakes in a warm oven on a tray before you're ready to eat.

70. African Peanut Soup

Prep Time: 15 min | **Cook Time:** 10 min | **Serve:** 3
- cup brown rice (uncooked)
- A few dashes hot sauce
- tbsp. Soy sauce

- clove garlic
- small carrot
- tbsp. tomato paste
- handful of peanuts
- 3-4 tbsp. peanut butter
- ½ medium courgette (zucchini)
- ½ red onion
- cups vegetable broth
- 0.2 inches ginger, fresh (0.2 inches = 0.5 cm = ½ tbsp. powdered ginger)

1. Prepare the brown rice.
2. Put to the boil 700ml of vegetable broth.
3. Split the cabbage, carrot, and courgette and add them to the broth
4. Garlic and gingeer are also added to the broth.
5. Put in the peanuts.
6. Add some peanut butter and tomato paste to your mixture.
7. Add some soy sauce last but ensure it's not still too salty.
8. Let the rice boil until it is done.

71. Zucchini Ravioli

Prep Time: 20 min | **Cook Time:** 25 min
- 1 cup 257 grams of sauce with marinara
- 3 Medium zucchini, washed + dried with cut off ends
- 1 Tbsp of olive oil
- 2 cups 60 grams of fresh and washed spinach
- 2 Cloves 1 Tsp of chopped garlic
- 1 cup of 250 grams of whole ricotta milk
- 2 Tbsps of sliced fresh basil for garnishing
- 1 cup of cherry tomatoes 150 grams
- 1/2 cup of 56 grams of mozzarella (shredded into chunks)
- 2 Tsps 10 grams Parmesan grated

1. Oven preheat to 425 ° F.
2. On the bottom of a broad roasting dish, spread out the marinara sauce.
3. Use a mandolin or vegetable peeler to make your zucchini noodles. Peel the zucchini into strips 1/4 of an inch wide. Spread them out and sprinkle with salt on a surface lined with a paper towel. Set aside the remaining ingredients as you prepare.
4. Apply the olive oil to a medium-sized skillet and bring low heat to medium. Add the spinach, then cook until it is wilted. Add the garlic to the saucepan and cook until fragrant, to prevent burning, for a minute or two, stirring all the time. Switch off the fire, and remove the fire burner from the pan.
5. Along with the ricotta and chopped basil, add the spinach and garlic to a dish. Stir to blend.
6. Give your sliced zucchini back and blot away the excess moisture.
7. Take three zucchini strips at a time, and lay them on a clean surface. Layout the first two strips to form a 't' minus case. Line the top stripe of the zucchini with the lower sheet. Apply about 1 tbsp of the ricotta mixture to the zucchini core. To make little 'ravioli' packets, fold the ends of the strips over the ricotta mixture. Continue with the rest of the cheese/zucchini.
8. Switch the folded zucchini to the roasting plate and put the marinara/tomatoes on top. Along with the mozzarella & parmesan, scatter the tomatoes over the top.
9. 20 Minutes to bake in the oven. Broil and blister the tomatoes for an additional 2 minutes and then remove.

10. It is necessary to wait for it to cool down for 5 minutes before serving and enjoy! If required, sprinkle with extra basil.

Nutrition: calories: 193; cholesterol: 35mg; sodium: 422mg; carbohydrates: 10g; fiber: 2g; sugar: 6g; protein: 11g

72.Lean & Green Tofu Stir-Fry

Prep Time: 10 min | **Cook Time:** 12 min

- Olive oil for 2 tbsp
- 1/4 cup of White oignon
- 1/2 cup Oyster champignon (cutted into large pieces)
- 1/2 Green bell pepper (cutted into large pieces)
- 3 Rapini stalk, broccoli raab, raw (cutted into large pieces)
- 1/3 cup of Edamame frozen (soybeans)
- Tofu 227 gm, standard, extra firm (pressed and cutted into bite size cubes)
- 1 (minced)Garlic clove
- 3 tsp Yeast nutrition
- Oyster Sauce 1 tbsp
- 1 Tbsp Soja sauce with low sodium
- 5 Cherry Tomatoes
- 4 Cup Spinach for Infant
- Hot sauce 1 tsp
- 1/4 cup of (cut) Peanuts

1. Over medium pressure, spray a non-stick skillet with cooking spray and pressure.
2. Add the onion and mushrooms and saute for around 2-3 minutes until the onions are translucent and the mushrooms have softened.
3. For 3-4 minutes, add the green pepper, rapini, and edamame and sauté.
4. Connect the tofu and garlic to your skillet now. Toss to mix and cook for another 1-2 minutes.
5. Fill the pan with your oyster sauce, soy sauce, and nutritional yeast. Remove until well concealed.
6. Add the tomatoes and spinach. Cook for another 2-3 minutes before the spinach begins to wilt slightly.
7. Place sriracha and chopped peanuts on top.

73.Zucchini Lasagna

Prep Time: 40 mins | **Cook Time:** 30 mins

For the zucchini layer:
- 5 Medium size zucchinis
- Cooking Spray With Olive Oil
- 1 1/2 tbsp kosher salt Diamond Crystal divided 1/2 tbsp split black pepper
- 1/2 tbsp powdered garlic

For the beef layer:
- Olive oil for 1 tbsp
- With 1 lb. Lean beef (85/15)
- 1 tbsp of garlic, minced
- 1 1/3 cup split marinara sauce

For the ricotta layer:
- 15 oz of room temperature whole milk ricotta cheese
- 2 large eggs
- 1/2 cup of chopped fresh basil

Topping:
- 8 oz of shredded part-skim split mozzarella cheese

Grill the zucchini slices:

1. Heat the grill and oven to 350 degrees F on medium heat. Long-slice the zucchinis into 1/4-inch-thick strips, get 6 slices out of each zucchini and discard the ends.
2. Spray olive oil on the zucchini slices and sprinkle with 1/2 tsp kosher salt, 1/8 tsp black-pepper, and 1/2 tsp garlic powder.
3. Grill the slices of zucchini, in lots, on each side for 2-3 minutes or until golden and firm, not browned and crisp. To soak up more humidity, spread them on clean kitchen towels.

Cook the beef:

1. In a large skillet over heat, heat the olive oil for about 2 minutes. Add the beef, minced garlic, kosher salt 1/2 tsp, and black pepper 1/4 tsp.
2. Cook, stirring to break up the beef with a spoon, until the meat is no longer raw, about five minutes. Return the meat to the pot and apply 1 cup of marinara sauce to the mixture, then drain in the colander. Turn off the flame and put yourself aside.

Prepare the ricotta layer:

1. In a medium bowl with a fork, combine the ricotta, eggs, basil, and the remaining kosher salt and black pepper together.

Assemble the lasagna:

1. Spread out the remaining 1/3 of a cup of marinara sauce on the bottom of a 9 X 13 baking dish. It is also possible to use a slightly smaller baking dish, such as a dish that measures 11 X 7 inches.
2. On top of the marinara sauce, add a layer of zucchini on top, then a third of the mixture of ricotta, a third of the mixture of meat, and a third of the shredded mozzarella cheese.
3. Repeat, in the opposite direction, arrange the zucchini slices: zucchini, 1/3 ricotta, 1/3 meat mixture, 1/3 mozzarella.
4. Add one extra layer of zucchini: zucchini, ricotta, meat mix, more zucchini, and mozzarella, and repeat for the last time.

Bake the lasagna:

1.Bake, uncovered, for about 31 minutes, until the cheese is golden. If desired and if your dish is broiler-safe, you can finish by broiling for 1-2 minutes on high to brown the cheese. For 10 minutes, Until serving, let stand.

74.Garlic Shrimp Zucchini Noodles

Prep Time: 15 mins | **Cook Time:** 15 mins

- 2 Medium zucchini
- Shrimp shelled and de-veined 1 pound
- 2 Tbsp butter
- 3 sliced Garlic cloves
- Parmesan cheese: 3/4 cup
- Kosher salt or sea salt
- Black chili
- (1/4 tsp) red chili flakes
- lemon wedges

1. Using the vegetable spiraliser or julienne peeler to cut the zucchini into spirals or noodle strands. Put the noodles aside.
2. Over medium-high heat, heat a wide pan. Melt the olive oil/butter, then add the garlic and shrimp. Cook the shrimp until it is cooked. Don't let it burn the garlic.
3. Add the zucchini noodles, and cook for around 3-5 minutes until tender. Zucchini noodles are very easy to cook, so taste a strand as you cook and determine how firm or "al-dente" the zucchini you want. Don't overcook the zucchini noodles, or they're going to turn into mush.

4. Remove the pan from the fire, add parmesan cheese, squeeze some lemon juice and sprinkle with salt and pepper to taste generous. Serve warm, then add chili flakes.

Nutrition: Calories: 257kcal | Carbohydrates: 4g | Protein: 31g | Fat: 12g| Cholesterol:313mg | Sodium: 1241mg | Potassium: 372mg | Sugar: 2g | Calcium: 406mg |Iron: 2.9mg

75. Tofu with Peas

Prep Time: 15 min | **Cook Time:** 8 min | **Serve:** 4
- 1¼ cups unsweetened coconut milk
- 2 tablespoons curry paste
- 14 ounces firm tofu, pressed, drained, and cubed
- 1 tablespoon olive oil
- ½ teaspoons garam masala powder
- ½ teaspoons ground cumin
- ¼ teaspoons cayenne pepper
- ¼ teaspoons ground turmeric
- 1½ cups frozen green peas, thawed
- Salt, as required

1. In a bowl, add coconut milk and curry paste and mix until smooth.
2. Add the oil in Instant Pot and select "Sauté". Then add the garam masala, cumin, cayenne and turmeric and cook for about 30 seconds.
3. Stir in tofu cubes and cook for about 2 minutes.
4. Press "Cancel" and stir in the coconut milk mixture, peas and salt.
5. Secure the lid and switch to the location of the "Seal".
6. Cook on "Manual" with "High Pressure" for about 5 minutes.
7. Press "Cancel" and carefully do a "Quick" release.
8. Remove the lid and serve hot.

Nutrition: Calories: 321 | fat: 24.8g | protein: 12.2g | carbs: 13g | net carbs: 9g | fiber: 4g

76. Barley Risotto

Prep Time: 15 min | **Cook Time:** 7 to 8 h | **Serve:** 8
- 21/4 cups hulled barley, rinsed
- 1 onion, finely chopped
- 4 garlic cloves, minced
- 1 (8-ounce) package button mushrooms, chopped
- 6 cups low-sodium vegetable broth
- 1/2 teaspoon dried marjoram leaves
- 1/8 teaspoon freshly ground black pepper
- 2/3 cup grated Parmesan cheese

1. In a 6-quart slow cooker, mix the barley, onion, garlic, mushrooms, broth, marjoram, and pepper.
2. Cook for 7/8 hours or until most of the liquid is absorbed and tender and the vegetables are tender, or until the barley is full.
3. Stir in the Parmesan cheese and serve.

Nutrition: Calories: 288 Cal, Carbohydrates: 45 g, Sugar: 2 g, Fiber: 9 g, Fat: 6 g, Saturated Fat: 3 g, Protein: 13 g, Sodium: 495 mg

77. Risotto with Green Beans, Sweet Potatoes, and Peas

Prep Time: 20 min | **Cook Time:** 4 to 5 h | **Serve:** 8
- 1 large sweet potato, peeled and chopped
- 1 onion, chopped
- 5 garlic cloves, minced
- 2 cups short-grain brown rice
- 1 teaspoon dried thyme leaves
- 7 cups low-sodium vegetable broth
- 2 cups green beans, cut in half crosswise
- 2 cups frozen baby peas
- 3 tablespoons unsalted butter
- 1/2 cup grated Parmesan cheese

1. In a 6-quart slow cooker, mix the sweet potato, onion, garlic, rice, thyme, and broth.
2. Cook on low heat for 3/4 hours, or until the rice is tender.
3. Stir in the green beans and frozen peas.
4. Cook on low heat for 30 to 40 minutes or until the vegetables are tender.
5. Stir in the butter and cheese. Cook for 20 minutes over low heat, then stir and serve.

Nutrition: Calories: 385 Cal, Carbohydrates: 52 g, Sugar: 4 g, Fiber: 6 g, Fat: 10 g, Saturated Fat: 5 g, Protein: 10 g, Sodium: 426 mg

78. Prawn Arrabbiata

Prep Time: 35 min | **Cook Time:** 30 min | **Serve:** 1
- Raw or cooked prawns, 1 cup
- Extra virgin olive oil, 1 tablespoon
- Buckwheat pasta, ½ cup
- Chopped parsley, 1 tablespoon
- Celery, ¼ cup (finely chopped)
- Tinned chopped tomatoes, 2 cups
- Red onion, 1/3 cup (finely chopped)
- Garlic clove, 1 (finely chopped)
- Extra virgin olive oil, 1 teaspoon
- Dried mixed herbs, 1 teaspoon
- Bird's eye chili, 1 (finely chopped)
- White wine, 2 tablespoons (optional)

1. Add the olive oil into your fry-pan and fry the dried herbs, celery, and onions over medium-low heat for about two minutes.
2. Increase the heat to low, add the wine and simmer for another minute.
3. Add the tomatoes to the pan and allow to simmer for about 30 minutes, over medium-low heat, until you get a good creamy consistency, over medium-low heat.
4. If the sauce gets too thick, add a bit of water.
5. Cook the pasta while the sauce is heating, following the packet's instructions. Drain the water once the pasta is done cooking, toss with the olive oil, and set aside until needed.
6. If using raw prawns, add them to your sauce and cook for another four minutes, until the prawns turn opaque and pink, then add the parsley. If using cooked prawns, add them at the same time with the parsley and allow the sauce to boil.
7. Add the already cooked pasta to the sauce and mix theme.

Nutrition: Calories: 321, Protein: 19 g, Fat: 2 g, Carbohydrate: 23 g

79. Mediterranean Baked Penne

Prep Time: 25 min | **Cook Time:** 1 h 20 min | **Serve:** 8
- Extra-virgin olive oil, 1 tablespoon
- Fine dry breadcrumbs, ½ cup
- Small zucchini, 2 (chopped)
- Medium eggplant, 1 (chopped)
- Medium onion, 1 (chopped)
- Red bell pepper, 1 (seeded and chopped)
- Celery, 1 stalk (sliced)

- Garlic, 1 clove (minced)
- Salt and freshly ground pepper to taste
- Dry white wine, ¼ cup
- Plum tomatoes, 28-ounces (drained and coarsely chopped, juice reserved)
- Freshly grated Parmesan cheese, 2 tablespoons
- Large eggs, 2 (lightly beaten)
- Coarsely grated part-skim mozzarella cheese, 1 ½ cups
- Dried penne rig ate or rigatoni, 1 pound

1. Preheat to 375 degrees F in your oven. Apply nonstick spray on a 3-quart baking dish. Then coat the dish with ¼ cup of breadcrumbs, tapping out the excess.
2. Heat the oil in a big non-stick skillet over medium to high heat. Then add the onion, celery, bell pepper, eggplant, and zucchini. Cook, stirring periodically, for about 10 minutes, until smooth.Then add the garlic and cook for another minute. Add the wine, stir and cook for about 2 minutes, long enough for the wine to almost evaporate. Then add the juice and tomatoes. Bring it to a boil for 10/15 minutes or so, until thickened, season with pepper and salt. Put it in a large bowl to let it cool.
3. Pour water into a pot and add some salt when then allow to boil. Add the penne into the boiling salted water to cook for about 10 minutes, until al dente. Drain the pasta under running water and rinse it. Toss the pasta with the vegetable mixture, then stir in the mozzarella.
4. Scoop the pasta mixture and place into the prepared baking dish. Drizzle the broken eggs evenly over the top. Mix the Parmesan and ¼ cups of breadcrumbs in a small bowl, then sprinkle evenly over the top of the dish.
5. Cook the dish in the oven for 40/50 minutes or so, until bubbly and golden.
6. Allow to rest for 10 min before you serve.
Nutrition: Calories: 372, Protein: 45 g, Fat: 8 g, Sugar: 2 g

80.Jalapeno Cheese Balls
Prep Time: 10 min | **Cook Time:** 8 min | **Serve:** 1
- 1-ounce cream cheese
- 1/6 cup shredded mozzarella cheese
- 1/6 cup shredded Cheddar cheese
- 1/2 jalapeños, finely chopped
- 1/2 cup breadcrumbs
- Two eggs
- 1/2 cup all-purpose flour
- Salt and Pepper
- Cooking oil

1. Combine the cream cheese, mozzarella, Cheddar, and jalapeños in a medium bowl. Mix well.
2. Form the cheese mixture into balls about an inch thick. You may also use a small ice cream scoop. It works well.
3. Arrange the cheese balls on a sheet pan and place in the freezer for 15 minutes. It will help the cheese balls maintain their shape while frying.
4. Spray the Instant Crisp Air Fryer basket with cooking oil.
5. Place the breadcrumbs in a small bowl. In another small bowl, beat the eggs. In the third small bowl, combine the flour with salt and pepper to taste, and mix well.
6. Remove the cheese balls from the freezer. Plunge the cheese balls in the flour, then the eggs, and then the breadcrumbs.
7. Place the cheese balls in the Instant Crisp Air Fryer. Spray with cooking oil. Lock the air fryer lid. Cook for 8 minutes.

8. Open the Instant Crisp Air Fryer and flip the cheese balls. I recommend flipping them instead of shaking, so the balls maintain their form. Cook an additional 4 minutes.
9. Cool before serving.
Nutrition: Calories: 96, Fat: 6 g, Protein: 4 g, Sugar: 0 g

81.Chicken with Spinach and Mushrooms
Prep Time: 10 min | **Cook Time:** 20 min | **Serve:** 4
- 1 tbsp. olive oil
- 4 6-oz boneless, skinless breasts of chicken Black pepper and kosher salt
- 1 lb. quartered button mushrooms
- 1 red-bell-pepper, sliced into 1/2-inch bits 2 garlic cloves, chopped
- One-half cup white dry wine
- 2 bunches of spinach, removal of thick stems (about 8 cups)

1.Heat 1 little-spoon of oil over medium to high heat in a large skillet. With a one-half teaspoon of salt and one-fourth teaspoon of pepper, season the poultry.
2.Cook the chicken, 6 to 7 minutes on each side until browned and cooked through. Move to a dish.
3.Send the skillet back to medium-high heat and heat the remaining oil tablespoon. Cook the mushrooms and pepper for 3 minutes, tossing.
4.Add the garlic and wine and cook for 2 to 3 minutes, until the mushrooms are tender and the wine has almost evaporated.
5.Toss the salt and pepper with the spinach, one-half teaspoon each, and eat with the chicken.
Nutrition: calories: 743 kcal Protein: 32.24 g Fat: 18.27 g Carbohydrates: 129.82 g Calcium, Ca227 mg Magnesium, Mg324 mg

82.Creamy Pesto Chicken
Prep Time: 10 min | **Cook Time:** 15 min | **Serve:** 2
- 1 tablespoon extra-virgin olive oil
- 4 chicken breast halves - cut into strips
- 4 large cloves garlic, sliced
- 3 1/2 tablespoons sherry
- 1/4 cup pine nuts
- 1/2 cup chopped fresh basil
- 1 (8 ounces) container reduced-fat sour cream
- 3 tablespoons grated Parmesan cheese
- ground black pepper to taste

1.In a frying contaniner, heat olive oil over medium heat and cook the chicken until turning light brown, about 5 minutes. Stir into the frying pan the sherry and garlic. Stir and cook until the juices run clear, the chicken is not pink anymore, and all the liquid has decreased.
2.Stir into the frying pan the pine nuts, and cook over medium heat for 2-3 minutes. Stir in the pepper, parmesan cheese, sour cream, and basil and lower the heat to mild. Until completely cooked, keep cooking.
Nutrition: Calories 312, Fat 6, Carbs 16, Protein 12, Sodium 645

83.Gnocchi With Chicken, Pesto And Fresh Mozzarella
Prep Time: 10 min | **Cook Time:** 30 min | **Serve:** 2
- 1 tablespoon olive oil
- 1 chicken breast half - cut into 1 1/2-inch cube
- salt and ground black pepper to taste

- 2 tablespoons chicken broth
- 1 (8 ounces) jar prepared pesto
- 1 (12 ounces) package potato gnocchi
- 4 ounces small fresh mozzarella balls

In a saucepan, bring olive oil to heat. Add pepper and salt to chicken pieces to season; cook, stirring, for 7-10 minutes in hot oil until no pink meat remains in the center. With a slotted spoon, bring the chicken to a bowl while reserving drippings in the pan.

Add chicken broth into the saucepan. Boil broth, using a wooden spoon to scrape browned bits off the bottom of the pan; keep boiling for another 7-10 minutes until broth is reduced by about half of its original volume. Put cooked chicken back into the saucepan. Whisk in pesto; turn off the heat.

Slightly boil lightly salted water in a large pot. Cook gnocchi for about 3 minutes in boiling water until they float to the top. With a slotted spoon, transfer gnocchi from the water to a big bowl while reserving water in the pot.

Set pesto and chicken saucepan over boiling water; cook, stirring, for about 5minutes above boiling water until completely warmed. Cover gnocchi with warmed pesto-chicken mixture; top with mozzarella and stir until combined evenly.

Nutrition: Calories 464, Fat 12, Carbs 16, Protein 23, Sodium 643

84.Instant Pot Gourmet Pesto Chicken

Prep Time: 10 min | **Cook Time:** 30 min | **Serve:** 2
- 5 bone-in chicken thighs, skinned
- salt and ground black pepper to taste
- 1 tablespoon all-purpose flour, or as needed
- 1 tablespoon olive oil
- 1 1/2 cups chicken broth
- 1 (8 ounces) package cream cheese
- 1 (12 ounces) package penne pasta
- 2 cups cut asparagus, 1-inch lengths
- 2 cups cut green beans, 1-inch pieces
- 4 ounces basil pesto (such as Classico® Traditional)
- 1/4 teaspoon onion powder
- 1/4 teaspoon garlic powder

1.Add salt and pepper to the chicken. Coat with flour and dust off the excess.

2.Turn on a pressure cooker that is multi-functional (such as the Instant Pot ®). Select its "Sauté" function. Add olive oil and chicken. Cook the chicken for about 3 minutes or until very lightly browned. Pour in the chicken broth. Close and lock the lid. Select the "Poultry" setting and set the cooker's timer for 30 minutes. Let the pressure build for about 10 to 15 minutes.

3.Refer to the manufacturer's instructions on the quick-release method and carefully release pressure for about 5 minutes. Carefully unlock and remove the lid.

4.Mix in the garlic powder, cream cheese, green beans, onion powder, penne pasta, pesto, and asparagus. Stir together until well combined. Close the lid, select the "Rice" function, and set the timer for 3 minutes. Let the pressure build for 10 to 15 minutes. Cook according to the manufacturer's instructions.

5.Refer to the manufacturer's instructions on the quick-release method and carefully release pressure for about 5 minutes. Unlock and remove the lid.

Nutrition: Calories 408, Fat 6, Carbs 16, Protein 18, Sodium 308

85.Italian Chicken With Pesto Potatoes

Prep Time: 10 min | **Cook Time:** 30 min | **Serve:** 2
- 3/4 cup balsamic vinegar
- 4 skinless, boneless chicken breast halves
- 4 1/2 ounces sliced mozzarella cheese
- salt and pepper to taste
- 4 slices Parma ham
- 1-pint cherry tomatoes
- 1 tablespoon olive oil
- 1 pound small potatoes
- 2 tablespoons prepared basil pesto

1.Turn the oven to 200 C. to preheat.

2.Boil vinegar in a saucepan. Lower the heat and simmer until thickened, often whisking, about 15 minutes.

3.In each chicken breast, slice a pocket. Fill an even amount of mozzarella cheese into each pocket and use pepper and salt to season. Wrap 1 ham slice around each chicken breast. In a baking dish, place the wrapped chicken breasts. Around the chicken, put tomatoes and sprinkle olive oil over everything; use pepper and salt to season.

4. Bake for 25 minutes in the preheated oven until the juices run clear and the chicken is no longer pink.

5.Pour a sufficient amount of lightly salted into the saucepan to cover, boil potatoes until soft, about 15 minutes. The strain put back into the pan, and add pesto to coat.

6.On serving dishes, put potatoes, tomatoes, and chicken breasts and drizzle the reduced balsamic vinegar over and enjoy.

Nutrition: Calories 464, Fat 14, Carbs 16, Protein 18, Sodium 620

86.Pesto Cheesy Chicken Rolls

Prep Time: 15 min | **Cook Time:** 50 min | **Serve:** 2
- chicken breast
- basil pesto
- cheese
- cooking spray

Set the oven to 175°C to preheat and use cooking spray to coat a baking dish.

Spread onto each flattened chicken breast with 2-3 tbsp. Of pesto sauce, then put over pesto with a slice of cheese. Roll up tightly and use toothpicks to secure, then arrange in a baking dish coated lightly with grease.

In the preheated oven, bake without a cover until juices run clear and chicken is browned beautifully about 45-50 minutes.

Nutrition: Calories 354, Fat 10, Carbs 19, Protein 21, Sodium 389

87.Chicken Squash Bake

Prep Time: 10 min | **Cook Time:** 30 min | **Serve:** 2
- 1 spaghetti squash
- 2 tablespoons olive oil, divided
- 1-1/2 pounds skinless, boneless chicken breast
- salt and ground black pepper to taste
- 1 pinch dried oregano
- 1 pinch garlic powder
- 1 cup pesto
- 1 cup ricotta cheese
- 1 egg yolk
- 1 tablespoon Italian seasoning
- 1 cup marinara sauce

- 1 cup shredded mozzarella cheese

1. Turn the oven to 175°C to preheat.

2. Drizzle over the squash with 1 tablespoon olive oil and put on a cookie sheet with the cut-side turning down.

3. Bake for 20 minutes in the preheated oven until fork-tender. Scrape a fork onto the squash on the inside into spaghetti strands. Evenly spread in a casserole dish.

4. Use garlic powder, oregano, black pepper, and salt to season the chicken breasts.

5. In a big frying pan, heat the leftover 1 tablespoon olive oil over medium heat. Add chicken, cook for 6 minutes each side until turning brown and an instant-read thermometer displays a minimum of 165°F (74°C) when you insert it into the middle.

6. Slice the cooked chicken into half an inch cubes and mix with pesto in a bowl.

7. In a small bowl, mix Italian seasoning, egg yolk, and ricotta cheese.

8. In the casserole dish, top the squash with pesto chicken, ricotta mixture, and 1/2 of the marinara sauce. Make another layer in the same manner. Sprinkle over the top with mozzarella cheese. Put on aluminum foil to cover.

9. Place the preheated oven in the oven and cook for 30 minutes. Until bubbling and the cheese melts. Take away the aluminum foil and broil for 5 minutes until turning golden brown.

Nutrition: Calories 320, Fat 3, Carbs 18, Protein 28, Sodium 520

88. Pesto Pasta With Chicken

Prep Time: 10 min | **Cook Time:** 30 min | **Serve:** 2
- pasta
- olive oil
- garlic
- 2 chicken breasts
- red pepper flakes
- tomatoes
- pesto sauce

1. Boil lightly salted water. Put in pasta and cook till al dente for 8 to 10 minutes; drain.

2. In a big skillet over medium heat, heat oil. Sauté garlic till soft, then mix in chicken. Put red pepper flakes to season. Cook till chicken is golden and cooked through.

3. Put together pesto, sun-dried tomatoes, chicken, and pasta in a big bowl. Coat equally by tossing.

Nutrition: Calories 645, Fat 18, Carbs 32, Protein 36, Sodium 534

89. Sheet Pan Chicken With Mozzarella, Pesto, And Broccoli

Prep Time: 10 min | **Cook Time:** 30 min | **Serve:** 2
- 2 pounds boneless chicken breasts
- 2 teaspoons garlic salt
- 1 pinch ground black pepper
- 6 tablespoons pesto
- 2 Roma (plum) tomatoes, thinly sliced
- 1 1/2 cups shredded mozzarella cheese
- 1 head broccoli, cut into florets
- 2 tablespoons olive oil
- salt to taste

1. Turn the oven to 425°F to preheat. Lightly coat a big rimmed cookie sheet with oil.

2. On the prepared cookie sheet, put the chicken and sprinkle black pepper and garlic salt over. Spread over the chicken with pesto and put cheese and tomatoes on top.

3. In a bowl, mix oil and broccoli. On the cookie sheet, put broccoli around the chicken. Sprinkle over the top with pepper and salt.

4. Put in the preheated oven and bake for 15-20 minutes until the middle of the chicken is not pink anymore, and the broccoli is soft. An instant-read thermometer should display a minimum of 165°F (74°C) when you insert it into the middle.

Nutrition: Calories 432, Fat 22, Carbs 26, Protein 19, Sodium 455

90. Chicken Breasts Covered With Parmesan Cheese

Prep time: 5 min | **Cook Time:** 12 min | **Serve:** 2
- ¼ cup panko breadcrumbs
- ¼ cup grated Parmesan cheese
- ¼ tsp. dried basil
- 1 tbsp. olive oil
- 1 tbsp. spicy mustard
- 1 tsp. Worcestershire sauce
- 2 boneless and skinless chicken breasts

1. Put the breadcrumbs, cheese, and basil in a small, shallow bowl. Add and stir the oil until completely mixed. Combine mustard with Worcestershire sauce in a small bowl. Put the mustard mixture on both sides of the breasts.

2. With the crumb mixture, place the chicken in the bowl and press the crumbs on both sides of the breasts to achieve a uniform and firm coating.

3. Put the chicken inside the basket. Cook at a temperature of 185 C. for 21 to 25 minutes, turning halfway through cooking.

Nutrition: Calories 409, Fat 13, Carbs 16, Protein 26, Sodium 534

91. Chicken in Wheat Cake with Aioli Sauce

Prep Time: 10 min | **Cook Time:** 35 min | **Serve:** 2
- 500g breaded chicken
- 4 wheat cakes
- Extra virgin olive oil
- 1 small lettuce
- Grated cheese
- Aioli sauce

1. Put the breaded chicken in the air fryer with a little extra virgin olive oil and fry at 180 degrees for 20 minutes.

2. Take out and reserve.

3. Chop the lettuce, put the wheat cakes on the worktable and distribute the chopped lettuce between them.

4. On the chopped lettuce, spread the pieces of breaded chicken.

5. Cover with grated cheese and add some aioli sauce.

6. Close the wheat cakes and place them on the baking sheet.

7. Take to the oven, 180 degrees, 15 minutes, or until the cheese is melted.

Nutrition: Calories 199, Fat 24, Carbs 21, Protein 18, Sodium 322

92. Soy Chicken and Sesame, Breaded and Fried

Prep Time: 10 min | **Cook Time:** 25 min | **Serve:** 2

- 1 large chicken breast
- Egg
- Breadcrumbs
- Extra virgin olive oil
- Salt
- Ground pepper
- Soy sauce
- Sesame

1. Cut the breast into fillets and put them in a bowl.
2. Season. Add soy sauce and sesame. Flirt well and leave 30 minutes.
3. Beat the eggs and pass all the steaks through the beaten egg and the breadcrumbs.
4. With a silicone brush, permeate the fillets well on both sides.
5. Place on the grill of the air fryer and select 180 degrees, 20 minutes.
6. Make the fillets in batches so that they pile against each other.

Nutrition: Calories 210, Fat 4, Carbs 26, Protein 6, Sodium 534

93. Chicken with Provencal Herbs and Potatoes

Prep Time: 10 min | **Cook Time:** 55 min | **Serve:** 2
- 4 potatoes
- 2 chicken hindquarters
- Provencal herbs
- Salt
- Ground pepper
- Extra virgin olive oil

1. Cut the potatoes into slices after peeling them pepper and put on the grid of the base air fryer.
2. Impregnate the chicken well with oil, salt, and pepper and put some Provencal herbs.
3. Place the chicken on the potatoes.
4. Take the grill to the bucket of the air fryer and put it inside.
5. Select 170 degrees for 40 minutes.
6. Turn the chicken and leave 15 more minutes.

Nutrition: Calories 321, Fat 12, Carbs 21, Protein 21, Sodium 543

94. Honey-Lemon Chicken

Prep Time: 10 min | **Cook Time:** 40 min | **Serve:** 2
- 2 large chicken thighs
- ½ cup lemon juice
- ¼ cup olive oil
- 1 clove garlic, minced
- 1 teaspoon salt
- ½ teaspoon dried oregano
- 1 Tablespoon honey
- Parsley, chopped, for garnish

1. Preheat broiler (about 450–500°F).
2. Place chicken, skin-side down, in cast iron pan.
3. Broil chicken for 30 minutes, flipping halfway through.
4. While broiling chicken, whisk together lemon juice, olive oil, garlic, salt, and oregano.
5. Brush some of the sauce over the chicken and broil until the chicken (about 3-5 minutes) appears brown and crisp.
6. Transfer skillet to stovetop.
7. Transfer chicken to serving dish, leaving drippings in skillet.

8. Remove any chicken bits from the skillet and drain out any drippings over a couple of tablespoons.
9. Stir in remaining sauce and honey to the skillet.
10. Bring the mixture to a boil and pour over the chicken.
11. Sprinkle with parsley and serve.

Nutrition: Calories 293, Fat 16, Carbs 8, Protein 22, Sodium 432

95. Greek-Style One Pan Chicken and Rice

Prep Time: 5 min | **Cook Time:** 55 min | **Serve:** 2
- 6 chicken thighs
- 2 Tablespoons olive oil, divided
- 1 Tablespoon fresh oregano, chopped
- 1 yellow onion, diced
- 1 cup basmati rice
- 2 cups chicken broth
- ¼ cup of water
- ½ cup cherry tomatoes
- ¼ cup pitted Kalamata olives
- ½–1 lemon, sliced thinly
- Freshly ground black pepper, to taste
- Chopped fresh parsley for garnish

Marinade:
- ¼ cup lemon juice
- Zest of 1 lemon
- 2 Tablespoons fresh oregano, chopped
- 4 cloves garlic, diced
- 1 teaspoon salt

1. Combine marinade ingredients in a shallow container or Ziploc bag.
2. Add the chicken, cover or seal, and let marinate for at least 1 hour to overnight.
3. Preheat oven to 350°F.
4. Heat cast-iron skillet over medium-high heat and swirl in a Tablespoon of oil.
5. Carefully remove the chicken from the marinade (reserving the marinade) and lay skin-side down in the skillet.
6. Cook until the skin is browned (about 3–5 minutes on each side).
7. Transfer chicken to a plate and set aside.
8. Remove any bits of chicken from the skillet and wipe clean with paper towels. (Do this carefully, as the skillet is hot!)
9. Swirl in remaining oil and onion. Cook until onion pieces begin to brown at the edges (about 5 minutes).
10. Stir in the reserved marinade, rice, broth, water, tomatoes, and olives.
11. Bring to a boil.
12. Reduce heat and let simmer briefly (30 seconds).
13. Using a fitted lid or aluminum foil to put chicken on top and cover.
14. Bake for 30 minutes.
15. Remove the lid and put the slices of lemon on top.
16. Bake until chicken is browned and liquid has evaporated (about 10 minutes).
17. Remove from the oven and allow 5-10 minutes to rest.
18. Fluff rice with a fork.
19. Sprinkle with black pepper and chopped parsley, which is freshly ground.

Nutrition: Calories 259, Fat 12, Carbs 10, Protein 18, Sodium 542

96. Harvest Chicken with Sweet Potatoes, Brussels Sprouts, and Apples

Prep Time: 5 min | **Cook Time:** 35 min | **Serve:** 2

- 1 Tablespoon olive oil
- 1 pound boneless, skinless chicken breasts, diced
- 1 teaspoon salt, divided
- ½ teaspoon black pepper
- 4 slices thick-cut bacon, chopped
- 3 cups Brussels sprouts, trimmed and quartered
- 1 medium sweet potato, peeled and diced
- 1 medium onion, chopped
- 2 Granny Smith apples, peeled, cored, and cubed
- 4 cloves garlic, minced
- 2 teaspoons chopped fresh thyme
- 1 teaspoon ground cinnamon
- 1 cup reduced-sodium chicken broth, divided

1. Season chicken with ½ teaspoon salt and pepper.
2. Heat the oil in a cooking pan until it almost starts to sizzle.
3. Add chicken and cook until browned (about 5 minutes).
4. Drain chicken over paper towels and set aside.
5. Reduce heat to medium-low and, using the same skillet, cook bacon until brown and crisp (about 8 minutes).
6. Reserving rendered fat, remove bacon and drain over paper towels.
7. Drain the unnecessary oil / fat from skillet, leaving about 1½ Tablespoons.
8. Add remaining broth and the drained chicken.
9. Let cook through (about 2 minutes).
10. Remove from heat and stir in bacon.

Nutrition: Calories 254, Fat 4, Carbs 26, Protein 6, Sodium 432

97. Chicken and Vegetable Roast with Dijon Au Jus

Prep Time: 35 min | **Cook Time:** 50 min | **Serve:** 2
- 16 fingerling or yellow new potatoes, scrubbed 3 large carrots, cut into 1-inch chunks, divided Salt and pepper, to taste
- 16 Brussels sprouts, halved
- 4 Tablespoons extra-virgin olive oil, divided
- 1 whole 4-pound chicken, cut into 8 serving pieces, backbone reserved 1 cup dry white wine
- 1 whole onion, halved
- 1 stalk celery, roughly chopped
- 3–4 sprigs fresh sage
- 2 bay leaves
- 2 cups low-sodium chicken stock
- 1 medium shallot, sliced thinly
- 2 Tablespoons fresh parsley leaves, minced
- 2 Tablespoons unsalted butter
- 1 Tablespoon Dijon mustard
- Juice of 1 lemon
- 2 teaspoons fish sauce

1. Place potatoes and 2 cups carrot chunks in a saucepan and cover with water. Add about ½ teaspoon of salt and bring to a boil. Let simmer until tender (about 10 minutes). Drain and transfer to a large bowl. Set aside an empty saucepan for later.
2. Add Brussels sprouts to carrots and potatoes. Season with salt and pepper.
3. Add 2 normal spoons olive oil and toss to coat. Set aside.
4. To the saucepan, add the chicken backbone, 1 cup carrots, onion, celery, sage, and bay leaves. Set aside.
5. Preheat oven to 450°F.

6. Clean the parts of chicken with paper towels and season with salt and pepper.
7. Heat 1 spoon oil in a cast-iron skillet over high heat.
8. When oil just begins to smoke, add chicken, skin-side down. Reduce the heat so that the oil does not burn.
9. Cook on the skin-side until golden brown (about 8 minutes), then flip over and brown the other side (about 3 minutes).
10. Transfer chicken to a plate.
11. In the same skillet, pour in white wine. Scrape any brown bits.
12. Carefully transfer white wine from skillet to saucepan with chicken backbone and veggies.
13. Wipe skillet clean.
14. Transfer any juices collected from chicken pieces to a saucepan with backbone and veggies.
15. Pour in chicken stock and bring mixture to a simmer.
16. Reduce heat to the lowest setting, cover, and cook as chicken and other ingredients roast in the oven.
17. Reheat cast iron skillet with remaining oil.
18. When oil just begins to smoke, add potato-carrot-Brussels sprouts mixture and spread evenly.
19. Place chicken pieces, skin-side up, on veggies.
19. Put in the oven e let roast until chicken pieces are done (about 20–45 minutes, with an internal temperature of 150°F for breasts and 165°F for other pieces).
20. Transfer chicken pieces to a serving plate.
21. Add shallot to veggies. Flipping occasionally, roast veggies until browned (about 10 minutes). Remove from the oven.
22. Sprinkle roasted vegetables with parsley and arrange chicken on top.
23. Make the Dijon sauce. Go back to the simmering mixture in the saucepan and drain the broth into a bowl. Whisk in butter, mustard, lemon juice, and fish sauce.

Nutrition: Calories 232, Fat 4, Carbs 26, Protein 6, Sodium 645

98. Cheesesteaks with Chipotle

Prep Time: 5 min | **Cook Time:** 15 min | **Serve:** 2
- 1–2 pieces (or to taste) chilies from canned chipotle chilies in adobo sauce, minced 1 Tablespoon adobo sauce
- 2 teaspoons olive oil, divided
- 12 ounces chicken cutlets, sliced thinly
- 1 cup onion, sliced thinly
- 1 cup red bell pepper, pitted and sliced
- 4 cloves garlic, minced
- ¼ teaspoon dried thyme or oregano
- ¼ teaspoon salt
- 1 cup shredded cheddar cheese
- 4 hotdog buns or flour tortillas
- Lime wedges (optional)

1. Heat 1 little spoon oil in a cast-iron skillet over medium-high heat.
2. Sauté chicken until done (about 4–5 minutes). Remove from skillet and set aside.
3. Add remaining oil to the still-hot skillet.
4. Sauté onion, garlic, bell pepper, and thyme/oregano until fragrant and tender (about 4 minutes)
5. Add minced chilies and adobo sauce and let heat through (about 30 seconds).
6. Stir in chicken and season with salt. Cook to heat through (about 1 minute).
7. Remove from heat.
8. Add cheese to the warm mixture and stir to melt.

9.Fill buns or tortillas and serve with lime wedges, if using.
Nutrition: Calories 254, Fat 4, Carbs 26, Protein 6, Sodium 654

99.Baked Eggs
Prep Time: 10 min | **Cook Time:** 9 min | **Serve:** 6
- 2 cups fresh spinach, chopped finely
- 12 large eggs
- ½ cup heavy cream
- ¾ cup low-fat Parmesan cheese, shredded Salt and ground black pepper, as required

1.Preheat your oven to 425 degrees F.
2.Grease a 12 cups muffin tin.
3.Divide spinach in each muffin cup.
4.Crack an egg over spinach into each cup and drizzle with heavy cream.
5.Sprinkle with salt and black pepper, followed by Parmesan cheese.
6.Bake for approximately 7-9 minutes or until desired doneness of eggs.

100.Eggs in Avocado Halves
Prep Time: 10 min | **Cook Time:** 15 min | **Serve:** 2
- 1 avocado, halved and pitted
- 2 eggs
- Salt and ground black pepper, as required
- ¼ cup cherry tomatoes, halved
- 2 cups fresh baby spinach

1.Preheat your oven to 425 degrees F.
2.Carefully remove about 2 tablespoons of flesh from each avocado half.
3.Place avocado halves into a small baking dish.
4.Carefully crack an egg in each avocado half and sprinkle with salt and black pepper.
5.Bake for about 15 minutes or until the eggs are cooked as desired.
6.Arrange 1 avocado half onto each serving plate and serve alongside the cherry tomatoes and spinach.

GREEN RECIPES

101.Pesto Zucchini Noodles
Time: 30 min | **Serve:** 4
- 4 zucchini, spiralized
- 1 tbsp avocado oil
- 2 garlic cloves, chopped
- 2/3 cup olive oil
- 1/3 cup parmesan cheese, grated
- 2 cups fresh basil
- 1/3 cup almonds
- 1/8 tsp black pepper
- ¾ tsp sea salt

1.Add zucchini noodles into a colander and sprinkle with ¼ teaspoon of salt. Cover and let sit for 30 minutes. Drain zucchini noodles well and pat dry.
2.Preheat the oven to 400 F.
3.Place almonds on a parchment-lined baking sheet and bake for 6-8 minutes. Transfer toasted almonds into the food processor and process until coarse.

4.Add olive oil, cheese, basil, garlic, pepper, and remaining salt in a food processor with almonds and process until pesto texture.
5.Heat the avocado-oil in a pan over medium to high heat. Add zucchini noodles and cook for 4-5 minutes.
6.Pour pesto over zucchini noodles, mix well and cook for 1 minute.
Nutrition: Calories 525 Fat 47.4 g Carbs 9.3 g Sugar 3.8 g Protein 16.6 g Cholesterol 30 mg

102.Baked Cod & Vegetables
Time: 30 min | **Serve:** 4
- 1 lb cod fillets
- 8 oz asparagus, chopped
- 3 cups broccoli, chopped
- ¼ cup parsley, minced
- ½ tsp lemon pepper seasoning
- ½ tsp paprika
- ¼ cup olive oil
- ¼ cup lemon juice
- 1 tsp salt

1.Preheat the oven to 410 F. Cover the pan with baking paper and set aside.
2.In a small bowl, mix lemon juice, paprika, olive oil, lemon pepper seasoning, and salt.
3.Place fish fillets in the middle of the parchment paper. Place broccoli and asparagus around the fish fillets.
4.Pour lemon juice mixture over the fish fillets and top with parsley.
5.Bake in preheated oven for 13-15 minutes.
Nutrition: Calories 240 Fat 14.1 g Carbs 7.6 g Sugar 2.6 g Protein 23.7 g Cholesterol 56 mg

103.Parmesan Zucchini
Time: 30 min | **Serve:** 4
- 4 zucchini, quartered lengthwise
- 2 tbsp fresh parsley, chopped
- 2 tbsp olive oil
- ¼ tsp garlic powder
- ½ tsp dried basil
- ½ tsp dried oregano
- ½ tsp dried thyme
- ½ cup parmesan cheese, grated
- Pepper and Salt

1.Preheat the oven to 355 F. Line baking sheet with parchment paper and set aside.
2.In a small bowl, mix parmesan cheese, garlic powder, basil, oregano, thyme, pepper, and salt.
3.Arrange zucchini onto the prepared baking sheet and drizzle with oil and sprinkle with parmesan cheese mixture.
4. Cook for 16 minutes in a preheated oven, then broil for 2 minutes or until lightly browned.
5.Garnish with parsley and serve immediately.
Nutrition: Calories 244 Fat 16.4 g Carbs 7 g Sugar 3.5 g Protein 14.5 g Cholesterol 30 mg

104.Chicken Zucchini Noodles
Time: 25 min | **Serve:** 2
- 1 large zucchini, spiralized
- 1 chicken breast, skinless & boneless
- ½ tbsp jalapeno, minced
- 2 garlic cloves, minced
- ½ tsp ginger, minced

- ½ tbsp fish sauce
- 2 tbsp coconut cream
- ½ tbsp honey
- ½ lime juice
- 1 tbsp peanut butter
- 1 carrot, chopped
- 2 tbsp cashews, chopped
- ¼ cup fresh cilantro, chopped
- 1 tbsp olive oil
- Pepper
- Salt

Heat the olive oil in a pan.

1.Season chicken breast with pepper and salt. Add the chicken breast to the pan once the oil is hot and cook for 3-4 minutes on each side or until cooked.

2.Remove chicken breast from pan. Shred chicken breast with a fork and set aside.

3.In a small bowl, mix peanut butter, jalapeno, garlic, ginger, fish sauce, coconut cream, honey, and lime juice. Set aside.

4.In a large mixing bowl, combine spiralized zucchini, carrots, cashews, cilantro, and shredded chicken.

5.Pour peanut butter mixture over zucchini noodles and toss to combine.

Nutrition: Calories 353 Fat 21.1 g Carbs 20.5 g Sugar 10.8 g Protein 24.5 g Cholesterol 54 mg

105.Tomato Cucumber Avocado Salad

Time: 15 min | **Serve:** 4
- 12 oz cherry tomatoes, cut in half
- 5 small cucumbers, chopped
- 3 small avocados, chopped
- ½ tsp ground black pepper
- 2 tbsp olive oil
- 2 tbsp fresh lemon juice
- ¼ cup fresh cilantro, chopped
- 1 tsp sea salt

1.Add cherry tomatoes, cucumbers, avocados, and cilantro into the large mixing bowl and mix well.

2.Mix olive oil, lemon juice, black pepper, and salt and pour over salad.

3.Toss well and serve immediately.

Nutrition: Calories 442 Fat 37.1 g Carbs 30.3 g Sugar 9.4 g Protein 6.2 g Cholesterol 0 mg

106.Creamy Cauliflower Soup

Time: 30 min | **Serve:** 6
- 5 cups cauliflower rice
- 8 oz cheddar cheese, grated
- 2 cups unsweetened almond milk
- 2 cups vegetable stock
- 2 tbsp water
- 1 small onion, chopped
- 2 garlic cloves, minced
- 1 tbsp olive oil
- Pepper and Salt

1.Heat olive-oil over medium heat in a big stockpot.

2.Add onion and garlic and cook for 1-2 minutes.

3.Add cauliflower rice and water. Cover and cook for 5-7 minutes.

3.Now add vegetable stock and almond milk and stir well. Bring to boil.

4.Turn heat to low and simmer for 5 minutes.

5.Turn off the heat. Slowly add cheddar cheese and stir until smooth.

6.Season soup with pepper and salt.

7.Stir well and serve hot.

Nutrition: Calories 214 Fat 16.5 g Carbs 7.3 g Sugar 3 g Protein 11.6 g Cholesterol 40 mg

107.Taco Zucchini Boats

Time: 70 min | **Serve:** 4
- 4 medium zucchinis, cut in half lengthwise
- ¼ cup fresh cilantro, chopped
- ½ cup cheddar cheese, shredded
- ¼ cup of water
- 4 oz tomato sauce
- 2 tbsp bell pepper, mined
- ½ small onion, minced
- ½ tsp oregano
- 1 tsp paprika
- 1 tsp chili powder
- 1 tsp cumin
- 1 tsp garlic powder
- 1 lb lean ground turkey
- ½ cup of salsa
- 1 tsp kosher salt

1.Preheat the oven to 400 F.

2.Add ¼ cup of salsa to the bottom of the baking dish.

3.Using a spoon, hollow out the center of the zucchini halves.

4.Chop the scooped-out flesh of zucchini and set aside ¾ of a cup of chopped flesh.

5.Add zucchini halves to the boiling water and cook for 1 minute. Remove zucchini halves from water.

6.Add ground turkey in a large pan and cook until meat is no longer pink. Add spices and mix well.

7.Add reserved zucchini flesh, water, tomato sauce, bell pepper, and onion. Stir well and cover, simmer over low heat for 20 minutes.

8.Stuff zucchini boats with taco meat and top each with one tablespoon of shredded cheddar cheese.

9.Place zucchini boats in a baking dish. Cover the dish with paper and bake in a preheated oven
   1. 35 minutes.
   2. Top with remaining salsa and chopped cilantro.

Nutrition: Calories 297 Fat 13.7 g Carbs 17.2 g Sugar 9.3 g Protein 30.2 g Cholesterol 96 mg

108.Healthy Broccoli Salad

Time: 25 min | **Serve:** 6
- 3 cups broccoli, chopped
- 1 tbsp apple cider vinegar
- ½ cup Greek yogurt
- 2 tbsp sunflower seeds
- 3 bacon slices, cooked and chopped
- 1/3 cup onion, sliced
- ¼ tsp stevia

1.In a mixing bowl, mix broccoli, onion, and bacon.

2.In a small bowl, mix yogurt, vinegar, and stevia and pour over broccoli mixture. Stir to combine.

3.Sprinkle sunflower seeds on top of the salad.

4.Store salad in the refrigerator for 30 minutes.

Nutrition: Calories 90 Fat 4.9 g Carbs 5.4 g Sugar 2.5 g Protein 6.2 g Cholesterol 12 mg

109.Delicious Zucchini Quiche

Time: 60 min | **Serve:** 8
- 6 eggs
- 2 medium zucchini, shredded
- ½ tsp dried basil
- 2 garlic cloves, minced
- 1 tbsp dry onion, minced
- 2 tbsp parmesan cheese, grated
- 2 tbsp fresh parsley, chopped
- ½ cup olive oil
- 1 cup cheddar cheese, shredded
- ¼ cup coconut flour
- ¾ cup almond flour
- ½ tsp salt

1. Preheat the furnace to 355 F. Grease a 9-inch dish of pie and set aside.
2. Squeeze out excess liquid from zucchini.
3. Into the cup, add all ingredients and blend until well mixed. Pour into the prepared pie dish.
4. Bake in preheated oven for 47-63 minutes or until set.
5. Remove it from the oven and let it cool down completely.
Nutrition: Calories 288 Fat 26.3 g Carbs 5 g Sugar 1.6 g Protein 11 g Cholesterol 139 mg

110. Turkey Spinach Egg Muffins

Time: 30 min | **Serve:** 3
- 5 egg whites
- 2 eggs
- ¼ cup cheddar cheese, shredded
- ¼ cup spinach, chopped
- ¼ cup milk
- 3 lean breakfast turkey sausage
- Pepper and Salt

1. Preheat the oven to 355 F. Grease muffin tray cups and set aside.
2. In a pan, brown the turkey sausage links over medium-high heat until the sausage is brown from all the sides.
3. Cut sausage into ½-inch pieces and set aside.
4. In a big bowl, whisk together eggs, egg whites, milk, pepper, and salt. Stir in spinach.
5. Pour egg mixture into the prepared muffin tray.
6. Divide sausage and cheese evenly between each muffin cup.
7. Bake in a preheated oven for 22 minutes or until muffins are set.
Nutrition: Calories 123 Fat 6.8 g Carbs 1.9 g Sugar 1.6 g Protein 13.3 g Cholesterol 123 mg

111. Chicken Casserole

Time: 40 min | **Serve:** 4
- 1 lb cooked chicken, shredded
- ¼ cup Greek yogurt
- 1 cup cheddar cheese, shredded
- ½ cup of salsa
- 4 oz cream cheese, softened
- 4 cups cauliflower florets
- 1/8 tsp black pepper
- ½ tsp kosher salt

1. Add cauliflower florets into the microwave-safe dish and cook for 10 minutes or until tender.
2. Add cream cheese and microwave for 35 seconds more. Stir well.
3. Add chicken, yogurt, cheddar cheese, salsa, pepper, and salt, and stir everything well.

4. Preheat the oven to 375 F.
5. Bake in preheated oven for 20 minutes.
Nutrition: Calories 429 Fat 23 g Carbs 9.6 g Sugar 4.7 g Protein 45.4 g Cholesterol 149 mg

112. Shrimp Cucumber Salad

Time: 20 minutes
Serve: 4
- 1 lb shrimp, cooked
- 1 bell pepper, sliced
- 2 green onions, sliced
- ½ cup fresh cilantro, chopped
- 2 cucumbers, sliced

For dressing:
- 2 tbsp fresh mint leaves, chopped
- 1 tsp sesame seeds
- ½ tsp red pepper flakes
- 1 tbsp olive oil
- ¼ cup rice wine vinegar
- ¼ cup lime juice
- 1 Serrano chili pepper, minced
- 3 garlic cloves, minced
- ½ tsp salt

1. In a little bowl, whisk together all dressing ingredients and set aside.
2. In a mixing bowl, mix shrimp, bell pepper, green onion, cilantro, and cucumbers.
3. Pour dressing over salad and toss well.
Nutrition: Calories 219 Fat 6.1 g Carbs 11.3 g Sugar 4.2 g Protein 27.7 g Cholesterol 239 mg

113. Asparagus & Shrimp Stir Fry

Time: 20 min | **Serve:** 4
- 1 lb asparagus
- 1 lb shrimp
- 2 tbsp lemon juice
- 1 tbsp soy sauce
- 1 tsp ginger, minced
- 1 garlic clove, minced
- 1 tsp red pepper flakes
- ¼ cup olive oil
- Pepper and Salt

1. Heat 2 normal spoons of oil in a large pan over medium-high heat.
2. Add shrimp to the pan and season with red pepper flakes, pepper, salt, and cook for 5 minutes.
3. Remove shrimp from pan and set aside.
4. Add remaining oil in the same pan. Add garlic, ginger, and asparagus, stir frequently, and cook until asparagus is tender about 5 minutes.
5. Return shrimp to the pan. Add lemon-juice and soy-sauce and stir until well combined.
Nutrition: Calories 274 Fat 14.8 g Carbs 7.4 g Sugar 2.4 g Protein 28.8 g Cholesterol 239 mg

114. Turkey Burgers

Time: 30 min | **Serve:** 4
- 1 lb lean ground turkey
- 2 green onions, sliced
- ¼ cup basil leaves, shredded
- 2 garlic cloves, minced

- 2 medium zucchini, shredded and squeeze out all the liquid
- ½ tsp black pepper
- ½ tsp sea salt

1. Heat grill to medium heat.
2. To the cup, add all the ingredients and combine until well blended.
3. Make four equal shapes of patties from the mixture.
4. Spray one piece of foil with cooking spray.
5. Place prepared patties on the foil and grill for 10 minutes. Turn patties to the other side and grill for 10 minutes more.

Nutrition: Calories 183 Fat 8.3 g Carbs 4.5 g Sugar 1.9 g Protein 23.8 g Cholesterol 81 mg

115. Broccoli Kale Salmon Burgers

Time: 30 min | **Serve:** 5
- 2 eggs
- ½ cup onion, chopped
- ½ cup broccoli, chopped
- ½ cup kale, chopped
- ½ tsp garlic powder
- 2 tbsp lemon juice
- ½ cup almond flour
- 15 oz can salmon, drained and bones removed
- ½ tsp salt

1. Line one plate with parchment paper and set aside.
2. Add all ingredients into the big bowl and mix until well combined.
3. Make five equal shapes of patties from the mixture and place them on a prepared plate.
4. Place plate in the refrigerator for 30 minutes.
5. Spray a big pan with cooking spray and heat over medium heat.
6. Once the pan is hot, then add patties and cook for 5-7 minutes per side.

Nutrition: Calories 221 Fat 12.6 g Carbs 5.2 g Sugar 1.4 g Protein 22.1 g Cholesterol 112 mg

116. Pan Seared Cod

Time: 25 min | **Serve:** 4
- 1 ¾ lbs cod fillets
- 1 tbsp ranch seasoning
- 4 tsp olive oil

1. Heat oil in a big pan over medium-high heat.
2. Season fish fillets with ranch seasoning.
3. Once the oil is hot, then place fish fillets in a pan and cook for 6-8 minutes on each side.

Nutrition: Calories 207 Fat 6.4 g Carbs 0 g Sugar 0 g Protein 35.4 g Cholesterol 97 mg

117. Quick Lemon Pepper Salmon

Time: 18 min | **Serve:** 4
- 1 ½ lbs salmon fillets
- ½ tsp ground black pepper
- 1 tsp dried oregano
- 2 garlic cloves, minced
- ¼ cup olive oil
- 1 lemon juice
- 1 tsp sea salt

1. In a big bowl, mix lemon-juice, olive-oil, garlic, oregano, black pepper, and salt.
2. Add fish fillets in the bowl and coat well with the marinade, and place in the refrigerator for 15 minutes.

3. Preheat the grill.
4. Brush grill grates with oil.
5. Place marinated salmon fillets on hot grill and cook for 4 minutes, then turn salmon fillets to the other side and cook for 4 minutes more.

Nutrition: Calories 340 Fat 23.3 g Carbs 1.2 g Sugar 0.3 g Protein 33.3 g Cholesterol 75 mg

118. Healthy Salmon Salad

Time: 20 min | **Serve:** 2
- 2 salmon fillets
- 2 tbsp olive oil
- ¼ cup onion, chopped
- 1 cucumber, peeled and sliced
- 1 avocado, diced
- 2 tomatoes, chopped
- 4 cups baby spinach
- Pepper and Salt

1. Heat the olive oil in a pan.
2. Season salmon fillets with pepper and salt. Place fish fillets in a pan and cook for 4-5 minutes.
3. Turn fish fillets and cook for 2-3 minutes more.
4. Divide remaining ingredients evenly between two bowls, then top with cooked fish fillet.

Nutrition: Calories 350 Fat 23.2 g Carbs 15.3 g Sugar 6.6 g Protein 25 g Cholesterol 18 mg

119. Pan Seared Tilapia

Time: 18 min | **Serve:** 2
- 18 oz tilapia fillets
- ¼ tsp lemon pepper
- ½ tsp parsley flakes
- ¼ tsp garlic powder
- 1 tsp Cajun seasoning
- ½ tsp dried oregano
- 2 tbsp olive oil

1. Heat the olive oil in a pan.
2. Season fish fillets with lemon pepper, parsley flakes, garlic powder, Cajun seasoning, and oregano.
3. Place fish fillets in the pan and cook for 3-4 minutes on each side.

Nutrition: Calories 333 Fat 16.4 g Carbs 0.7 g Sugar 0.1 g Protein 47.6 g Cholesterol 124 mg

120. Creamy Broccoli Soup

Time: 35 min | **Serve:** 8
- 20 oz frozen broccoli, thawed and chopped
- ¼ tsp nutmeg
- 4 cups vegetable broth
- 1 potato, peeled and chopped
- 2 garlic cloves, peeled and chopped
- 1 large onion, chopped
- 1 tbsp olive oil
- Pepper and Salt

1. Heat the olive oil in a pan.
2. Add the onion, garlic and sauté until the onion is tender.
3. Add potato, broccoli, and broth and bring to boil. Turn heat to low and simmer for 15 minutes or until vegetables are tender.
4. Using a blender, puree the soup until smooth. Season soup with nutmeg, pepper, and salt.

Nutrition: Calories 84 Fat 2.7 g Carbs 10.9 g Sugar 2.6 g Protein 5.1 g Cholesterol 0 mg

121.Tuna Muffins

Time: 35 min | **Serve:** 8
- 2 eggs, lightly beaten
- 1 can tuna, flaked
- 1 tsp cayenne pepper
- 1/4 cup mayonnaise
- 1 celery stalk, chopped
- 1 1/2 cups cheddar cheese, shredded
- 1/4 cup sour cream
- Pepper and Salt

1.Preheat the oven to 355 F. Grease muffin tin and set aside.
2.Add all ingredients into the big bowl and mix until well combined, and pour into the prepared muffin tin.
3.Bake for 25 minutes.
Nutrition: Calories 185 Fat 14 g Carbs 2.6 g Sugar 0.7 g Protein 13 g Cholesterol 75 mg

122.Chicken Cauliflower Rice

Time: 25 min | **Serve:** 4
- 1 cauliflower head, chopped
- 2 cups cooked chicken, shredded
- 1 tsp olive oil
- 1 tsp garlic powder
- 1 tsp chili powder
- 1 tsp cumin
- 1/4 cup tomatoes, diced
- Salt

1.Add cauliflower into the food processor and process until you get rice size pieces.
2.Heat oil in a pan over high heat.
3.Add cauliflower rice and chicken in a pan and cook for 5-7 minutes.
4.Add garlic powder, chili powder, cumin, tomatoes, and salt. Stir well and cook for 7-10 minutes more.
Nutrition: Calories 140 Fat 3.6 g Carbs 5 g Sugar 2 g Protein 22 g Cholesterol 54 mg

123.Easy Spinach Muffins

Time: 25 min | **Serve:** 12
- 10 eggs
- 2 cups spinach, chopped
- 1/4 tsp garlic powder
- 1/4 tsp onion powder
- 1/2 tsp dried basil
- 1 1/2 cups parmesan cheese, grated
- Salt

1.Preheat the oven to 410 F. Grease muffin tin and set aside.
2.In a large bowl, whisk eggs with basil, garlic powder, onion powder, and salt.
3.Add cheese and spinach and stir well.
4.Pour egg-mixture into the prepared muffin tin and bake 15 minutes.
Nutrition: Calories 110 Fat 7 g Carbs 1 g Sugar 0.3 g Protein 9 g Cholesterol 165 mg

124.Healthy Cauliflower Grits

Time: 2 h 10 min | **Serve:** 8
- 6 cups cauliflower rice
- 1/4 tsp garlic powder

- 1 cup cream cheese
- 1/2 cup vegetable stock
- 1/4 tsp onion powder
- 1/2 tsp pepper
- 1 tsp salt

1. Add all the ingredients to the slow-cooker and blend well.
2.Cover and cook on low for 2 hours.
Nutrition: Calories 126 Fat 10 g Carbs 5 g Sugar 2 g Protein 4 g Cholesterol 31 mg

125.Spinach Tomato Frittata

Time: 30 min | **Serve:** 8

- 12 eggs
- 2 cups baby spinach, shredded
- 1/4 cup sun-dried tomatoes, sliced
- 1/2 tsp dried basil
- 1/4 cup parmesan cheese, grated
- Pepper and Salt

1.Preheat the oven to 425 F. Grease oven-safe pan and set aside.
2.In a large bowl, whisk eggs with pepper and salt. Add remaining ingredients and stir to combine.
3.Pour egg-mixture into the prepared pan and bake for 20 minutes.
Nutrition: Calories 116 Fat 7 g Carbs 1 g Sugar 1 g Protein 10 g Cholesterol 250 mg

126.Tofu Scramble

Time: 17 min | **Serve:** 2
- 1/2 block firm tofu, crumbled
- 1 cup spinach
- 1/4 cup zucchini, chopped
- 1 tbsp olive oil
- 1 tomato, chopped
- 1/4 tsp ground cumin
- 1 tbsp turmeric
- 1 tbsp coriander, chopped
- 1 tbsp chives, chopped
- Pepper and Salt

1.Heat the oil in a pan.
2.Add tomato, zucchini, and spinach and sauté for 2 minutes.
3.Add tofu, turmeric, cumin, pepper, and salt, and sauté for 5 minutes.
4.Garnish with chives and coriander.
Nutrition: Calories 102 Fat 8 g Carbs 5 g Sugar 2 g Protein 3 g Cholesterol 0 mg

127.Shrimp & Zucchini

Time: 30 min | **Serve:** 4
- 1 lb shrimp, peeled and deveined
- 1 zucchini, chopped
- 1 summer squash, chopped
- 2 tbsp olive oil
- 1/2 small onion, chopped
- 1/2 tsp paprika
- 1/2 tsp garlic powder
- 1/2 tsp onion powder
- Pepper and Salt

1.In a bowl, mix paprika, garlic powder, onion powder, pepper, and salt. Add shrimp and toss well.
2.Heat 1 normal spoon of oil in a pan over medium heat,

3.Add shrimp and cook for 2 minutes on each side or until shrimp turns pink.
4.Transfer shrimp on a plate.
5.Add remaining oil to a pan.
6.Add onion, summer squash, and zucchini, and cook for 6-8 minutes or until vegetables are softened.
7. Place the shrimp-back in the pan and cook for 1 minute.
Nutrition: Calories 215 Fat 9 g Carbs 6 g Sugar 2 g Protein 27 g Cholesterol 239 mg

128.Baked Dijon Salmon

Time: 30 min | **Serve:** 5
- 1 1/2 lbs salmon
- 1/4 cup Dijon mustard
- 1/4 cup fresh parsley, chopped
- 1 tbsp garlic, chopped
- 1 tbsp olive oil
- 1 tbsp fresh lemon juice
- Pepper and Salt

1.Preheat the oven to 385 F. Line baking sheet with parchment paper.
2.Arrange salmon fillets on a prepared baking sheet.
3.In a small bowl, mix garlic, oil, lemon juice, Dijon mustard, parsley, pepper, and salt.
4.Brush salmon top with garlic mixture.
5.Bake for 18-20 minutes.
Nutrition: Calories 217 Fat 11 g Carbs 2 g Sugar 0.2 g Protein 27 g Cholesterol 60 mg

129.Cauliflower Spinach Rice

Time: 15 min | **Serve:** 4
- 5 oz baby spinach
- 4 cups cauliflower rice
- 1 tsp garlic, minced
- 3 tbsp olive oil
- 1 fresh lime juice
- 1/4 cup vegetable broth
- 1/4 tsp chili powder
- Pepper and Salt

1.Heat the olive oil in a pan.
2.Add garlic and sauté for 30 seconds. Add cauliflower rice, chili powder, pepper, and salt and cook for 2 minutes.
3.Add broth and lime juice and stir well.
4.Add spinach and stir until spinach is wilted.
Nutrition: Calories 147 Fat 11 g Carbs 9 g Sugar 4 g Protein 5 g Cholesterol 23 mg

130.Cauliflower Broccoli Mash

Time: 22 min | **Serve:** 3
- 1 lb cauliflower, cut into florets
- 2 cups broccoli, chopped
- 1 tsp garlic, minced
- 1 tsp dried rosemary
- 1/4 cup olive oil
- Salt

1.Add broccoli and cauliflower into the instant pot.
2.Pour enough water into the instant pot to cover broccoli and cauliflower.
3.Seal pot and cook on high-pressure for 12 minutes.
4.Once done, allow to release pressure naturally. Remove lid.
5.Drain broccoli and cauliflower and clean the instant pot.

6.Add oil into the instant pot and set the pot on sauté mode.
7.Add broccoli, cauliflower, rosemary, garlic, and salt, and cook for 10 minutes.
8.Mash the broccoli and cauliflower mixture using a masher until smooth.
Nutrition: Calories 205 Fat 17 g Carbs 12 g Sugar 5 g Protein 5 g Cholesterol 0 mg

131.Italian Chicken Soup

Time: 35 min | **Serve:** 6
- 1 lb chicken breasts, boneless and cut into chunks
- 1 1/2 cups salsa
- 1 tsp Italian seasoning
- 2 tbsp fresh parsley, chopped
- 3 cups chicken stock
- 8 oz cream cheese
- Pepper and Salt

1.Add all ingredients except cream cheese and parsley into the instant pot and stir well.
2.Seal pot and cook on high-pressure for 25 minutes.
3.Release pressure using quick release. Remove lid.
4.Remove chicken from pot and shred using a fork.
5.Return shredded chicken to the instant pot.
6.Add cream cheese and stir well and cook on sauté mode until cheese is melted.
Nutrition: Calories 300 Fat 19 g Carbs 5 g Sugar 2 g Protein 26 g Cholesterol 109 mg

132.Tasty Tomatoes Soup

Time: 15 min | **Serve:** 2
- 14 oz can fire-roasted tomatoes
- 1/2 tsp dried basil
- 1/2 cup heavy cream
- 1/2 cup parmesan cheese, grated
- 1 cup cheddar cheese, grated
- 1 1/2 cups vegetable stock
- 1/4 cup zucchini, grated
- 1/2 tsp dried oregano
- Pepper and Salt

1.Add tomatoes, stock, zucchini, oregano, basil, pepper, and salt into the instant pot and stir well.
2.Seal pot and cook on high-pressure for 5 minutes.
3.Release pressure using quick release. Remove lid.
4.Set pot on sauté mode. Add heavy cream, parmesan cheese, and cheddar cheese and stir well and cook until cheese is melted.
Nutrition: Calories 460 Fat 35 g Carbs 13 g Sugar 6 g Protein 24 g Cholesterol 117 mg

133.Cauliflower Spinach Soup

Time: 20 min | **Serve:** 2
- 3 cups spinach, chopped
- 1 cup cauliflower, chopped
- 2 tbsp olive oil
- 3 cups vegetable broth
- 1/2 cup heavy cream
- 1 tsp garlic powder
- Pepper
- Salt

1.Add all ingredients except cream into the instant pot and stir well.
2.Seal pot and cook on high-pressure for 11 minutes.

3.Release pressure using quick release. Remove lid.
4.Stir in cream and blend soup using a blender until smooth.
Nutrition: Calories 310 Fat 27 g Carbs 7 g Sugar 3 g Protein 10 g Cholesterol 41 mg

134.Delicious Chicken Salad

Time: 15 min | **Serve:** 4
- 1 1/2 cups chicken breast, skinless, boneless, and cooked
- 2 tbsp onion, diced
- 1/4 cup olives, diced
- 1/4 cup roasted red peppers, diced
- 1/4 cup cucumbers, diced
- 1/4 cup celery, diced
- 1/4 cup feta cheese, crumbled
- 1/2 tsp onion powder
- 1/2 tbsp fresh lemon juice
- 1 tbsp fresh parsley, chopped
- 1 tbsp fresh dill, chopped
- 2 1/2 tbsp mayonnaise
- 1/4 cup Greek yogurt
- 1/4 tsp pepper
- 1/2 tsp salt

1.In a bowl, mix yogurt, onion powder, lemon juice, parsley, dill, mayonnaise, pepper, and salt.
2.Add chicken, onion, olives, red peppers, cucumbers, and feta cheese and stir well.
Nutrition: Calories 172 Fat 7.9 g Carbs 6.7 g Sugar 3.1 g Protein 18.1 g Cholesterol 52 mg

135.Baked Pesto Salmon

Time: 30 min | **Serve:** 5
- 1 3/4 lbs salmon fillet
- 1/3 cup basil pesto
- 1/4 cup sun-dried tomatoes, drained
- 1/4 cup olives, pitted and chopped
- 1 tbsp fresh dill, chopped
- 1/4 cup capers
- 1/3 cup artichoke hearts
- 1 tsp paprika
- 1/4 tsp salt

1.Preheat the oven to 410 F. Cover the pan with parchment paper.
2.Arrange salmon fillet on a prepared baking sheet and season with paprika and salt.
3.Add remaining ingredients on top of salmon and spread evenly.
4.Bake for 20 minutes.
Nutrition: Calories 228 Fat 10.7 g Carbs 2.7 g Sugar 0.3 g Protein 31.6 g Cholesterol 70 mg

136.Easy Shrimp Salad

Time: 15 min | **Serve:** 6
- 2 lbs shrimp, cooked
- 1/4 cup onion, minced
- 1/4 cup fresh dill, chopped
- 1/3 cup fresh chives, chopped
- 1/2 cup fresh celery, chopped
- 1/4 tsp cayenne pepper
- 1 tbsp fresh lemon juice
- 1 tbsp olive oil
- 1/4 cup mayonnaise

- 1/4 tsp pepper
- 1/4 tsp salt

1.In a big-bowl, add all ingredients except shrimp and mix well.
2.Add shrimp and toss well.
Nutrition: Calories 248 Fat 8.3 g Carbs 6.7 g Sugar 1.1 g Protein 35.2 g Cholesterol 321 mg

137.Simple Haddock Salad

Time: 15 minutes
Serve: 6
- 1 lb haddock, cooked
- 1 tbsp green onion, chopped
- 1 tbsp olive oil
- 1 tsp garlic, minced
- Pepper and Salt

1.Cut cooked haddock into bite-size pieces and place on a plate.
2.Season with oil, pepper, and salt
3.Sprinkle garlic and green onion over haddock.
Nutrition: Calories 106 Fat 3 g Carbs 0.2 g Sugar 0 g Protein 18.4 g Cholesterol 56 mg

138.Baked White Fish Fillet

Time: 40 min | **Serve:** 1
- 8 oz frozen white fish fillet
- 1 tbsp roasted red bell pepper, diced
- 1/2 tsp Italian seasoning
- 1 tbsp fresh parsley, chopped
- 1 1/2 tbsp olive oil
- 1 tbsp lemon juice

1.Preheat the oven to 410 F. Line baking sheet with foil.
2.Place a fish fillet on a baking sheet.
3.Drizzle oil and lemon juice over fish. Season with Italian seasoning.
4.Top with roasted bell pepper and parsley and bake for 30 minutes.
Nutrition: Calories 383 Fat 22.5 g Carbs 0.8 g Sugar 0.6 g Protein 46.5 g Cholesterol 2 mg

139.Air Fry Salmon

Time: 25 min | **Serve:** 4
- 1 lbs salmon, cut into 4 pieces
- 1 tbsp olive oil
- 1/2 tbsp dried rosemary
- 1/4 tsp dried basil
- 1 tbsp dried chives
- Pepper and Salt

1.Place salmon-pieces skin side down into the air fryer basket.
2.In a small bowl, mix olive oil, basil, chives, and rosemary.
3.Brush salmon with oil mixture and air fry at 400 F for 15 minutes.
Nutrition: Calories 182 Fat 10.6 g Carbs 0.3 g Sugar 0 g Protein 22 g Cholesterol 50 mg

140.Baked Salmon Patties

Time: 30 min | **Serve:** 4
- 2 eggs, lightly beaten
- 14 oz can salmon, drained and flaked with a fork
- 1 tbsp garlic, minced
- 1/4 cup almond flour

- 1/2 cup fresh parsley, chopped
- 1 tsp Dijon mustard
- 1/4 tsp pepper
- 1/2 tsp kosher salt

1. Preheat a 410 F microwave. Line a baking sheet and set it aside with parchment paper.
2. Add all ingredients into the bowl and mix until well combined.
3. Make small patties from the mixture and place on a prepared baking sheet.
4. Bake patties for 10 minutes.
5. Turn patties and bake for 10 minutes more.

Nutrition: Calories 216 Fat 11.8 g Carbs 3 g Sugar 0.5 g Protein 24.3 g Cholesterol 136 mg

141. Peanut Butter Banana Sandwich

Prep Time: 2 min | **Cook Time:** 6 min | **Serve:** 1
- 1 banana
- 1 tbsp. olive oil (or coconut oil)
- ½ tbsp. cinnamon
- 1 tbsp. peanut butter
- slices bread

1. On both slices of toast, smear the peanut butter.
2. Slice the banana into thin slices about 8 mm thick and spread them on just ONE toast slice.
3. Over them, add cinnamon.
4. Place all slices on each other's top.
5. For 2-3 minutes, apply oil to the pan and cook both faces until crispy and brown and yummy and delicious, and boom! Now, back to bed.

142. Tuna Pate

Prep Time: 15 min | **Cook Time:** 45 min | **Serve:** 6
- 1/4 teaspoon pepper
- 1/4 teaspoon salt
- Grated rind of half an orange
- 2 tablespoons fresh parsley
- 1 can (6 ounces) tuna, drained
- 1 package (8 ounces) cream cheese, softened
- 1 can (4 ounces) mushrooms, drained
- 1/2 teaspoon orange extract
- 1 tablespoon Splendor
- 1/2 medium onion, chopped
- 2 cloves garlic, crushed
- 2 tablespoons butter

1. Melt the butter and stir-fry the onion and garlic, and mushrooms in a thin, heavy skillet over low heat until the onion is floppy. Connect the orange and Splendor extract and blend well.
2. With the S blade in, put the tuna, cream cheese, orange rind, parsley, salt, and pepper in a food mixer. Pulse for mixing. Add the sautéed mixture, and pulse until well combined and smooth.
3. Cool and spoon into a mixing dish. Serve with (for carb-eaters) pepper strips, cucumber rounds, celery sticks, and crackers.

Nutrition: 3 g. carb. | 1 g. fib. for a total of 2 g. of usable carbs and 11 grams of protein.

143. Arugula Lentil Salad

Prep Time: 5 min | **Cook Time:** 7 min | **Serve:** 2
- 1-2 tbsp. balsamic vinegar

- ¾ cups cashews (¾ cups = 100 g)
- 1 handful arugula/rocket (1 handful = 100 g)
- 1 cup brown lentils, cooked (1 cup = 1 / 15oz. / 400 g)
- slices bread (whole wheat)
- 5-6 sun-dried tomatoes in oil
- 1 chili / jalapeño
- tbsp. olive oil
- 1 onion
- salt and pepper to taste
- Optional
- 1 tbsp. honey
- 1 small handful of raisins

1. To optimize the scent, toast the cashews in a pan over low heat for about three to four minutes. Then dump them into a pot of salad.
2. Dice and fry the onion in one-third of the olive oil over low heat for around 3 minutes.
3. In the meantime, cut your chili / jalapeño and dried tomatoes. In the grill, add them and fry for the next 1-2 minutes.
4. Slice the bread into large croutons.
5. Shift the mixture of onions into a large container. Now add the remaaining oil to the pan and cook the sliced bread until it's crispy with salt and pepper seasoning.
6. Now clean the arugula and put it in the bowl.
7. Bring in the lentils, too, and blend everything over. Using salt, pepper, and balsamic vinegar to season. With the croutons, eat.

144. Tomato Avocado Toast

Prep Time: 5 min | **Cook Time:** 5 min | **Serve:** 1
- 1 slice bread (ideally whole grain)
- ½ medium avocado (½ avocado = about 50g)
- 1 tbsp. lemon juice
- 1 tbsp. olive oil
- salt and pepper to taste
- cherry tomatoes

1. Split in half your cherry tomatoes.
2. Dump them in a pan and let them cook until tender (about 5 minutes) with olive oil.
3. In the meantime, mash and add some lemon with your avocado. Put it all together now, and season with salt and pepper.

145. Classic Tofu Salad

Prep Time: 5 min | **Cook Time:** 15 min | **Serve:** 2
- 1 small tin pineapple (small tin = 8 oz. = 225g = ¼)
- 1 handful spinach
- ½ bunch radishes
- ½ medium cucumber
- 1 cup bean sprouts
- 14 oz. firm tofu (ideally get fresh tofu from the supermarket)

For the dressing
- tbsp. olive oil
- salt and pepper to taste
- 1 small handful of peanuts
- ½ chili pepper (e.g., jalapeño)
- ½ lime (juiced; lemon also works)
- 1 tbsp. sriracha (or equivalent)
- 1 tbsp. maple syrup

1. Squeeze out some of the tofu block's excess moisture, split it (about one square centimeter) into tiny cubes, heat some oil in a pan over low to medium heat, and add it to your tofu. Fry until golden brown for approximately 15 minutes. Challenge for multitasking: make sure that you stir every once in a while (and put some salt). When preparing the rest of the salad, you should do it, get it on!
2. Next step: rinse the vegetables!
3. Chop the radishes.
4. Lengthwise, slice the cucumber in half, scrape the seeds with a big spoon, and cut what's left.
5. Also, cut the pineapple into smaller pieces.
6. Put all together with the bean sprouts and spinach into a dish.

Now to the dressing
1. Put the sugar, the olive oil, the sriracha, the lime juice, the salt, and the pepper together and toss in the salad
2. Get the pieces of tofu and put them in a separate bowl. Mix them to every
3. Serving of salad. (They'll get mushy easily if you put them straight into the salad).
4. Cut the chili and slightly crush or chop the peanuts for garnish as well. When served, dust them over the salad.

146. Two Ingredient Peanut Butter
Prep Time: 3 min | **Cook Time:** None | **Serve:** 8
- 2 tbsp. olive oil
- 1 tbsp. maple syrup
- 1¼ cup peanuts

1. In a blender/food processor, add chunks of peanuts and oil (add maple syrup if desired).
2. Mix more for smooth texture, less for a crunchy blend.

147. Avocado Toast with Cottage Cheese
Prep Time: 5 min | **Cook Time:** None | **Serve:** 1
- 1 green onion
- 2 tbsp. cottage cheese
- 1 tbsp. lemon
- ½ medium avocado
- 1 slice bread (ideally whole grain)
- salt and pepper to taste

1. Mash the avocado; add the lemon and some salt.
2. On the toast, put a layer of cottage cheese.
3. Garnish with fresh pepper and sliced green onion.

148. Creamy Corn Soup
Prep Time: 5 min | **Cook Time:** 15 min | **Serve:** 3
- 1 pinch pepper (preferably freshly ground black pepper)
- 1 pinch salt
- 2 handfuls cilantro/coriander, fresh
- 2 tbsp. olive oil
- 2 cups vegetable broth (2 cups = ½ liter)
- 1 thumb ginger, fresh (or 1 tbsp. ground ginger)
- 2 cloves garlic
- 1 red pepper *
- 2 onion
- cans sweet corn (ca. 14oz. or 350-400g cans)

Optional and highly recommended:
- 1 tbsp. lemon juice (as an extra twist before serving)
- 2 stalks lemongrass (or 1 tbsp. ground lemongrass)

1. Heat the oven to a temperature of 430 ° F/220 ° C.
2. Flush the sweet corn in a different bowl, but save the water from the can!
3. To the baking tray, add 1/3 of the corn (without the water). Sprinkle with salt, pepper, and oil. Put it on for about 10 minutes in the oven. Stir periodically to make sure the maize is not burning.
4. Meanwhile, heat the remaining spoon of oil in a pan over medium heat.
5. Chop and sauté the onion (slowly fry it).
6. Peel the fresh ginger and chop it and transfer it to the onion. (Keep off a moment if dried ginger is used). For a moment, stir.
7. The garlic is sliced and added to the onion. Stir for around 30-60 seconds when the heat is low.
8. Now's the time to apply that to the mix and swirl for around 30-60 seconds if you're using freshly grated ginger (and optional: ground lemongrass).
9. Put the other 2 cans of corn and the liquid you set aside earlier (with the water / moist / broth from the can). The vegetable broth is also added and brought to a boil.
10. Make tiny slits in the lemongrass and apply them to the soup if you're using fresh lemongrass. Or, to slap the lemongrass a few times, use a wooden spoon. Later, as a whole, you can pull them out, so make sure that they remain in one piece.
11. Let the soup-boil on medium heat for around 10 minutes.
12. Regularly check on your oven-roasted corn. Meanwhile, cut the cilantro and slice the red pepper into small bits. If you don't want it hot, you want the red pepper first.
13. When the roasted corn is done (superbly golden, piping hot, popping here and there), put in the red pepper and coriander together to a cup. Just blend it well.
14. Remove the soup from the heat after ten minutes of boiling and mix it (a hand blender is ideal) until it's (kind of) smooth.
15. Serve the soup with the corn-coriander-red pepper mix in a teaspoon (or two!) of it.

149. Egg on Avocado Toast
Prep Time: 3 min | **Cook Time:** 5 min | **Serve:** 1
- slice bread
- salt and pepper to taste
- 1 tbsp. olive oil
- Sriracha
- 1 egg
- 1 tbsp. lemon
- ½ medium avocado

1. On medium-high heat, fry the egg and the toast in the pan with the olive oil.
2. In the meantime, mash the avocado, add salt and pepper, and put some lemon to the mixture.
3. Now add an egg to your toast.
4. Put a little bit of Sriracha and munches (or your favorite spicy sauce).

150. Moroccan Couscous Salad
Prep Time: 30 min | **Cook Time:** None | **Serve:** 6
- 2 tbsp. olive oil
- fig, fresh (don't worry if you can't find one)
- ½ orange's zest
- orange
- 1 medium zucchini
- 1 pomegranate

- 1 tbsp. ginger powder (fresh is fine too. Chop it finely.)
- tbsp. cumin
- 1 tbsp. paprika powder
- 1 bell pepper, red
- ½ cup parsley, fresh
- 1 tbsp. salt
- salt and pepper to taste
- 1 cup of water
- ¼ cup raisins
- 1 cup instant couscous
- Optional
- bunch radish (thinly sliced)

1.Boil water in a wide serving bowl and apply it to the couscous.
2.Cover a tea towel or lid with the couscous and leave for 5 minutes.
3.Gently loosen the couscous with a fork and add the cumin, ginger, olive oil, and paprika powder. You want it dry and cool, no big clumps.
4.Wash the cherry, rub the zest.
5.Peel and chop the orange and, along with the zest, add it to the salad.
6.Deseed and apply the seeds to the pomegranate.
7.Finely cut the zucchini and thinly slice the red pepper. To the salad, add them.
8.Cut it upp and add it to the salad if you've managed to find a fig.
9.Clean the parsley and any other optional herbs, chop them, and then return them to the salad again.
10. Give a decent toss to it. It's that easy!

151.Chicken Breast with Asparagus
Prep Time: 15 min | **Cook Time:** 16 min | **Serve:** 5
For Chicken:
- ¼ cup extra-virgin olive oil
- ¼ cup fresh lemon juice
- 2 tablespoons maple syrup
- 1 garlic clove, minced
- Salt and ground black pepper, as required
- 5 (6-ounce) boneless, skinless chicken breasts

For Asparagus:
- 1½ pounds fresh asparagus
- 2 tablespoons extra-virgin olive oil

1.For marinade: in a large bowl, add oil, lemon juice, Erythritol, garlic, salt and black pepper and beat until well combined.
2.In a large-resealable plastic-bag, place the chicken and ¾ cup of marinade.
3.Seal the bag and shake to coat well.
4.Refrigerate overnight.
5.Cover the bowl of remaining marinade and refrigerate before serving.
6.Preheat the grill to medium heat. Grease the grill grate.
7.Remove the chicken from bag and discard the marinade.
8.Place the chicken onto grill grate and grill, covered for about 5-8 minutes per side.
9.Meanwhile, in a pan of boiling water, arrange a steamer basket.
10. Place the asparagus in steamer basket and steam, covered for about 5-7 minutes.
11. Drain the asparagus well and transfer into a bowl.
12. Add oil and toss to coat well.

13. Divide the chicken breasts and asparagus onto serving plates and serve.

152.Chicken with Zoodles
Prep Time: 15 min | **Cook Time:** 18 min | **Serve:** 4
- 2 cups zucchini, spiralized with Blade
- Salt, to taste
- 1½ pounds boneless, skinless chicken breasts Freshly ground black pepper, to taste
- 1 tablespoon olive oil
- 1 cup low-fat plain Greek yogurt
- ¼ cup low-fat Parmesan cheese, shredded ½ cup low-sodium chicken broth
- ½ teaspoon Italian seasoning
- ½ teaspoon garlic powder
- 1 cup fresh spinach, chopped
- 3-6 slices sun-dried tomatoes
- 1 tablespoon garlic, chopped

1.Preheat your oven to 350 degrees F.
2.Line a large-baking-sheet with a parchment paper.
3.Place the zucchini noodles and salt onto the prepared baking sheet and toss to coat well.
4.Arrange the zucchini-noodles in an even layer and Bake for approximately 15 minutes.
5.Meanwhile, season the chicken breasts with salt and black pepper.
6.In a large-skillet, heat the oil over medium-high heat and cook the chicken breasts for about 4-5 minutes per side or until cooked through.
7.With a slotted spoon, transfer the cooked chicken onto a plate and set aside.
8.In the same skillet, add the yogurt, Parmesan cheese, broth, Italian seasoning and garlic powder and beat until well combined.
9.Place the skillet over medium-high-heat and cook for about 2-3 minutes or until it starts to thicken, stirring continuously.
10.Stir in the spinach, sun-dried tomatoes and garlic and cook for about 2-3 minutes.
11. Attach the chicken breasts, then cook for 1-2 minutes or so.
12.Divide the zucchini noodles onto serving plates and top each with chicken mixture.

153.Chicken with Yellow Squash
Prep Time: 15 min | **Cook Time:** 17 min | **Serve:** 6
- 2 tablespoons olive oil, divided
- 1½ pounds skinless, boneless-chicken breasts, cut into bite-sized pieces
- Salt and freshly ground black-pepper, to taste 2 garlic cloves, minced
- 1½ pounds yellow squash, sliced
- 2 tablespoons fresh lemon juice
- 1 teaspoon fresh lemon zest, grated finely
- 2 tablespoons fresh parsley, minced

1.Heat 1 normal spoon of oil in a large skillet over medium heat and fry the chicken for around 6-8 minutes, or until golden brown on all sides.
2.Transfer the chicken onto a plate.
3.Heat the remaining oil over medium heat in the same skillet and sauté the garlic for approximately 1 minute.
4.Add the squash slices and cook for about 5-6 minutes,
5.Stir in the chicken and cook for about 2 minutes.

6. Remove from heat and apply-lemon juice to whisk, zest and parsley.

154. Chicken with Bell Peppers

Prep Time: 15 min | **Cook Time:** 20 min | **Serve:** 6
- 3 tablespoons olive oil, divided
- 1 yellow bell pepper, seeded and sliced
- 1 red bell pepper, seeded and sliced
- 1 green bell pepper, seeded and sliced
- 1 medium onion, sliced
- 1-pound boneless, skinless chicken breasts, sliced thinly1 teaspoon dried oregano, crushed
- ¼ teaspoon garlic powder
- ¼ teaspoon ground cumin
- Salt and freshly ground black-pepper, to taste
- ¼ cup low-sodium chicken broth

1.In a skillet, heat 1 normal spoon of oil over medium-high heat and cook the bell peppers and onion slices for about 4-5 minutes.
2.With a slotted spoon, transfer the peppers mixture onto a plate.
3.In the same skillet, heat the remaining oil over medium-high heat and cook the chicken for about 8 minutes, stirring frequently.
4.Stir in the thyme, spices, salt, black pepper, and broth, and bring to a boil.
5.Add the peppers mixture and stir to combine.
6. Reduce the heat to medium and cook, stirring periodically, for around 3-5 minutes or until all the liquid is absorbed.

155. Chicken with Mushrooms

Prep Time: 15 min | **Cook Time:** 20 min | **Serve:** 4
- 2 tablespoons almond flour
- Salt and freshly ground black-pepper, to taste
- 4 (4-ounce) skinless, boneless chicken breasts
- 2 tablespoons olive oil
- 6 garlic cloves, chopped
- ¾ pound fresh mushrooms, sliced
- ¾ cup low-sodium chicken broth
- ¼ cup balsamic vinegar
- 1 bay leaf
- ¼ teaspoon dried thyme

1. Mix the rice, salt and black pepper together in a dish.
2.Coat the chicken breasts with flour mixture evenly.
3.In a skillet, heat the olive-oil over medium-high heat and stir fry chicken for about 3 minutes.
4.Add the garlic and flip the chicken breasts.
5.Spread mushrooms over chicken and cook for about 3 minutes, shaking the skillet frequently.
6.Add the broth, vinegar, bay leaf and thyme and stir to combine.
7. Lower the heat to medium-low, cover and simmer for about 10 minutes, occasionally tossing the chicken.
8. Move the chicken with a slotted spoon to a warm serving platter and cover it with a piece of foil to keep it warm.
9.Place the pan of sauce over medium-high heat and cook, uncovered for about 7 minutes.
10.Remove the pan from heat and discard the bay leaf.
11.Place mushroom sauce over chicken and serve hot.

156. Chicken with Broccoli

Prep Time: 15 min | **Cook Time:** 22 min | **Serve:** 4
- 2 tablespoons olive oil, divided

- 4 (4-ounce) boneless, skinless chicken breasts, cut into small-pieces
- Salt and freshly ground black-pepper, 1 onion to taste, finely chopped
- 1 teaspoon fresh ginger, grated
- 1 teaspoon garlic, minced
- 1 cup broccoli florets
- 1½ cups fresh mushrooms, sliced
- 8 ounces low-sodium chicken broth

1.In a large skillet, heat 1 normal spoon of oil over medium-high heat and stir fry the chicken pieces, salt, and black pepper for about 4-5 minutes or until golden brown.
2.With a grooved spoon, transfer the chicken onto a plate.
3.In the same skillet, heat the remaining-oil over medium-high heat and sauté the onion, ginger, and garlic for about 4-5 minutes.
4.Add in mushrooms and cook for about 4-5 minutes, stirring frequently.
5.Add the broccoli and stir fry for about 3 minutes.
6.Add the cooked chicken and broth and stir fry for about 3-5 minutes
7.Add in the salt and black-pepper and remove from the heat.

157. Chicken & Veggies Stir Fry

Prep Time: 15 min | **Cook Time:** 15 min | **Serve:** 6
- 2 tablespoons fresh lime juice
- 2 tablespoons fish sauce
- 1½ teaspoons arrowroot starch
- 4 teaspoons olive oil, divided
- 1-pound skinless, boneless chicken tenders, cubed
- 1 teaspoon fresh ginger, minced
- 2 garlic cloves, minced
- ¾ teaspoon red pepper flakes, crushed
- ¼ cup water
- 4 cups broccoli, cut into bite-sized pieces
- 3 cup red-bell-pepper, seeded and sliced
- ¼ cup pine nuts

1.In a bowl, add lime juice, fish sauce, and arrowroot starch and mix until well combined. Set aside.
2.In a large non-stick sauté pan, heat 2 teaspoons of oil over high heat and cook chicken about 6-8 minutes, stirring frequently.
3. Move the chicken and set it aside in a dish.
4.In the same sauté pan, heat remaining oil over medium heat and sauté ginger, garlic and red pepper flakes for about 1 minute.
5.Add water, broccoli and bell pepper and stir fry for about 2-3 minutes.
6.Stir in chicken and lime juice mixture and cook for about 2-3 minutes.
7.Stir in pine nuts and immediately remove from heat.

158. Chicken & Broccoli Bake

Prep Time: 15 min | **Cook Time:** 24 min | **Serve:** 6
- Olive oil cooking spray
- 6 (6-ounce) skinless, boneless chicken thighs
- 3 broccoli heads, cut into florets
- 4 garlic cloves, minced
- ¼ cup extra-virgin olive oil
- 1 teaspoon dried oregano, crushed
- 1 teaspoon dried rosemary
- Salt and freshly ground black-pepper, to taste

1.Preheat your oven to 375 degrees F.
2.Grease a large-baking dish with cooking spray.
3.In a big-bowl, add all the ingredients and toss to coat well.
4.In the bottom of the prepared baking-dish, arrange the broccoli florets and top with chicken breasts in a single layer.
5.Bake for approximately 45 minutes.

159.Balsamic Chicken Breast

Prep Time: 10 min | **Cook Time:** 14 min | **Serve:** 4
- ¼ cup balsamic vinegar
- 2 tablespoons olive oil
- 1½ teaspoons fresh lemon juice
- ½ teaspoon lemon-pepper seasoning
- 4 (6-ounce) boneless, skinless-chicken breast halves, pounded slightly
- 6 cups fresh baby kale

1.In a glass baking dish, place the vinegar, oil, lemon juice and seasoning and mix well.
2.Add the chicken breasts and coat with the mixture generously.
3.Refrigerate to marinate for about 25-30 minutes.
4.Preheat the grill to medium heat.
5.Grease the grill grate.
6.Remove the chicken from bowl and discard the remaining marinade.
7.Place the chicken breasts onto the grill and cover with the lid.
8.Cook for about 5-7 minutes per side or until desired doneness.
9.Serve hot alongside the kale.

160.Lemony Chicken Thighs

Prep Time: 10 min | **Cook Time:** 16 min | **Serve:** 4
- 2 tablespoons olive oil, divided
- 1 tablespoon fresh lemon juice
- 1 tablespoon lemon zest, grated
- 2 teaspoons dried oregano
- 1 teaspoon dried thyme
- Salt and ground black pepper, to taste
- 1½ pounds bone-in chicken thighs
- 6 cups fresh baby spinach

1.Preheat your oven to 420 degree F.
2.Add 1 tablespoon of the oil, lemon juice, lemon zest, dried herbs, salt, and black pepper in a big-mixing bowl and mix well.
3.Add the chicken thighs and coat with the mixture generously.
4.Refrigerate to marinate for at least 20 minutes.
5.In an oven-proof wok, heat the remaining oil over medium-high heat and sear the chicken thighs for about 2–3 minutes per side.
6.Immediately transfer the wok into the oven and Bake for approximately 10 minutes.
7.Serve hot alongside the spinach.

161.Spicy Chicken Drumsticks

Prep Time: 10 min | **Cook Time:** 40 min | **Serve:** 5
- 2 tablespoons avocado oil
- 1 tablespoon fresh lime juice
- 1 teaspoon red chili powder
- 1 teaspoon garlic powder
- Salt, as required
- 5 (8-ounce) chicken drumsticks

- 8 cups fresh baby arugula

1.In a mixing bowl, mix avocado oil, lime juice, chili powder and garlic powder and mix well.
2.Add the chicken-drumsticks and coat with the marinade generously.
3.Cover the bowl and refrigerate for about 30-60 minutes to marinate.
4.Preheat your grill to medium-high heat.
5.Place the chicken drumsticks onto the grill and cook for about 30-40 minutes, flipping after every 5 minutes.
6.Serve hot alongside the arugula.

162.Baked Chicken & Bell Peppers

Prep Time: 15 min | **Cook Time:** 25 min | **Serve:** 4
- 1-pound boneless, skinless chicken breasts, cut into thin strips ½ of green bell pepper, seeded and cut into strips
- ½ of red bell pepper, seeded and cut into strips 1 medium onion, sliced 2 tablespoons olive oil
- ½ teaspoon dried oregano
- 2 teaspoons chili powder
- 1½ teaspoons ground cumin
- 1 teaspoon garlic powder
- Salt, to taste

1. Preheat your oven to 400 degrees F.
2. In a tub, add all of the ingredients and mix well.
3.Place the chicken mixture into a 9x13-inch baking dish and spread in an even layer.
4.Bake for about 22-25 minutes, or until the chicken is completely cooked.

163.Tofu & Veggie Salad

Prep Time: 20 min | **Serve:** 8
For Dressing:
- ¼ cup balsamic vinegar
- ¼ cup low-sodium soy sauce
- 2 tablespoons water
- 1 teaspoon sesame oil, toasted
- 1 teaspoon Sriracha
- 3-4 drops liquid stevia
For Salad:
- 1½ pounds baked firm tofu, cubed
- 2 large zucchinis, sliced thinly
- 2 large-yellow bell-peppers, seeded and sliced thinly
- 3 cups cherry tomatoes, halved
- 2 cups radishes, sliced thinly
- 2 cups purple cabbage, shredded
- 10 cups fresh baby spinach

1.For Dressing: in a bowl, add all the ingredients and beat until well combined.
2.Divide the chickpeas, tofu and vegetables into serving bowls.
3.Drizzle with dressing and serve immediately.

164.Blueberries & Spinach Salad

Prep Time: 15 min | **Serve:** 4
For Salad:
- 6 cups fresh baby spinach
- 1½ cups fresh blueberries
- ¼ cup onion, sliced
- ¼ cup almond, sliced
- ¼ cup feta cheese, crumbled

For Dressing:
- 1/3 cup olive oil
- 2 tablespoons fresh lemon juice
- ¼ teaspoon liquid stevia
- 1/8 teaspoon garlic powder
- Salt, as required

1. For Salad: in a bowl, add the spinach, berries, onion and almonds and mix.
2. For Dressing: in another small bowl, add all the ingredients and beat until well blended.
3. Place the dressing over salad and gently toss to coat well.

165. Mixed Berries Salad

Prep Time: 15 min | **Serve:** 4
- 1 cup fresh strawberries, hulled and sliced ½ cups fresh blackberries
- ½ cup fresh blueberries
- ½ cup fresh raspberries
- 6 cup fresh arugula
- 2 tablespoons extra-virgin olive oil
- Salt and ground black pepper, as required

1. Place all the ingredients in a salad-bowl and toss to coat them well.

166. Kale & Citrus Fruit Salad

Prep Time: 15 min | **Serve:** 2
For Salad:
- 3 cups-fresh kale, tough ribs removed and torn
- 1 orange, peeled and segmented
- 1 grapefruit, peeled and segmented
- 2 tablespoons unsweetened dried cranberries ¼ teaspoon white sesame seeds

For Dressing:
- 2 tablespoons extra-virgin olive oil
- 2 tablespoons fresh orange juice
- 1 teaspoon Dijon mustard
- ½ teaspoon raw honey
- Salt and ground black pepper, as required

1. For Salad: in a salad bowl, place all ingredients and mix.
2. For Dressing: place all ingredients in another bowl and beat until well combined.
3. Place dressing on top of salad and toss to coat well.

167. Kale, Apple & Cranberry Salad

Prep Time: 15 min | **Serve:** 4
- 6 cups fresh baby kale
- 3 large apples, cored and sliced
- ¼ cup unsweetened dried cranberries
- ¼ cup almonds, sliced
- 2 tablespoons extra-virgin olive oil
- 1 tablespoon raw honey
- Salt and ground black pepper, as required

1. Place all the ingredients in a salad-bowl and toss to coat them well.

168. Rocket, Beat & Orange Salad

Prep Time: 15 min | **Serve:** 4
- 3 large oranges, peeled, seeded and sectioned
- 2 beets, trimmed, peeled and sliced
- 6 cups fresh rocket
- ¼ cup walnuts, chopped

- 3 tablespoons olive oil
- Pinch of salt

1. In a salad bowl, place all ingredients and gently, toss to coat.

169. Cucumber & Tomato Salad

Prep Time: 15 min | **Serve:** 6
For Salad:
- 3 large English cucumbers, sliced thinly sliced
- 2 cups tomatoes, chopped
- 6 cup lettuce, torn

For Dressing:
- 4 tablespoons olive oil
- 2 tablespoons balsamic vinegar
- 1 tablespoon fresh lemon juice
- Salt and ground black pepper, as required

1. For Salad: in a big-bowl, add the cucumbers, onion and dill and mix.
2. For Dressing: in a small bowl, add all the ingredients and beat until well combined.
3. Place the dressing over the salad and toss to coat well.

170. Mixed Veggie Salad

Prep Time: 20 min | **Serve:** 6
For Dressing:
- 1 small avocado, peeled, pitted and chopped
- ¼ cup low-fat plain Greek yogurt
- 1 small yellow onion, chopped
- 1 garlic clove, chopped
- 2 tablespoons fresh parsley
- 2 tablespoons fresh lemon juice

For Salad:
- 6 cups fresh spinach, shredded
- 2 medium zucchinis, cut into thin slices
- ½ cup celery, sliced
- ½ cup red bell pepper, seeded and sliced thinly
- ½ cup yellow onion, sliced thinly
- ½ cup cucumber, sliced thinly
- ½ cup cherry tomatoes, halved
- ¼ cup Kalamata olives, pitted
- ½ cup feta cheese, crumbled

1. For Dressing: in a food processor, add all the ingredients and pulse until smooth.
2. For Salad: in a salad bowl, add all the ingredients and mix well.
3. Pour the dressing over the salad, throw it gently and cover it well.

171. Eggs & Veggie Salad

Prep Time: 15 min | **Serve:** 8
For Salad:
- 2 large English cucumbers, sliced thinly sliced
- 2 cups tomatoes, chopped
- 8 hard-boiled eggs, peeled and sliced
- 8 cups fresh baby spinach

For Dressing:
- 4 tablespoons olive oil
- 2 tablespoons balsamic vinegar
- 1 tablespoon fresh lemon juice
- Salt and ground black pepper, as required

1. For Salad: in a salad bowl, add the cucumbers, onion and dill and mix.

2.For Dressing: in a small bowl, add all the ingredients and beat until well blended.
3.Place the dressing over the salad and toss to coat well.

172.Chicken & Orange Salad

Prep Time: 15 min | **Cook Time:** 16 min | **Serve:** 5
For Chicken:

- 4 (6-ounce) boneless, skinless-chicken breast halves Salt and ground black pepper, as required 2 tablespoons extra-virgin olive oil

For Salad:

- 8 cups fresh baby arugula
- 5 medium oranges, peeled and sectioned
- 1 cup onion, sliced

For Dressing:

- 2 tablespoons extra-virgin olive oil
- 2 tablespoons fresh orange juice
- 2 tablespoons balsamic vinegar
- 1½ teaspoons shallots, minced
- 1 garlic clove, minced
- Salt and ground black pepper, as required

1.For chicken: season each chicken breast half with salt and black pepper evenly.
2.Place chicken over a rack set in a rimmed baking sheet.
3.Refrigerate for at least 30 minutes.
4.Remove the baking sheet from refrigerator and pat dry the chicken breast halves with paper towels.
5.Heat the oil in a 12-inch sauté pan over medium-low heat.
6.Place the chicken breast halves, smooth-side down, and cook for about 9-10 minutes, without moving.
7.Flip the chicken breasts and cook for about 6 minutes or until cooked through.
8.Remove the sauté pan from heat and let the chicken stand in the pan for about 3 minutes.
9.Transfer the chicken breasts onto a cutting board for about 5 minutes.
10.Cut each chicken breast half into desired-sized slices.
11.For Salad: place all ingredients in a salad bowl and mix.
12.Add chicken slices and stir to combine.
13.For Dressing: place all ingredients in another bowl and beat until well combined.
14.Place the salad onto each serving plate.
15.Drizzle with dressing.

173.Chicken & Strawberry Salad

Prep Time: 20 min | **Cook Time:** 16 min | **Serve:** 8

- 2 pounds boneless, skinless chicken breasts ½ cup olive oil
- ¼ cup fresh lemon juice
- 2 tablespoons Erythritol
- 1 garlic clove, minced
- Salt and ground black pepper, as required 4 cups fresh strawberries
- 8 cups fresh spinach, torn

1.For marinade: in a large bowl, add oil, lemon juice, Erythritol, garlic, salt and black pepper and beat until well combined.
2.In a big-resealable plastic bag, place chicken and ¾ cup marinade.
3.Seal bag and shake to coat well.
4.Refrigerate overnight.
5.Cover the bowl of remaining marinade and refrigerate before serving.
6.Preheat the grill to medium heat. Grease the grill grate.

7.Remove the chicken from bag and discard the marinade.
8.Place the chicken onto grill grate and grill, covered for about 5-8 minutes per side.
9.Remove chicken from grill and cut into bite sized pieces.
10.In a large bowl, add the chicken pieces, strawberries and spinach and mix.
11.Place the reserved marinade and toss to coat.

174.Chicken & Fruit Salad

Prep Time: 15 min | **Serve:** 4
For Vinaigrette:

- 2 tablespoons apple cider vinegar
- 2 tablespoons extra-virgin olive-oil
- Salt and freshly ground black-pepper, to taste
- For Salad:
- 2 cup cooked chicken, cubed
- 4 cup lettuce, torn
- 1 large apple, peeled, cored and chopped
- 1 cup fresh strawberries, hulled and sliced

1.For vinaigrette: in a small bowl, add all ingredients and beat well.
2.For Salad: in a big-salad bowl, mix together all ingredients.
3.Place vinaigrette over chicken mixture and toss to coat well.

175.Chicken, Tomato & Arugula Salad

Prep Time: 15 min | **Cook Time:** 15 min | **Serve:** 4
For Chicken:

- 3 (6-ounce) skinless, boneless chicken breast halves
- 2 teaspoons orange zest, grated finely
- 1/3 cup fresh orange juice
- 4 garlic cloves, minced
- 2 tablespoons maple syrup
- 1½ teaspoons dried thyme, crushed

For Salad:

- 6 cups fresh baby arugula
- 2 cups cherry tomatoes, quartered
- 3 tablespoons extra-virgin olive oil
- 2 tablespoons fresh lime juice
- Salt and ground black pepper, as required

1.For chicken: in a zip lock bag, all the ingredients.
2.Seal the bag and shake to coat well.
3.Refrigerate to marinate for about 6-8 hours, flipping occasionally.
4.Preheat the oven to broiler.
5.Line a broiler pan with a piece of foil.
6.Arrange the oven rack about 6-inch away from heating element.
7.Remove the chicken breasts from bag and discard the marinade.
8.Arrange the chicken breasts onto the prepared pan in a single layer.
9.Broil for about for 15 minutes, flipping once halfway through.
10.Remove the chicken breasts from oven and place onto a cutting board for about 10 minutes.
11.Cut the chicken breasts into desired sized slices.
12.For Salad: in a bowl, add all ingredients and toss to coat well.
13.Add chicken slices and stir to combine.

176.Chicken, Cucumber & Tomato Salad

Prep Time: 15 min | **Cook Time:** 16 min | **Serve:** 4

- 4 (6-ounce) boneless, skinless chicken breast halves
- Salt and freshly ground black-pepper, to taste 2 normale spoons olive oil
- 1 tomato, chopped
- 1 cucumber, chopped
- 3 cup fresh baby greens
- 3 cup lettuce, torn

1. Season each half of each chicken breast evenly with salt and black pepper.
2. Place chicken over a rack set in a rimmed baking sheet.
3. Refrigerate for at least 30 minutes.
4. Remove from refrigerator and with paper towels, pat dry the chicken breasts.
5. In a 11-inch skillet, heat the oil over medium-low heat.
6. Place the chicken breast halves, smooth-side down, and cook for about 9-10 minutes, without moving.
7. Flip the chicken breasts and cook for about 6 minutes or until cooked through.
8. Remove the skillet from heat and let the chicken stand in the pan for about 3 minutes.
9. Divide greens, lettuce, cucumber and tomatoes onto serving plates.
10. Top each plate with 1 breast half and serve.

177.Chicken, Kale & Olives Salad

Prep Time: 15 min | **Serve:** 4

For Dressing:
- 2 tablespoons fresh orange juice
- 2 tablespoons fresh lemon juice
- 3 tablespoons extra-virgin olive oil
- 1 tablespoon red wine vinegar
- 1 tablespoon honey
- 1 tablespoon fresh orange zest, grated
- ¾ tablespoon Dijon mustard
- Salt and ground black pepper, as required

For Salad:
- 3 cups cooked chicken, chopped
- 2 cups mixed olives, pitted
- 1 cup red onion, chopped
- 6 cups fresh kale, tough ribs removed and torn

1. For Dressing: in a small bowl, add all ingredients and beat well.
2. For Salad: in a big-salad bowl, mix together all ingredients.
3. Place dressing over salad and toss to coat well.

178.Chicken, Kale & Cucumber Salad

Prep Time: 15 min | **Cook Time:** 18 min | **Serve:** 4

For Chicken:
- 1 teaspoon dried thyme
- ½ teaspoon garlic powder
- ½ teaspoon onion powder
- ¼ teaspoon cayenne pepper
- ¼ teaspoon ground turmeric
- Salt and ground black pepper, as required
- 2 (7-ounce) boneless, skinless chicken breasts, pounded into ¾-inch thickness
- 1 tablespoon extra-virgin olive oil

For Salad:
- 5 cups fresh kale, tough ribs removed and chopped
- 1 cup cucumber, chopped

- ½ cup red onion, sliced
- ¼ cup pine nuts

For Dressing:
- 1 small garlic clove, minced
- 2 tablespoons fresh lemon juice
- 2 tablespoons extra-virgin olive oil
- 1 teaspoon maple syrup
- Salt and ground black pepper, as required

1. Preheat your oven to 429 degrees F. Line a baking dish with parchment paper.
2. For chicken: in a bowl, mix together the thyme, spices, salt and black pepper.
3. Drizzle the chicken breasts with oil and then rub with spice mixture generously and drizzle with the oil.
4. On the prepared baking platter, arrange the chicken breasts.
5. Bake for approximately 16-18 minutes.
6. Remove pan from oven and place the chicken breasts onto a cutting board for about 5 minutes.
7. For Salad: place all ingredients in a salad bowl and mix.
8. For Dressing: place all ingredients in another bowl and beat until well combined.
9. Cut each chicken breast into desired sized slices.
10. Place the salad onto each serving plate and top each with chicken slices.
11. Drizzle with dressing and serve.

179.Turkey & Veggie Salad

Prep Time: 15 min | **Serve:** 4

For Salad:
- 3 cups cooked turkey meat, chopped
- 2 cups, cucumber, chopped
- 1 cup cherry tomatoes, halved
- 1 cup radishes, trimmed and sliced
- 6 cups fresh baby arugula
- 4 tablespoons scallion greens, chopped
- 4 tablespoons fresh parsley leaves, chopped

For Dressing:
- 1 garlic clove, minced
- 3 tablespoons extra-virgin olive oil
- 1 tablespoon balsamic vinegar
- 1 tablespoon fresh lemon juice
- Salt and ground black pepper, as required

1. For Salad: in a large serving bowl, add all the ingredients and mix.
2. For Dressing: in another bowl, add all the ingredients and beat till well combined.
3. Pour dressing over salad and gently toss to coat well.

180.Ground Turkey Salad

Prep Time: 20 min | **Cook Time:** 13 min | **Serve:** 6

- 1-pound ground turkey
- 1 tablespoon olive oil
- Salt and ground black pepper, as required
- ¼ cup water
- ½ of English cucumber, chopped
- 4 cups green cabbage, shredded
- ½ cup fresh mint leaves, chopped
- 2 tablespoons fresh lime juice
- ¼ cup walnuts, chopped

1. Heat the oil in a big-skillet over medium-high heat and cook the turkey for around 6-8 minutes, using a spatula to break up the bits.

2.Stir in the water and cook for about 4-5 minutes or until almost all the liquid is evaporated.
3.Remove from the heat and transfer the turkey into a bowl.
4.Set the bowl aside to cool completely.
5.In a big-serving bowl, add the vegetables, mint and lime juice and mix well.
6.Add the cooked turkey and stir to combine.

181.Steak & Tomato Salad

Prep Time: 15 min | **Cook Time:** 15 min | **Serve:** 5
For Steak:
- 2 tablespoons fresh oregano, chopped
- ½ tablespoon garlic, minced
- 1 tablespoon fresh lemon peel, grated ½ teaspoon red pepper flakes, crushed Salt and ground black pepper, as required
- 1 (1-pound) (1-inch thick) boneless beef top sirloin steak

For Salad:
- 6 cups fresh salad greens
- 2 cups cherry tomatoes, halved
- 2 tablespoons olive oil
- 2 tablespoons fresh lime juice
- Salt and ground black pepper, as required

1.Preheat the gas grill to medium heat.
2.Lightly grease the grill grate.
3.For steak: in a bowl, add the oregano, garlic, lemon peel, red pepper flakes, salt and black pepper and mix well.
4.Rub the steak with garlic mixture evenly.
5. Put the steak on the grill and cook, covered, sometimes flipping, for about 12-17 minutes.
6.Remove the steak from the grill and position it for approximately 10 minutes on a cutting board.
7.Meanwhile, For Salad: in a large serving bowl, place all ingredients and toss to coat well.
8.Cut the steak into bite-sized pieces.
9.Add the steak pieces into the bowl of salad and toss to coat well.

182.Steak, Egg & Veggies Salad

Prep Time: 20 min | **Cook Time:** 9 min | **Serve:** 4
For Steak:
- 2 tablespoons extra-virgin olive oil
- 1-pound flank steak, sliced thinly
- Salt and ground black pepper, as require

For Salad:
- 4 hard-boiled eggs, peeled and halved
- 1 cup radishes, cut into matchsticks
- 1 cup cucumber, cut into matchsticks
- 1 cup tomato, chopped
- ½ cup scallion greens, chopped

For Dressing:
- ¼ cup fresh orange juice
- 3 tablespoons extra-virgin olive oil
- 2 tablespoons low-sodium soy sauce
- 2 tablespoons white vinegar
- 1 tablespoon fresh lime juice
- 1 tablespoon maple syrup
- 1 teaspoon fresh lime zest, grated
- 1 garlic clove, minced

1.Heat oil in a big-heavy-bottomed pan over medium-high heat and sear the beef slices with salt and black-pepper for about 3-6 minutes or until cooked through.

2.Transfer the beef slices onto a plate and set aside.
3.Meanwhile, in a pan of the lightly salted boiling water, cook the noodles for about 5 minutes.
4.Drain well with the noodles and rinse under cold water.
5.Drain the noodles again.
6.For Dressing: in a bowl, add all ingredients and beat until well combined.
7.Divide beef slices, noodles, veggies and scallion into serving bowls and drizzle with dressing.

183.Steak & Kale Salad

Prep Time: 15 min | **Cook Time:** 8 min | **Serve:** 2
For Steak:
- 2 teaspoons olive oil
- 2 (4-ounce) strip steaks
- Salt and ground black pepper, as required

For Salad:
- ½ cup carrot, peeled and shredded
- ½ cup cucumber, peeled, seeded and sliced
- 3 cups-fresh kale, tough ribs removed and chopped

For Dressing:
- 1 tablespoon extra-virgin olive oil
- 1 tablespoon fresh lemon juice
- Salt and ground black pepper, as required

1.For steak: in a large heavy-bottomed skillet, heat the oil over high heat and cook the steaks with salt and black pepper for about 3-4 minutes per side.
2.Transfer the steaks onto a cutting board for about 5 minutes before slicing.
3.For Salad: place all ingredients in a salad bowl and mix.
4.For Dressing: place all ingredients in another bowl and beat until well combined.
5.Cut the steaks into desired sized slices against the grain.
6.Place the salad onto each serving plate.
7.Top each plate with steak slices.
8.Drizzle with dressing.

184.Steak & Veggie Salad

Prep Time: 20 min | **Cook Time:** 16 min | **Serve:** 8
For Steak:
- 2 garlic cloves, crushed
- 1 teaspoon fresh ginger, grated
- 1 tablespoon honey
- 2 normal spoons olive oil
- Salt and freshly ground black-pepper, to taste
- 1½ pounds flank steak, trimmed

For Dressing:
- 1 garlic clove, minced
- 4 tablespoons extra-virgin olive oil
- 3 tablespoons fresh lime juice
- ¼ little spoon red-pepper flakes, crushed
- Salt and freshly ground black-pepper, to taste

For Salad:
- 3 cup cucumber, sliced
- 3 cup cherry tomatoes, halved
- 1 cup red onion, sliced thinly
- 4 tablespoons fresh mint leaves
- 8 cup fresh spinach, torn

1.For steak: in a large sealable bag, mix together all ingredients except steak.
2.Add steak and coat with marinade generously.
3.Seal the bag and refrigerate to marinate for about 24 hours.

4.Remove from the refrigerator and set aside in room temperature for about 15 minutes.
5.Heat a Lightly-greased grill pan over-medium-high heat and cook the steak for about 6-8 minutes per side.
6.Remove the steak from grill pan and place onto a cutting board for about 10 minutes before slicing.
7.For Dressing: in a small bowl, add all ingredients and beat well.
8.For Salad: in a large-salad bowl, mix together all ingredients.
9.With a sharp knife, cut into desired slices.
10.On serving plates, divide the salad and top with steak slices.
11.Drizzle with dressing and serve immediately.

185. Chicken & Bell Pepper Muffins

Prep Time: 15 min | **Cook Time:** 20 min | **Serve:** 4
- 8 eggs
- Salt and ground black-pepper, as required 2 tablespoons water
- 8 ounces cooked chicken, chopped finely
- 1 cup green-bell-pepper, seeded and chopped
- 1 cup onion, chopped

1.Preheat your oven to 350 degrees F.
2.Grease 8 cups of a muffin tin.
3.In a bowl, add eggs, black pepper and water and beat until well combined.
4.Add the chicken, bell-pepper and onion and stir to combine.
5.Transfer the mixture in prepared muffin cups evenly.
6.Bake for approximately 17-21 minutes or until golden brown.
7.Remove the muffin tin from oven and place onto a wire rack to cool for about 10 minutes.
8.Carefully invert the muffins onto a platter and serve warm.

186. Chicken & Kale Muffins

Prep Time: 15 min | **Cook Time:** 20 min | **Serve:** 4
- 8 eggs
- Freshly ground black pepper, as required
- 2 tablespoons water
- 7 ounces cooked chicken, chopped finely
- 1½ cups fresh kale, tough ribs removed and chopped
- 1 cup onion, chopped
- 2 tablespoons fresh parsley, chopped

1.Preheat your oven to 350 degrees F.
2.Grease 8 cups of a muffin tin.
3.In a bowl, add eggs, black pepper and water and beat until well combined.
4.Add chicken, kale, onion and parsley and stir to combine.
5.Transfer the mixture in prepared muffin cups evenly.
6.Bake for approximately 17-21 minutes or until golden brown.
7.Remove the muffin tin from oven and place onto a wire rack to cool for about 10 minutes.
8.Carefully invert the muffins onto a platter.

187. Eggs with Kale & Tomatoes

Prep Time: 15 min | **Cook Time:** 25 min | **Serve:** 4
- 2 tablespoons olive oil
- 1 yellow onion, chopped
- 2 garlic cloves, minced
- 1 cup tomatoes, chopped
- ½ pound fresh kale, tough ribs removed and chopped 1 teaspoon ground cumin
- ¼ teaspoon red pepper flakes, crushed
- Salt and ground black pepper, as required 4 eggs
- 2 tablespoons fresh parsley, chopped

1.In a large nonstick wok, heat the olive oil over medium heat and sauté the onion for about 4-5 minutes.
2. Add the garlic and sauté for approximately 1 minute.
3.Add the tomatoes, spices, salt and black pepper and cook for about 2-3 minutes, stirring frequently.
4.Attach the kale and cook for 4-5 minutes or so.
5.Carefully crack eggs on top of kale mixture.
6.With the lid, cover the wok and cook for about 10 minutes or until desired doneness of eggs.
7.Serve hot with the garnishing of parsley.

188. Eggs with Veggies

Prep Time: 10 min | **Cook Time:** 15 min | **Serve:** 4
- 2 tablespoons olive oil, divided
- ¾ pound zucchini, quartered and sliced thinly
- 1 red bell pepper, seeded and chopped
- 1 medium onion, chopped
- 1 teaspoon fresh rosemary, chopped finely
- Salt and ground black pepper, as required 4 large egg

1.In a large skillet, heat 1 tablespoon of oil over medium-high heat and sauté the zucchini, bell pepper and onion for about 5-8 minutes.
2.Add the rosemary, salt and black pepper and stir to combine.
3.With a wooden spoon, make a large well in the center of skillet by moving the veggie mixture towards the sides.
4.Reduce the heat to medium and pour the remaining oil in the well.
5.Carefully crack the eggs in the well and sprinkle the eggs with salt and black pepper.
6.Cook for about 1-2 minutes.
7.Cover the skillet and cook for about 1-2 minutes more.
8.For serving, carefully scoop the veggie mixture onto 4 serving plates.
9.Top each serving with an egg.

189. Chicken & Veggie Frittata

Prep Time: 45 min | **Cook Time:** 15 min | **Serve:** 8
- 1 teaspoon olive oil
- ½ cup yellow onion, sliced
- 2 garlic cloves, minced
- 2 cups fresh spinach, chopped
- 1 cup red-bell-pepper, seeded and chopped
- 2 cups cooked chicken, chopped
- 2 large eggs
- 4 large egg whites
- 1¼ cups unsweetened almond milk
- 1 cup low-fat cheddar cheese, shredded Freshly ground black pepper, as required 1 tablespoon Parmesan cheese, shredded

1.Preheat your oven to 350 degrees F.
2.Grease a 9-inch pie plate.
3.In a skillet, heat-oil over medium heat and sauté onion and garlic for about 2-3 minutes.
4.Add spinach and bell pepper and sauté for about 1-2 minutes.

5.Stir in chicken and transfer the mixture into the prepared pie dish evenly.

6.Add eggs, egg whites, almond milk, cheddar cheese, salt, and black pepper in a mixing bowl and beat until well combined.

7.Pour egg mixture over the chicken mixture evenly and top with Parmesan cheese.

8.Bake for approximately 40 minutes or until top becomes golden brown.

9.Remove the pie-dish from oven and set aside for about 5 minutes.

10. Cut into 8 equal-sized wedges and serve.

190.Broccoli Frittata

Prep Time: 15 min | **Cook Time:** 13 min | **Serve:** 6

- 8 eggs
- 1 tablespoon fresh cilantro, chopped
- 1 tablespoon fresh basil, chopped
- ¼ teaspoon red pepper flakes, crushed
- Salt and ground-black-pepper, as required 2 tablespoons olive oil
- 1 bunch scallions, chopped
- 1 cup broccoli, chopped finely
- ½ cup goat cheese, crumbled

1.Preheat the broiler of oven.

2.Arrange the upper third of the oven on a stand.

3.In a bowl, add eggs, fresh herbs, red pepper flakes, salt and black pepper and beat well.

4.In an ovenproof-skillet, heat the oil over medium heat and sauté scallion and broccoli for about 1-2 minutes.

5.Add the egg mixture over the broccoli mixture evenly and lift the edges to let the egg mixture flow underneath.

6.Cook for about 2-3 minutes.

7.Place the cheese on top in the form of dots.

8.Now, transfer the skillet under broiler and broil for about 2-3 minutes.

9.Remove the skillet from oven and set aside for about 5 minutes.

10. Cut the frittata into desired size slices and serve.

191.Chicken & Veggie Quiche

Prep Time: 15 min | **Cook Time:** 20 min | **Serve:** 4

- 6 eggs
- ½ cup unsweetened almond milk
- Freshly ground black pepper, to taste
- 1 cup cooked chicken, chopped
- ½ cup fresh baby spinach, chopped
- ½ cup fresh baby kale, chopped
- ¼ cup fresh mushrooms, sliced
- ¼ cup green bell-pepper, seeded and chopped 1 scallion, chopped
- ¼ cup fresh cilantro, chopped
- 1 tablespoon fresh chives, minced

1.Preheat the oven to 400 degrees F.

2.Lightly grease a pie dish.

3.In a big-bowl, add the eggs, almond milk, salt and black pepper and beat well. Set aside.

4.In another bowl, add the chicken, vegetables, scallion and herbs and mix well.

5.Place the chicken mixture in the bottom of prepared pie dish.

6.Place the egg mixture over chicken mixture evenly.

7.Bake for approximately 20 minutes or until a toothpick inserted in the center comes out clean.

8. Take it out of the oven and set-aside for about 5-10 minutes to cool before slicing.

9.Cut into desired size wedges and serve.

192.Kale & Mushroom Frittata

Prep Time: 15 min | **Cook Time:** 30 min | **Serve:** 5

- 8 eggs
- ½ cup unsweetened almond milk
- Salt and ground black pepper, as required
- 1 tablespoon extra-virgin olive oil
- 1 onion, chopped
- 1 garlic clove, minced
- 1 cup fresh mushrooms, chopped
- 1½ cups fresh kale, tough ribs removed and chopped

1.Preheat your oven to 350 degrees F.

2.In a large bowl, place the eggs, almond milk, salt and black pepper and beat well. Set aside.

3.In a large ovenproof wok, heat the oil over medium heat and sauté the onion and garlic for about 3-4 minutes.

4.Add the mushrooms, kale, salt and black pepper and cook for about 8-10 minutes.

5.Stir in the mushrooms, then cook for 3-4 minutes or so.

6.Add the kale and cook for about 5 minutes.

7.Place the egg mixture on top evenly and cook for about 4 minutes, without stirring.

8.Transfer the wok in the oven and Bake for approximately 12-15 minutes or until desired doneness.

9.Remove from the oven and place the frittata side for about 3-5 minutes before serving.

10. Cut into desired sized wedges and serve.

193.Kale & Bell Pepper Frittata

Prep Time: 10 min | **Cook Time:** 17 min | **Serve:** 3

- 6 eggs
- Salt, as required
- 1 tablespoon olive oil
- ½ teaspoon ground turmeric
- 1 small red-bell-pepper, seeded and chopped
- 1 cup fresh kale, trimmed and chopped
- ¼ cup fresh chives, chopped

1.In a bowl, add the eggs and salt and beat well. Set aside.

2.In a cast-iron skillet, heat the oil over medium-low heat and sprinkle with turmeric.

3.Immediately stir in the bell pepper and kale and sauté for about 2 minutes.

4.Place the beaten eggs over bell pepper mixture evenly and immediately reduce the heat to low.

5.Cover the skillet and bake for 10-15 minutes or so.

6.Remove from the heat and set aside for about 5 minutes.

7.Cut into equal-sized wedges and serve.

194.Mushroom & Tomato Omelet

Prep Time: 15 min | **Cook Time:** 36 min | **Serve:** 2

- 2 poblano peppers
- Olive oil cooking spray
- 1 small tomato
- ½ teaspoon dried oregano
- ½ teaspoon chicken bouillon seasoning 4 eggs, separated
- 2 tablespoons sour cream
- ½ cup fresh white mushrooms, sliced

- 2/3 cups part-skim mozzarella cheese, shredded and divided

1.Preheat your oven to broiler.

2.Line a sheet with a piece of foil for baking.

3.Spray the poblano peppers with cooking spray lightly.

4.Arrange the peppers onto the prepared baking sheet in a single layer and broil for about 5-10 minutes per side or until skin becomes dark ad blistered.

5.Remove from the oven to cool and set aside.

6.After cooking, remove the stems, skin and seeds from peppers and then cut each into thin strips.

7.Meanwhile, for sauce: with a knife, make 2 small slits in a crisscross pattern on the top of tomato.

8.In a microwave-safe plate, place the tomato and microwave on High for about 2-3 minutes.

9.In a blender, add the tomato, oregano and chicken bouillon seasoning and pulse until smooth.

10.Move the sauce and set it aside in a bowl.

11.In a bowl, add the egg yolks and sour cream and beat until well combined.

12.In a clean glass bowl, add egg whites and with an electric mixer, beat until soft peaks form

13.Gently gold the egg yolk mixture into whipped egg whites

14.Heat a lightly greased skillet over medium-low heat and cook half of the egg mixture cook for about 3-5 minutes or until bottom is set

15.Place half of the mushrooms and pepper strips over one half of omelet and sprinkle with half of the cheese

16.Cover the skillet and cook for about 2-3 minutes

17.Uncover the skillet and fold in the omelet

18.Transfer the omelet onto a plate

19.Repeat with the remaining egg mixture, mushrooms, pepper strips and cheese.

20.Top each omelet with sauce.

195.Tomato & Egg Scramble

Prep Time: 10 min | **Cook Time:** 5 min | **Serve:** 2

- 4 eggs
- ¼ teaspoon red pepper flakes, crushed Salt and ground black pepper, as required ¼ cup fresh basil, chopped
- ½ cup tomatoes, chopped
- 1 tablespoon olive oil

1.In a large bowl, add eggs, red pepper flakes, salt and black pepper and beat well.

2.Add the basil and tomatoes and stir to combine.

3.In a large non-stick skillet, heat th oil over medium-high heat.

4.Add the egg mixture and cook for about 3-5 minutes, stirring continuously.

196.Tofu & Spinach Scramble

Prep Time: 10 min | **Cook Time:** 8 min | **Serve:** 2

- 1 tablespoon olive oil
- 1 garlic clove, minced
- ¼ pound medium-firm tofu, drained, pressed and crumbled 1/3 cup low-sodium vegetable broth 2¾ cups fresh baby spinach
- 2 teaspoons low-sodium soy sauce
- 1 teaspoon ground turmeric
- 1 teaspoon fresh lemon juice

1.In a frying pan, heat the olive oil over medium-high heat and sauté the garlic for about 1 minute

2.Add the tofu and cook for about 3-4 minutes, slowly adding the broth.

3.Add the spinach, soy sauce and turmeric and stir fry for about 3-4 minutes or until all the liquid is absorbed

4.Remove and whisk in the lemon juice from the sun.

197.Tofu & Veggie Scramble

Prep Time: 15 min | **Cook Time:** 15 min | **Serve:** 2

- ½ tablespoon olive oil
- 1 small onion, chopped finely
- 1 small red-bell-pepper, seeded and chopped finely
- 1 cup cherry tomatoes, chopped finely
- 1½ cups firm tofu, crumbled and chopped Pinch of cayenne pepper
- Pinch of ground turmeric
- Sea salt, to taste

1.In a skillet, heat-oil over medium-heat and sauté the onion and bell pepper for about 4-5 minutes.

2.Add the tomatoes and cook for about 1-2 minutes.

3.Add the tofu, turmeric, cayenne pepper and salt and cook for about 6-8 minutes.

198.Chicken & Zucchini Pancakes

Prep Time: 15 min | **Cook Time:** 32 min | **Serve:** 4

- 4 cups zucchinis, shredded
- Salt, as required
- ¼ cup cooked chicken, shredded
- ¼ cup scallion, chopped finely
- 1 egg, beaten
- ¼ cup coconut flour
- Salt and ground-black-pepper, as required 1 tablespoon extra-virgin olive oil

1.In a colander, place the zucchini and sprinkle with salt.

2.Set aside for about 8-10 minutes.

3.Squeeze the zucchinis well and transfer into a bowl.

4.In the bowl of zucchini, add the remaining ingredients and mix until well combined.

5.Heat the oil in a big-nonstick skillet over normal heat.

6.Add ¼ cup of zucchini mixture into the preheated skillet and spread in an even layer.

7.Cook for about 3-4 minutes per side.

8.Repeat with the remaining mixture.

199.Broccoli Waffles

Prep Time: 10 min | **Cook Time:** 8 min | **Serve:** 2

- 1/3 cup broccoli, chopped finely
- ¼ cup low-fat Cheddar cheese, shredded 1 egg
- ½ teaspoon garlic powder
- ½ teaspoon dried onion, minced
- Salt and ground black pepper, as required

1.Preheat a mini waffle iron and then grease it.

2.In a normal bowl, place all ingredients and mix until well combined.

3.Place ½ of the mixture into preheated waffle iron and cook for about 3-4 minutes or until golden brown.

4.Repeat with the remaining mixture.

200.Cheesy Spinach Waffles

Prep Time: 10 min | **Cook Time:** 20 min | **Serve:** 4

- 1 large egg, beaten
- 1 cup ricotta cheese, crumbled
- ½ cup part-skim Mozzarella cheese, shredded
- ¼ cup low-fat Parmesan cheese, grated
- 4 ounces frozen-spinach, thawed and squeezed dry
- 1 garlic clove, minced
- Salt and ground black pepper, as required

1. Preheat a mini waffle iron and then grease it.
2. Stir in all the ingredients in a bowl and beat until well mixed.
3. Place ¼ of the mixture into preheated waffle iron and cook for about 4-5 minutes or until golden brown. Repeat with the remaining mixture.

FIRST COURSES AND SOUP RECIPES

201.Tomatillo and Green Chili Pork Stew

Prep Time: 15 min | **Cook Time:** 30 min | **Serve:** 1
- 1/2 scallions, chopped
- 1/2 cloves of garlic
- 1/4 pound tomatillos, trimmed and chopped
- 2 large romaine or green lettuce leaves, divided
- 1/2 serrano chilies, seeds, and membranes
- ½ teaspoon dried Mexican oregano (or you can use regular oregano)
- 1/4 pound of boneless pork loin, to be cut into bite-sized cubes
- ¼ cup coriander, chopped
- ¼ tablespoon (each) salt and paper
- 1/4 jalapeno, seeds, and membranes to be removed and thinly sliced
- 1/4 cup sliced radishes
- 1 lime wedge

1. Combine scallions, garlic, tomatillos, four lettuce leaves, serrano chilies, and oregano in a blender. Then puree until smooth.
2. Put pork and tomatillo mixture in a medium pot. 1-inch of puree should cover the pork; if not, add water until it covers it. Season with pepper & salt, and cover it simmers. For 20 minutes, let it simmer on low heat.
3. Now, finely shred the remaining lettuce leaves.
4. When the stew is done cooking, garnish with coriander, radishes, finely shredded lettuce, sliced jalapenos, and lime wedges.

Nutrition: Calories: 370, Protein: 36g, Carbohydrates: 14g, Fats: 19g

202.Cloud Bread

Prep Time: 30 min | **Cook Time:** 30 min | **Serve:** 1
- 1/4 cup fat-free 0%
- Plain Greek yogurt (4.4 oz)
- 1 egg, separated
- 1/32 teaspoon cream of tartar
- 1/2 packet sweetener (a granulated sweetener just like stevia)

1. For about 30 minutes before making this meal, place the Kitchen Aid Bowl and the freezer's whisk attachment.
2. Preheat your oven to 30 degrees.
3. Eliminate the bowl and whisk attachment from the freezer.
4. Separate the eggs. Now put the egg whites in the Kitchen Aid Bowl, and they should be in a different medium-sized bowl.

5. In the medium-sized bowl containing the yolks, mix in the sweetener and yogurt.
6. In the bowl containing the egg white, add in the cream of tartar. Beat this mixture until the egg whites turn to stiff peaks.
7. Now, take the egg yolk mixture and carefully fold it into the egg whites. Be cautious and avoid over-stirring.
8. On a parchment paper, place it on a baking tray and spray with cooking spray.
9. Scoop out six equally sized "blobs" of the "dough" onto the parchment paper.
10. Bake for about 25–35 minutes (make sure you check when it is 25 minutes, in some ovens, they are done at this timestamp). You will know they are done as they will get brownish at the top and have some crack.
11. Most people like them cold against being warm.
12. Most people like to re-heat in a toast oven or toaster to get them a little bit crispy.
Nutrition: Calories: 0, Protein: 0g, Carbohydrates: 0g, Fats: 0g

203.Rosemary Cauliflower Rolls

Prep Time: 15 min | **Cook Time:** 30 min | **Serve:** 1 (3 biscuits per serving)
- 1/12 cup almond flour
- 1 cup grated cauliflower
- 1/12 cup reduced-fat, shredded mozzarella or cheddar cheese
- 1/2 eggs
- 1/2 tablespoons fresh rosemary, finely chopped
- ½ teaspoon salt

1. Preheat your oven to 4000F.
2. Into a medium-sized dish, pour all the ingredients.
3. Scoop cauliflower mixture into 12 evenly sized rolls/biscuits onto a lightly greased and foil-lined baking sheet.
4. Bake until it turns golden brown, which should be achieved in about 30 minutes.
5. Note: if you want to have the outside of the rolls/biscuits crisp, then broil for some minutes before serving.
Nutrition: Calories: 138, Protein: 11g, Carbohydrates: 8g, Fats: 7g

204.Tomato Braised Cauliflower with Chicken

Prep Time: 15 min | **Cook Time:** 30 min | **Serve:** 1
- 1 garlic clove, sliced
- ¾ scallions, to be trimmed and cut into 1-inch pieces 1/8 teaspoon dried oregano
- 1/8 teaspoon red pepper flakes
- ¼ cups cauliflower
- ¾ cups diced canned tomatoes
- ¼ cup fresh basil, gently torn
- 1/8 teaspoon each of pepper and salt, divided
- ¾ teaspoon olive oil
- ¾ pound boneless, skinless chicken breasts

1. Get a saucepan and combine the garlic, scallions, oregano, crushed red pepper, cauliflower, tomato, and add ¼ cup of water. Get everything boil together, add ¼ teaspoon of pepper and salt for seasoning, and then cover the pot with a lid. Let it simmer for 10 minutes and stir as often as possible until you observe that the cauliflower is tender. Now, wrap up the seasoning with the remaining ¼ teaspoon of pepper and salt.

2. Using olive oil, toss the chicken breast and let it roast in the oven with the heat of 4500F for 20 minutes and an internal temperature of 1650F. Allow the chicken to rest for like 10 minutes.

3. Now slice the chicken and serve on a bed of tomato-braised cauliflower.

Nutrition: Calories: 290, Fats: 10g, Carbohydrates: 13g, Protein: 38g

205.Cheeseburger Soup

Prep Time: 15 min | **Cook Time:** 30 min | **Serve:** 1
- 1/16 cup chopped onion
- 1 quantity of (14.5 oz) can dice a tomato
- ¼ pound 90% lean ground beef
- 3/16 cup chopped celery
- 1/4 teaspoons Worcestershire sauce
- 1/2 cup chicken broth
- 1/8 teaspoon salt
- 1/4 teaspoon dried parsley
- 2/3 cups of baby spinach
- 1/8 teaspoon ground pepper
- 1 oz. reduced-fat shredded cheddar cheese

1. Get a large soup pot and cook the beef until it becomes brown. Add the celery, onion, and sauté until it becomes tender. Make sure to drain the excess liquid.

2. Stir in the broth, tomatoes, parsley, Worcestershire sauce, pepper, and salt. Cover and wait for it to simmer on low heat for about 20 minutes.

3. Add spinach and leave it to cook until it becomes wilted in about 1–3 minutes. Top each of your servings with 1 oz of cheese.

Nutrition: Calories: 400, Carbohydrates: 11g, Protein: 44g, Fats: 20g

206.Braised Collard Beans in Peanut Sauce with Pork Tenderloin

Prep Time: 25 min | **Cook Time:** 35 min | **Serve:** 1
- 1/2 cups chicken stock
- 3 cups chopped collard greens
- 1 1/2 tablespoons powdered peanut butter
- 3/4 cloves of garlic, crushed
- 1/4 teaspoon salt
- 1/8 teaspoon allspice
- 1/8 teaspoon black pepper
- 1/2 teaspoons lemon juice
- 3/8 teaspoon hot sauce
- 1/8 pound pork tenderloin

1. Get a pot with a tight-fitting lid and combine the collards with the garlic, chicken stock, hot sauce, and half of the pepper and salt. Cook on low heat for about 1 hour or until the collards become tender.

2. Once the collards are tender, stir in the allspice, lemon juice. And they have powdered peanut butter. Keep warm.

3. Season the pork tenderloin with the remaining pepper and salt, and broil in a toaster oven for 10 minutes when you have an internal temperature of 1450F. Make sure to turn the tenderloin every 2 minutes to achieve an even browning all over. After that, you can take away the pork from the oven and allow it to rest for like 5 minutes.

4. Slice the pork as you will like and serve it on top of the braised greens.

Nutrition: Calories: 320, Fats: 10g, Carbohydrates: 15g, Protein: 45g

207.Zucchini Pizza Casserole

Prep Time: 15 min | **Cook Time:** 50–60 min | **Serve:** 1
- ¼ teaspoon salt
- ¼ cup grated parmesan cheese
- 1/2 eggs
- 2/3 cups shredded unpeeled zucchini (this is about two medium zucchinis)
- 1 oz. reduced-fat, shredded cheddar cheese, divided
- 1 oz. reduced-fat, shredded mozzarella cheese, divided 1/8 pound 90–94% of lean ground beef
- Cooking spray
- 1 quantity 14.5 oz. can petite diced Italian tomatoes
- 1/8 cup chopped onion
- 1/2 small green bell pepper, chopped

1. Preheat your oven to over 4000F.

2. Place zucchini in a strainer and sprinkle it with salt. Let it stand for about 10 minutes, and after that, press it to drain its moisture.

3. Combine zucchini with eggs, parmesan, and half of cheddar cheese and mozzarella.

4.In a lightly greased baking dish, press the mixture and bake for about 20 minutes when uncovered.

5. Cook the onion and beef in a medium skillet until it becomes done. Drain any leftover liquid, and then stir in the tomatoes.

6. Pour the beef mixture over the zucchini and sprinkle with the remaining mozzarella cheese and cheddar. Top with green pepper

7. Bake for an extra 20 minutes or until it becomes heated all through.

Nutrition: Calories: 478, Protein: 30g, Carbohydrates: 22g, Fats: 29g

208.Tofu Power Bowl

Prep Time: 10 min | **Cook Time:** 15–20 min | **Serve:** 1
- 15 oz. extra-firm tofu
- 1 teaspoon rice vinegar
- 2 tablespoons soy sauce
- 1 teaspoon sesame oil
- ½ cup grated cauliflower
- ½ cup grated eggplant
- ½ cup chopped kale

1. Press tofu. Place tofu strips in multiple layers of paper towel or a clean dishcloth on top of a cutting board or plate. On top of the tofu, put another clean dish towel or paper towel. Place a weight on top of this second layer (this can be a large plate with canned foods on top or hardcover books, or a stack of leaves). Let it sit for not less than 16 minutes, and then cut the tofu into 1-inch cubes.

2. Combine both the vinegar and soy sauce in a small bowl and whisk together.

3. Get a large skillet and heat the sesame oil in it. Place cubed tofu to cover one half of the skillet, and the cubed eggplant should cover the other half. Cook both together until they become slightly brown and tender in about 10–12 minutes. Remove from skillet and keep aside. Now, add kale and sauté until they become wilted in about 3–5 minutes.

4. Microwave the already grated cauliflower in a small bowl with one teaspoon of water for about 3–4 minutes until it becomes tender.

5. Arrange the cauliflower "rice" with tofu, eggplant, and kale in a bowl.

Nutrition: Calories: 117, Protein: 14g, Carbohydrates: 2.2g, Fats: 7g

209. Grilled Veggie Kabobs

Prep Time: 15 min | **Cook Time:** 12 to 15 min | **Serve:** 1

Marinade:
- ½ cup balsamic vinegar
- 1/3 tablespoons minced thyme
- 1/4 tablespoons minced rosemary
- 1/2 cloves garlic, peeled and minced
- Sea salt, to taste (optional)
- Freshly ground black pepper, to taste

Veggies:
- 1/3 cups cherry tomatoes
- 1/3 red bell pepper, it should be seeded and cut into 1-inch pieces 1/3 green bell pepper, without seeds and cut into 1-inch pieces 1/3 medium yellow squash, cut into 1-inch rounds
- 1/3 medium zucchini, cut into 1-inch rounds
- 1/3 medium red onion skinned and cut into large chunks

Special Equipment:
- Two bamboo skewers, make sure to soak it in water for 30 minutes.

1. Preheat the grill to medium heat.

2. In making the marinade: In a small bowl, stir together the balsamic vinegar, thyme, rosemary, garlic, salt (if desired), and pepper.

3. Thread veggies onto skewers, alternating between different-colored veggies.

4. Grill the veggies for 12 to 15 minutes until softened, and lightly it was charred, brushing the veggies with the marinade and flipping the skewers every 4 to 5 minutes.

5. Remove from the grill and serve hot.

Nutrition: Calories: 98,   Fat: 0.7g,   Carbs: 19.2g, Protein: 3.8g, Fiber: 3.4g

210. Grilled Cauliflower Steaks

Prep Time: 10 min | **Cook Time:** 57 min | **Serve:** 1
- 1/2 medium heads cauliflower
- 1/2 medium shallots, peeled and minced Water, as needed
- 1/2 clove garlic, peeled and minced
- ½ teaspoon ground fennel
- ½ teaspoon minced sage
- ½ teaspoon crushed red pepper flakes
- ½ cup green lentils, rinsed
- 1/2 cups low-sodium vegetable broth
- Salt, to taste (optional)
- Freshly ground black pepper, to taste
- Chopped parsley, for garnish

1. On a flat work surface, cut each of the cauliflower heads in half through the stem, then trim each half, so you get a 1-inch-thick steak.

2. Arrange each piece on a baking sheet and set aside. You can reserve the extra cauliflower florets for other uses.

3. Sauté the shallots in a medium saucepan over medium heat for 10 minutes, stirring occasionally. Add water, 1 to 3 tablespoons at a time, to keep the shallots from sticking.

4. Stir in the garlic, fennel, sage, red pepper flakes, and lentils and cook for 3 minutes.

5. Pour into the vegetable broth and bring to a boil over high heat.

6. Reduce the heat to medium, cover, and cook for 45 to 50 minutes, or until the lentils are very soft, adding more water as needed.

7. Using an immersion blender, purée the mixture until smooth. Sprinkle with salt (if desired) and pepper. Keep warm and set aside.

8. Preheat the grill to medium heat.

9. Grill the cauliflower steaks for about 7 minutes per side until evenly browned.

10. Transfer the cauliflower steaks to a plate and spoon the purée over them. Serve garnished with the parsley.

Nutrition: Calories: 105,   Fat: 1.1g,   Carbs: 18.3g, Protein: 5.4g, Fiber: 4.9g

212. Vegetable Hash with White Beans

Prep Time: 15 min | **Cook Time:** 23 min | **Serve:** 1
- 1 leek (white part only), finely chopped
- 1 red bell pepper, deseeded and diced
- Water, as needed
- 2 teaspoons minced rosemary
- 3 cloves garlic, peeled and minced
- 1 medium sweet potato, peeled and diced
- 1 enormous turnip, peeled and diced
- 2 cups cooked white beans
- Zest and juice of 1 orange
- 1 cup chopped kale
- Salt, to taste (optional)
- Freshly ground black pepper, to taste

1. Put the leek and red pepper in a large saucepan over medium heat and sauté for 8 minutes, stirring occasionally. Add water, 1 to 3 tablespoons at a time, to keep them from sticking to the bottom of the pan.

2. Stir in the rosemary and garlic and sauté for 1 minute more.

3. Add the sweet potato, turnip, beans, and orange juice and zest, and stir okay—heat until the vegetables are softened.

4. Add the kale and sprinkle with salt (if desired) and pepper. Cook for about 5 minutes or more until the kale is wilted.

Nutrition: Calories: 245,   Fat: 0.6g,   Carbs: 48.0g, Protein: 11.9g, Fiber: 9.3g

213. Ratatouille

Prep Time: 20 min | **Cook Time:** 25 min | **Serve:** 1
- 1 medium red onion, peeled and diced
- Water, as needed
- 4 cloves garlic, peeled and minced
- 1 medium red bell pepper, without seeds and diced
- 1 small zucchini, diced
- 1 medium eggplant stemmed and diced
- 1 large tomato, diced
- ½ cup chopped basil
- Salt, to taste (optional)
- Freshly ground black pepper, to taste

1. Put the onion in a medium saucepan over medium heat and sauté for 10 minutes, stirring occasionally, or until the onion is tender. Add water 1 to 3 tablespoons at a time to keep it from sticking.

2. Add the garlic, red pepper, zucchini, and eggplant and stir well. Lid the saucepan and cook for 12 to 15 minutes, stirring occasionally.

3. Mix in the tomatoes and basil, then sprinkle with salt (if desired) and pepper. Serve immediately.

Nutrition: Calories: 76, Fat: 0.5g, Carbs: 15.3g, Protein: 2.7g, Fiber: 5.9g

214.Baingan Bharta (Indian Spiced Eggplant)

Prep Time: 15 min | **Cook Time:** 25 min | **Serve:** 1
- 1/2 medium onions, peeled and diced
- 1/4 medium red bell pepper, deseeded and diced Water, as needed
- 1/2 large tomatoes, finely chopped
- 1/2 medium eggplants, stemmed, peeled, and cut into ½-inch dices
- 3/4 tablespoons grated ginger
- 1/4 teaspoon coriander seed, toasted and ground
- 1/2 teaspoons cumin seeds, toasted and ground
- ½ teaspoon crushed red pepper flakes
- Pinch cloves
- Salt, to taste (optional)
- 1/2 coriander, leaves, and tender stems, finely sliced

1. Combine the onions and red pepper in a large saucepan and cook over medium heat for about 10 to 12 minutes. Include water 1 to 2 tablespoons now to keep them from sticking to the pan.

2. Stir in the tomatoes, eggplant, ginger, coriander, cumin, crushed red pepper flakes, and cloves and cook for just about 12 to 15 minutes, or until the vegetables are tender.

3. Sprinkle with the salt, if desired. Garnish with the coriander.

Nutrition: Calories: 140, Fat: 1.1g, Carbs: 27.9g, Protein: 4.7g, Fiber: 10.9g

215.Kale and Pinto Bean Enchilada Casserole

Prep Time: 10 min | **Cook Time:** 30 min | **Serve:** 1
- 1/2 teaspoon olive oil (optional)
- 1/2 yellow onion, diced
- 1/2 bunch kale stemmed and chopped
- 1/4 teaspoons taco seasoning
- 1/2 to 2/3 cups cooked pinto beans, or 2 (15-oz./425-g) cans pinto beans, drained and rinsed
- Sea salt, to taste (optional)
- Black pepper, to taste
- 1/2 (16-oz./454-g) jar salsa (any variety), divided
- 2 corn tortillas
- ½ cup cashew cheese, or more to taste

1. Preheat the oven to 350°F (205°C). Grease a baking dish with the olive oil, if desired.

2. Place the onion, kale, taco seasoning, and beans in the dish. Then sprinkle with salt (if desired) and pepper. Drizzle half the salsa over the beans. Next, place the tortillas on top. Scatter with the remaining salsa and cashew cheese.

3. Before baking, cover the dish with aluminum foil in the preheated oven for about 30 minutes or until the vegetables are warm and the salsa bubbles.

4. Let it cool for 10 minutes before slicing and serving.

Nutrition: Calories: 194, Fat: 3.8g, Carbs: 29.0g, Protein: 10.9g, Fiber: 9.4g

216.Potato and Zucchini Casserole

Prep Time: 10 min | **Cook Time:** 1 h | **Serve:** 1
- 1/2 large russet potatoes halved lengthwise and thinly sliced
- 1/2 medium zucchinis halved lengthwise and thinly sliced 1/4 cup nutritional yeast
- 1/4 cup diced green or red-bell-pepper (about one small bell pepper)
- 1/4 cup diced red, white, or yellow onion (about one small onion) 1/8 cup dry breadcrumbs
- 1/8 cup olive oil (optional)
- 2/3 teaspoons minced garlic (about three small cloves)
- Pepper, to taste
- Sea salt, to taste (optional)

1. Preheat the oven to 400°F.

2. Mix all the ingredients.

3. Place the mixture in a large cooking pot dish.

4.Bake in the preheated oven for 55 minutes until heated through, stirring once halfway through.

5. Remove and allow to cool from the oven before serving for 5 minutes.

Nutrition: Calories: 352, Fat: 10.0g, Carbs: 51.5g, Protein: 14.1g, Fiber: 5.5g

217.Broccoli Casserole with Beans and Walnuts

Prep Time: 10 min | **Cook Time:** 35–40 min | **Serve:** 1
- 1/4 cup vegetable broth
- 1/2 broccoli heads, crowns, and stalks finely chopped 1/3 teaspoon salt (optional)
- 2/5 cups cooked pinto or navy beans
- 1/2 to 2/3 tablespoons brown rice flour or arrowroot flour
- 1/4 cup chopped walnuts

1. Preheat the oven to 410°F (205°C).

2. Warm the vegetable broth in a large ovenproof pot over medium heat.

3. Add the broccoli and season with salt, if desired, then cook for 6 to 8 minutes, stirring occasionally, or until the broccoli is light green.

4. Add the pinto beans and brown rice flour to the skillet and stir well. Sauté for another 5 to 7 minutes, or until the liquid thickens slightly. Scatter the top with the walnuts.

5. Transfer the pot to the oven. Bake it until the walnuts are toasted, 20 to 25 minutes.

6. Let the casserole cool for 8 to 10 minutes in the pot before serving.

Nutrition: Calories: 412, Fat: 20.2g, Carbs: 43.3g, Protein: 21.6g, Fiber: 13.1g

218.Pistachio Crusted Tofu

Prep Time: 10 min | **Cook Time:** 20 min | **Serve:** 1
- 1/8 cup roasted, shelled pistachios
- 1/8 cup whole-wheat breadcrumbs
- 1/4 garlic clove, minced
- 1/4 shallot, minced

- 1/8 teaspoon dried tarragon
- 1/4 teaspoon grated lemon zest
- Sea salt, to taste (optional)
- Black pepper, to taste
- 1/4 (16-oz./454-g) package sprouted or extra-firm tofu, drained and sliced lengthwise into eight pieces
- 1/8 tablespoon dijon mustard
- 1/8 tablespoon lemon juice

1. Warm up the oven to 400°F (205°C). Line a baking sheet with parchment paper.
2. Then, place the pistachios in a food processor until they are about the breadcrumbs' size. Mix the pistachios, breadcrumbs, garlic, shallot, tarragon, and lemon zest in a shallow dish. Sprinkle with salt (if desired) and pepper. Set aside.
3. Sprinkle the tofu with salt (if desired) and pepper. Mix the mustard and lemon juice in a small bowl and stir well.
4. Brush all over the tofu with the mustard mixture, then coat each slice with the pistachio mixture.
5. Arrange the tofu on the baking sheet. Scatter any remaining pistachio mixture over the slices.
6. Bake in the warmed oven for about 18 to 20 minutes, or until the tofu is browned and crispy.
Nutrition: Calories: 159, Fat: 9.3g, Carbs: 8.3g, Protein: 10.4g, Fiber: 1.6g

219.Air Fryer Asparagus
Prep Time: 5 min | **Cook Time:** 8 min | **Serve:** 1
- Nutritional yeast
- Olive oil non-stick spray
- 1 bunch of asparagus

1. Prepare the ingredients. Wash asparagus. Do not forget to trim off thick, woody ends.
2. Spray asparagus with olive oil spray and sprinkle with yeast.
3. Air Frying. In your Instant Crisp Air Fryer, lay asparagus in a singular layer. Set the temperature to 360°F. While the time limit to 8 minutes.
Nutrition: Calories: 17, Fat: 4g, Protein: 9g

220.Avocado Fries
Prep Time: 10 min | **Cook Time:** 7 min | **Serve:** 1
- 1 avocado
- 1/8 teaspoon salt
- 1/4 cup panko breadcrumbs
- Bean liquid (Aquafaba) from a 15- oz. can of white or garbanzo beans

1. Prepare the ingredients. Peel, pit, and slice up avocado.
2. In a tub, toss the salt and breadcrumbs together. Put the aquafaba in a separate tub.
3. First in Aquafaba and then in panko, dredge slices of avocado, ensuring you can also cover them.
4. Air Frying. Place coated avocado slices into a single layer in the Instant Crisp Air Fryer. Set temperature to 390°F and set time to 5 minutes.
5. Serve with your favorite Keto dipping sauce!
Nutrition: Calories: 102, Fat: 22g, Protein: 9g, Sugar: 1g

221.Cauliflower Rice
Prep Time: 5 min | **Cook Time:** 20 min | **Serve:** 1
Round 1:
- 1/2 teaspoon turmeric
- 1/2 cup diced carrot
- 1/8 cup diced onion
- 1/2 tablespoon low-sodium soy sauce
- 1/8 block extra firm tofu

Round 2:
- ½ cup frozen peas
- 1/4 minced garlic cloves
- ½ cup chopped broccoli
- 1/2 tablespoon minced ginger
- 1/4 tablespoon rice vinegar
- 1/4 teaspoon toasted sesame oil
- 1/2 spoon reduced-sodium soy sauce 1/2 cup riced cauliflower

1. Prepare the ingredients. Crush tofu in a large bowl and toss with all the round one ingredient.
2. Air Frying. Lock the air fryer lid. Preheat the Instant Crisp Air Fryer to 370 degrees. Also, set the temperature to 370°F, set the time to 10 minutes, and cook 10 minutes, making sure to shake once.
3. In another bowl, toss ingredients from round 2 together.
4. Add round 2 mixture to Instant Crisp Air Fryer and cook another 10 minutes to shake 5 minutes.
Nutrition: Calories: 67, Fat: 8g, Protein: 3g, Sugar: 0g

222.Stuffed Mushrooms
Prep Time: 7 min | **Cook Time:** 8 min | **Serve:** 1
- 1/2 rashers bacon, diced
- ½ onion, diced
- ½ bell pepper, diced
- 1/2 small carrot, diced
- 2 medium-size mushrooms (Separate the caps & stalks)
- 1/4 cup shredded cheddar plus extra for the top 1/4 cup sour cream

1. Prepare the ingredients. Chop the mushrooms stalks finely and fry them up with the bacon, onion, pepper, and carrot at 350F° for 8 minutes.
2. Also, check when the veggies are tender, stir in the sour cream & the cheese. Keep on the heat until the cheese has melted and everything is mixed nicely.
3. Now grab the mushroom caps and heap a plop of filling on each one.
4. Place in the fryer basket and top with a little extra cheese.
Nutrition: Calories: 285, Fat: 20.5g, Protein: 8.6g

223.Zucchini Omelet
Prep Time: 10 min | **Cook Time:** 10 min | **Serve:** 1
- 1/2 teaspoon butter
- 1/2 zucchini, julienned
- 1 egg
- 1/8 teaspoon fresh basil, chopped
- 1/8 teaspoon red pepper flakes, crushed Salted and newly ground black pepper, to taste

1. Prepare the ingredients. Preheat the Instant Crisp Air Fryer to 355°F.
2. Melt butter on medium heat using a skillet.
3. Add zucchini and cook for about 3–4 minutes.
4. In a bowl, add the eggs, basil, red pepper flakes, salt, and black pepper and beat well.
5. Add cooked zucchini and gently stir to combine.
6. Air Frying. Transfer the mixture into the Instant Crisp Air Fryer pan. Lock the air fryer lid.
7. Cook for about 10 minutes. Also, you may opt to wait until it is done thoroughly.

Nutrition: Calories: 285, Fat: 20.5g, Protein: 8.6g

224.Cheesy Cauliflower Fritters

Prep Time: 10 min | **Cook Time:** 7 min | **Serve:** 1
- ½ cup chopped parsley
- 1 cup Italian breadcrumbs
- 1/3 cup shredded mozzarella cheese
- 1/3 cup shredded sharp cheddar cheese
- 1 egg
- 2 minced garlic cloves
- 3 chopped scallions
- 1 head of cauliflower

1. Prepare the ingredients. Cut the cauliflower up into florets. Wash well and pat dry. Place into a food processor and pulse 20–30 seconds until it looks like rice.
2. Place the cauliflower rice in a bowl and mix with pepper, salt, egg, cheeses, breadcrumbs, garlic, and scallions.
3. With hands, form 15 patties of the mixture, then add more breadcrumbs if needed.
4. Air Frying. With olive oil, spritz patties, and put the fitters into your Instant Crisp Air Fryer. Pile it in a single layer. Lock the air fryer lid. Set temperature to 390°F, and set time to 7 minutes, flipping after 7 minutes.
Nutrition: Calories: 209, Fat: 17g, Protein: 6g, Sugar: 0.5

225.Zucchini Parmesan Chips

Prep Time: 10 min | **Cook Time:** 8 min | **Serve:** 1
- ½ teaspoon paprika
- ½ cup grated parmesan cheese
- ½ cup Italian breadcrumbs
- 1 lightly beaten egg
- 2 thinly sliced zucchinis

1. Prepare the ingredients. Use a very sharp knife or mandolin slicer to slice zucchini as thinly as you can. Pat off extra moisture.
2. Beat egg with a pinch of pepper and salt and a bit of water.
3. Combine paprika, cheese, and breadcrumbs in a bowl.
4. Dip slices of zucchini into the egg mixture and then into the breadcrumb mixture. Press gently to coat.
5. Air Frying. With olive oil cooking spray, mist encrusted zucchini slices. Put into your Instant Crisp Air Fryer in a single layer. Latch the air fryer lid. Set temperature to 350°F and set time to 8 minutes.
6. Sprinkle with salt and serve with salsa.
Nutrition: Calories: 211, Fat: 16g, Protein: 8g, Sugar: 0g

226.Crispy Roasted Broccoli

Prep Time: 10 min | **Cook Time:** 8 min | **Serve:** 1
- ¼ teaspoon masala
- ½ teaspoon red chili powder
- ½ teaspoon salt
- ¼ teaspoon turmeric powder
- 1 tablespoon chickpea flour
- 1 tablespoon yogurt
- ½ pound broccoli

1. Prepare the ingredients. Cut broccoli up into florets. Immerse in a bowl of water with two teaspoons of salt for at least half an hour to remove impurities.
2. Take out broccoli florets from water and let drain. Wipe down thoroughly.
3. Mix all other ingredients to create a marinade.
4. Toss broccoli florets in the marinade. Cover and chill for 15–30 minutes.

5. Air Frying. Preheat the Instant Crisp Air Fryer to 390 degrees. Place marinated broccoli florets into the fryer, lock the air fryer lid, set the temperature to 350°F, and set the time to 10 minutes. Florets will be crispy when done.
Nutrition: Calories: 96, Fat: 1.3g, Protein: 7g, Sugar: 4.5g

227.Coconut Battered Cauliflower Bites

Prep Time: 5 min | **Cook Time:** 20 min | **Serve:** 1
- Salt and pepper to taste
- 1 flax egg or one tablespoon flaxseed meal + 3 tablespoon water
- 1 small cauliflower, cut into florets
- 1 teaspoon mixed spice
- ½ teaspoon mustard powder
- 2 tablespoons maple syrup
- 1 clove of garlic, minced
- 2 tablespoons soy sauce
- 1/3 cup oats flour
- 1/3 cup plain flour
- 1/3 cup desiccated coconut

1. Prepare the ingredients.
2. In a mixing bowl, mix oats, flour, and desiccated coconut. Season with salt and pepper to taste. Set aside.
3. In another bowl, place the flax egg and add a pinch of salt to taste. Set aside.
4. Season the cauliflower with mixed spice and mustard powder.
5. Dredge the florets in the flax egg first, then in the flour mixture.
6. Air Frying. Place inside the Instant Crisp Air Fryer, lock the air fryer lid and cook at 400°F or 15 minutes.
7. Meanwhile, place the maple syrup, garlic, and soy sauce in a saucepan and heat over medium flame. Wait for it to boil and adjust the heat to low until the sauce thickens.
8. After 15 minutes, take out the florets from the Instant Crisp Air Fryer and place them in the saucepan.
9. Toss to coat the florets and place inside the Instant Crisp Air Fryer and cook for another 5 minutes.
Nutrition: Calories: 154, Fat: 2.3g, Protein: 4.69g

228.Crispy Jalapeno Coins

Prep Time: 10 min | **Cook Time:** 5 min | **Serve:** 1
- 1 egg
- 2–3 tablespoon coconut flour
- 1 sliced and seeded jalapeno
- Pinch garlic powder
- Pinch onion powder
- Bit cajun seasoning (optional)
- Pinch pepper and salt

1. Prepare the ingredients. Ensure your Instant Crisp Air Fryer is preheated to 400 degrees.
2. Mix all dry ingredients.
3. Pat jalapeno slices dry. Dip coins into the egg wash and then into the dry mixture. Toss to coat thoroughly.
4. Add coated jalapeno slices to Instant Crisp Air Fryer in a singular layer. Spray with olive oil.
5. Air Frying. Lock the air fryer lid. Set temperature to 350°F and set time to 5 minutes. Cook just till crispy.
Nutrition: Calories: 128, Fat: 8g, Protein: 7g, Sugar: 0g

229.Buffalo Cauliflower

Prep Time: 5 min | **Cook Time:** 15 min | **Serve:** 1
Cauliflower

- 1 cup panko breadcrumbs
- 1 teaspoon salt
- 2 cup cauliflower florets

Buffalo Coating
- ¼ cup vegan buffalo sauce
- ¼ cup melted vegan butter

1. Prepare the ingredients. Melt butter in microwave and whisk in buffalo sauce.
2. Dip each cauliflower floret into a buffalo mixture, ensuring it gets coated well. Holdover a bowl till the floret is done dripping.
3. Mix breadcrumbs with salt.
4. Air Frying. Dredge dipped florets into breadcrumbs and place them into Instant Crisp Air Fryer. Lock the air fryer lid. Set temperature to 350°F and set time to 15 minutes. When slightly browned, they are ready to eat!
5. Serve with your favorite Keto dipping sauce!

Nutrition: Calories: 194, Fat: 17g, Protein: 10g, Sugar: 3

230.Cream of Cauliflower

Prep Time: 1 h | **Cook Time:** 1 h | **Serve:** 4
- Salt and pepper
- ½ cup (120 ml) heavy cream
- ½ teaspoon guar or xanthan (optional)
- 1 package or 285 g frozen cauliflower
- 1 quart (960 ml) chicken broth
- ¾ cup (90 g) diced celery
- ¾ cup (120 g) diced onion
- tablespoons (42 g) butter

1. Melt the buutter and sauté the onion and celery in it until they are floppy. Incorporate this in a large saucepan with the cauliflower and chicken broth and cook until the cauliflower is soft.
2. Using a slotted spoon to pass the vegetables to a blender, and add in the broth as much as you want. Add (if using) guar or xanthan and purée the ingredients.
3. Pour back the paste into the saucepan. Add salt and some pepper into the mix with some cream.

Nutrition: 9,5 g. carbo. and 3 g. fiber, for a total of 6,5 grams of usable carbs and 7 grams of protein.

231.California Soup

Prep Time: 10 min | **Cook Time:** 10 min | **Serve:** 3
- 1 quart (960 ml) chicken broth, heated
- 1 large or 2 small, very ripe black avocados, pitted, peeled, and cut into chunks

1. Add the avocados with the broth in a blender puree until very smooth and serve.

Nutrition: 3,5 g. carbo. and 1,5 g. fiber, total of 2,5 grams of usable carbs and 4 grams of protein.

232.Cheesy Cauliflower Soup

Prep Time: 15 min | **Cook Time:** 1 h | **Serve:** 5
- 1 tablespoon (6 g) minced scallion
- slices bacon, cooked and drained
- Guar or xanthan (optional)
- 1½ cups (180 g) shredded cheddar cheese
- 1½ cups (360 ml) Carb Countdown dairy beverage or half-and-half
- teaspoons white vinegar
- 1 teaspoon salt
- cups (720 ml) chicken broth

- 1 tablespoon (7 g) grated carrot
- 2 tablespoons (20 g) finely chopped celery
- 1 tablespoon (10 g) finely chopped onion
- cups (600 g) cauliflower, diced small

1. In a big, heavy-bottomed pan, placed the cauliflower, onion, celery, and carrot. Add the broth, salt, and vinegar to the chicken; bring it to a simmer and cook for about 30 to 45 minutes.
2. Stir in the Carb Countdown or half-and-half and then whisk in the cheese a bit at a time before adding more, allowing each additional time to melt. With guar or xanthan, thicken it a bit if you think it needs it.
3. Cover each serving with slightly crumbled bacon and hazelnuts.

Nutrition: 17 g protein; 7 g carbohydrate; 2 g dietary fiber; 5 g usable carbs.

233.Egg drop Soup

Prep Time: 10 min | **Cook Time:** 10 min | **Serve:** 3
- eggs
- 1 scallion, sliced
- ½ teaspoon grated fresh ginger
- 1 tablespoon (15 ml) rice vinegar
- 1 tablespoon (15 ml) soy sauce
- ¼ teaspoon guar (optional)
- 1 quart (960 ml) chicken broth

1. Put 1 cup (240 ml) or so of the chicken stock in your processor, turn it on medium, and add the guar (if using). Let it mix for a moment, and then put it in a big saucepan with the broth's rest. (If you're not using the guar, then put all the liquid directly in a saucepan.)
2. Put in the rice vinegar, soy sauce, ginger, and scallion. Heat over medium-high heat and let it boil for 5-10 minutes to let the flavors mix.
3. Beat the eggs in a glass mixing cup or small pitcher — something with a pouring edge. Using a fork to stir the soup's surface in a gradual circle and pour in about ¼ of the eggs, stirring while cooking and turning into shreds (which can occur almost instantly). Do three more times, using up half the egg.

Nutrition: 2 g. carbo. | a trace of fiber, and 8 grams of protein.

234.Cauliflower, Spinach, and Cheese Soup

Prep Time: 6 h | **Cook Time:** 1 1/2 h | **Serve:** 8
- 1 cup (240 ml) Carb Countdown dairy beverage
- Gouda cheese
- cups (675 g) shredded smoked
- cloves garlic, crushed
- ¼ teaspoon pepper
- ½ teaspoon salt or Vega-Sal
- ¼ teaspoon cayenne
- ounces (140 g) bagged baby spinach leaves, pre-washed
- ½ cup (80 g) minced red onion
- 1 quart (960 ml) chicken broth
- Guar or xanthan
- cups (900 g) cauliflower florets, cut into ½-inch (1.3-cm) pieces

1. Combine the broth, cauliflower, onion, spinach, cayenne, or Vega-Sal salt, pepper, and garlic in your slow cooker. Close

the slow cooker, set it to low, and let simmer for 6 hours or until tender.

2.Stir in the Gouda when the time's up, a little at a time, and then the Carb Timer. Cover the slow cooker again and steam for another 15 minutes or until the cheese has melted completely. Slightly thicken the broth with guar or xanthan.

Nutrition: 17 g protein, 7 g carbohydrate, 2 g dietary fiber, 5 g usable carbs.

235.Corner-Filling Soup

Prep Time: 1/2 h | **Cook Time:** 1/2 h | **Serve:** 6
- ¼ teaspoon pepper
- tablespoons (30 ml) dry sherry
- 1 quart (960 ml) beef broth
- 1 small onion, sliced paper-thin
- ounces (115 g) sliced mushrooms
- 2 tablespoons (28 g) butter

1. In a pot, heat the butter and sauté the mushrooms and onions into the butter until they're soft.

2. Apply the broth, sherry, and pepper over the meat. For 5-10 minutes or so, let it steam, just to change the flavors a bit.

Nutrition: 5,5 grams of carbohydrates and 1,1 gram of fiber, for a total of 4,5 grams of usable carbs and 8 grams of protein.

236.Stracciatella

Prep Time: 15 min | **Cook Time:** 45 min | **Serve:** 4-6
- ½ teaspoon dried marjoram
- Pinch of nutmeg
- ½ teaspoon lemon juice
- ½ cup (50 g) grated Parmesan cheese
- eggs
- 1 quart (960 ml) chicken broth, divided

1.In a glass measuring cup or large pitcher, place ¼ cup (60 ml) of the broth. Over medium heat, spill the remainder into a large saucepan.

2.In a measuring cup, add the eggs to the broth and beat them with a fork. Apply the lemon juice, Parmesan, and nutmeg, and then beat until well mixed using a fork.

3.Stir it using a fork as you add small quantities of the egg and cheese mixture until it is all mixed in while the broth in the saucepan is boiling. (Don't allow this to create long scraps like Chinese egg drop soup; instead, it makes small, fluffy particles because of the Parmesan.)

4.Apply the marjoram, smash it between your fingers a little bit, and steam the soup for a minute or two before serving.

Nutrition: 2 grams of carbohydrates, a trace of fiber, and 12 grams of protein.

237.Peanut Soup

Prep Time: 15 min | **Cook Time:** 45 min | **Serve:** 5-7
- Salted peanuts, chopped
- cups (420 ml) half-and-half or heavy cream
- 1 teaspoon guar gum (optional)
- 1¼ cups (325 g) natural peanut butter (Here, we used smooth.)
- ½ teaspoon salt or Vega-Sal
- quarts (1.9 L) chicken broth
- 1 medium onion, finely chopped
- 2 or 3 ribs celery, finely chopped
- tablespoons (42 g) butter

1.Melt the butter in a pot, then sauté the butter with the celery and onion.

2.Stir in the broth, salt, and peanut butter.

3.Cover and cook for at least 60 minutes at the lowest temperature, stirring now and then.

4.If you are using guar gum (without adding carbohydrates, it makes the soup thicker; scoop 1 cup (245 ml) of the soup out of the pot about 16 minutes before serving.

5.to this cup, apply the guar gum, run the mixture for a couple of seconds through the blender and whisk it back into the broth.

6.Stir in half-and-a-half and cook for 15 minutes more. Connect the peanuts to the garnish.

Nutrition: 19 grams of carbohydrates and 3 grams of fiber in each serving, with 16 grams of available carbohydrates and 29 grams of protein.

238.Soap De Frijoles Negros

Prep Time: 15 min | **Cook Time:** 45 min | **Serve:** 6-8
- ¼ cup (16 g) chopped cilantro
- ½ cup (115 g) plain yogurt
- ½ teaspoon salt or Vega-Sal
- ½ teaspoon red pepper flakes
- 1 tablespoon (6.3 g) ground cumin
- tablespoons (30 ml) lime juice
- 1 cup (130 g) salsa
- cloves garlic, crushed
- ½ cup (80 g) chopped onion
- 1 tablespoon (15 ml) olive oil
- 1 can (14½ ounces, or 411 ml) chicken broth
- 1 can (15 ounces, or 420 g) black beans
- 2 cans (15 ounces, or 420 g) Eden brand black soybeans

1.With the S-blade in place, bring half of the beans and half of the chicken broth into your blender or in your food processor. Run the unit before it purées the beans. Transfer the mixture and purée the other half of the beans and the other half of the chicken broth into a bowl that contains at least 2 quarts (1.9 L). To the first batch, add it.

2.Heat the olive oil over medium-low-heat in a heavy-bottomed saucepan and put in the onion. Sauté until the onion becomes transparent. Add the garlic and bean purée. Now incorporate sauce, lime juice, cumin, flakes of red pepper, and salt or Vega-Sal. Once the soup is cooked through, turn the heat up a little and then turn it back down to the lowest level and let it boil for 30 to 45 minutes. Serve with a dollop of plain-yogurt and a sprinkle of minced cilantro (or sour cream, if you prefer).

Nutrition: 18 g of protein, 25 g of fiber, 13 g of dietary fiber, 13 g of available carbohydrates.

239.Artichoke Soup

Prep Time: 15 min | **Cook Time:** 45 min | **Serve:** 6
- Juice of ½ lemon
- 1 cup (240 ml) half-and-half
- ½ teaspoon guar or xanthan
- cups (0.9 L) chicken broth, divided
- 1 can (14 ounces, or 410 g) quartered artichoke hearts, drained
- 1 clove garlic, crushed
- stalks celery, finely chopped
- 1 small onion, finely chopped
- to 4 tablespoons (42 to 56 g) butter
- Salt or Vega-Sal
- Pepper

1. Melt the butter in a big skillet, then sauté the celery, onion, and garlic over low to medium heat. Shake from time to time.

2. Drain the hearts of the artichoke and pick off any rough leaf pieces left on.

3. Placed the heart of the artichoke in a food processor with the S-blade in place. Add ½ cup (120 ml) of chicken broth and guar gum and strain until a fine purée is made from the artichokes. In a saucepan, scrape the artichoke mixture, add the remaining chicken broth, and boil over medium-high heat.

4. Stir the onion and celery into the artichoke mixture until tender. Whisk on the half-and-half when it comes to a boil. Take it back to a boil, push in the juice of a lemon and stir again. To taste, apply salt and pepper. You can eat this right now, hot, or you can eat it cooled in summers.

Nutrition: 10 grams of carbohydrates and 3 grams of fiber each, with 7 grams of carbohydrates and 4 grams of protein, respectively.

240. Curried Pumpkin Soup

Prep Time: 30 min | **Cook Time:** 30 min | **Serve:** 6

- teaspoons curry powder
- ½ cup (120 ml) Carb Countdown dairy beverage
- 1½ cups (240 g) canned pumpkin
- 1 quart (960 ml) chicken broth
- 1 tablespoon (14 g) butter
- 1 clove garlic
- ¼ cup (40 g) minced onion
- Salt and pepper to taste

1. In a big saucepan, saute the garlic and onion in butter, heavy-bottomed saucepan with medium-low heat until only softened. Put in the broth of the chicken and cook for half an hour.

2. Mix in the dairy beverage Carb Countdown, canned pumpkin, and Curry Powder. Adjust to a boil and cook softly for a further 15 minutes.

3. To taste, incorporate salt and pepper, and then eat.

Nutrition: 6 servings, Each with 5 g protein; 7 g carbohydrate; 2 g dietary fiber; 5 g usable carbs.

241. Soap Aguacate

Prep Time: 30 min | **Cook Time:** 30 min | **Serve:** 4

- ½ teaspoon salt or Vega-Sal
- tablespoons (8 g) chopped cilantro
- Canned green chilies or 1 or 2 canned jalapeños, if you like it hot!
- 2 scallions
- 1 ripe black avocado
- 1 quart (960 ml) chicken broth

1. Begin heating the broth. You can put it on the burner in a pan or put it in the microwave in a big microwaveable bowl.

2. Scrape the avocado out of its skin and into a food mixer with the S-blade in place as the broth is heating up.

3. Add the chilies, cilantro, scallions, and salt. Pulse all to cut together — you can add any bits of avocado or purée it flat, whatever you want.

4. Split the avocado mixture into 4 tiny soup bowls when the broth is hot. Spoon over the avocado mixture with the heated broth and eat.

Nutrition: 6 grams of carbohydrates and 3 grams of fiber, respectively, with 3 grams of available carbohydrates and 6 grams of protein.

242. Cheesy Onion Soup

Prep Time: 1 h | **Cook Time:** 1 h | **Serve:** 4

- ½ cup (120 ml) Carb Countdown dairy beverage
- 1 medium onion
- 1 quart (960 ml) beef broth
- ½ cup (120 ml) heavy cream
- Guar or xanthan (optional)
- 1½ cups (180 g) shredded sharp cheddar cheese
- Salt and pepper to taste

1. In a large saucepan, add the beef broth and start heating it over a medium-high flame. Cut the paper-thin onion and apply it to the broth. Switch the heat down to low as the broth begins to boil and let the entire thing steam for 1 hour. You should do this ahead of time if you like; turn off the heat, let the entire thing cool, refrigerate it, and later do the rest. If you do this, before moving, lift the broth from heating again.

2. Stir in the cream and the dairy beverage Carb Timer softly. Now stir in the cheese, a little at a time, until all of it has melted in. If you want to thicken with guar or xanthan, stir with a ladle or spoon instead of a whisk, you don't want to sever the onion threads.

3. Garnish with salt and pepper and serve.

Nutrition: 24 g protein; 8 g carbohydrate; trace dietary fiber; 8 g usable carbs.

243. Cream of Potato Soup

Prep Time: 1 h | **Cook Time:** 5 h | **Serve:** 6

- ½ cup (120 ml) Carb Countdown dairy beverage
- ½ cup (120 ml) heavy cream
- ½ cup (50 g) Ketones mix
- ½ cup (50 g) chopped onion
- ½ head cauliflower, chunked
- 1 quart (960 ml) chicken broth Guar or xanthan (optional)
- 5 scallions, sliced

1. in your slow cooker, put cauliflower, broth, and onion. Close and set the slow cooker to low and run for about 4 to 5 hours.

2. We used a hand mixer to purée the soup right in the slow cooker; so alternatively, you should pass the cauliflower and onion into your blender or food processor, along with 1 cup (240 ml) of broth. Purée until entirely smooth, and then blend into the Ketatoes, either way. If the cauliflower has been withdrawn from the slow cooker for purée, add the purée back in and whisk it back into the remaining broth.

3. Stir in the Carb Countdown and cream. If you believe it needs it, thicken it a little more with guar or xanthan.

4. To taste, apply salt and pepper and mix in the sliced scallions. Serve instantly hot or chill and serve as Vichyssoise.

Nutrition: 12 g protein, 13 g carbohydrate, 6 g dietary fiber, 7 g usable carbs.

244. Swiss cheese and Broccoli Soup

Prep Time: 10 min | **Cook Time:** 1 h | **Serve:** 6-8

- Guar or xanthan
- cups (360 g) shredded Swiss cheese
- 1 cup (240 ml) heavy cream
- cup (500 ml) Carb Countdown dairy beverage

- 10 ounces (560 g) frozen chopped broccoli, thawed
- 28 ounces (400 ml) chicken broth
- tablespoon (28 g) butter
- tablespoons (420 g) minced onion

1. Sauté the onion into the butter in a big, heavy-bottomed saucepan until it is transparent. Put the broccoli and the chicken broth in the pan and cook for 20 to 30 minutes until the broccoli is very soft.

2. Mix in the Countdown Carb and some cream. Brought it to a simmer again.

3. Now mix in the cheese, a little at a time, allowing each batch to melt before adding any more. Thicken a bit with guar or xanthan when all the cheese is melted if you think it needs it.

Nutrition: 20 g protein; 7 g carbohydrate; 2 g dietary fiber; 5 g usable carbs.

245. Tavern Soup

Prep Time: 8-10 h | **Cook Time:** 1 h | **Serve:** 8
- 1/2 teaspoon hot pepper sauce
- 1 teaspoon salt or Vega-Sal
- 24 ounces (500 ml) light beer
- pound (900 g) sharp cheddar cheese, shredded
- 1 teaspoon pepper
- 1/2 cup (30.4 g) chopped fresh parsley
- 1/2 cup (60 g) shredded carrot
- 1/2 cup (60 g) finely diced green bell pepper
- 1/2 cup (60 g) finely diced celery
- Guar or xanthan
- quarts (3 L) chicken broth

1. Mix in your slow cooker celery, broth, green pepper, onion, parsley, and pepper. Close the slow cooker, set it to low, and let it steam for 6 to 8 hours (it won't hurt for a little longer).

2. To purée the vegetables in the slow cooker right there until the time is up, use a handheld blender to scoop them out with a slotted spoon, and purée them in the blender, and add them to the slow cooker.

3. Now swirl a little at a time in the cheese until it's all melted. Add the hot pepper sauce, beer, salt, or Vega-Sal, and mix until the foaming ends.

4. To thicken the broth, use guar or xanthan until it is about sour cream thickness. Cover the pot again, turn it too heavy, and simmer for an additional 20 minutes before eating.

Nutrition: 18 g protein, 3 g carbohydrate, trace dietary fiber, 3 g usable carbs.

246. Broccoli Blue Cheese Soup

Prep Time: 1 h | **Cook Time:** 1 h | **Serve:** 6-8
- 1 cup (120 g) crumbled blue cheese
- 1/4 cup (60 ml) heavy cream
- 1 pound (455 g) frozen broccoli, thawed
- 1½ quarts (1.4 L) chicken broth
- 1 cup (240 ml) Carb Countdown dairy beverage
- 1 turnip, peeled and diced
- tablespoons (28 g) butter
- cup (160 g) chopped onion

1. Sauté the onion in the butter over medium-low heat in a broad saucepan — you don't want it to tan.

2. Until the onion is soft and transpaarent, add the chicken broth and the turnip to your pot. Brought the blend to a boil and let it cook for 20 to 30 minutes over medium to low heat.

3. Put in the thawed broccoli and cook for the next 20 minutes.

4. With a slotted spon, scoop the vegetables out and put them in a Mixer. A ladleful broth is added to the mix, and the blender runs until the vegetables are finely puréed. Shift the mixture back to your pot. Stir in the Countdown Carbohydrate, the heavy cream, and the blue cheese. Simmer for the next 5 to 10 minutes stirring periodically, and serve.

Nutrition: 14 g protein; 9 g carbohydrate; 3 g dietary fiber; 6 g usable carbs.

247. Cream of Mushroom Soup

Prep Time: 6 h | **Cook Time:** 1 1/2 h | **Serve:** 5-7
- ½ cup (120 g) light sour cream
- ½ cup (120 ml) heavy cream
- 1 quart (960 ml) chicken broth
- tablespoons (28 g) butter
- ¼ cup (25 g) chopped onion
- 8 ounces (225 g) mushrooms, sliced
- Guar or xanthan (optional)

1. Sauté the onion and mushrooms in the butter in a large, heavy skillet until the mushrooms soften and change color. Move them to a slow cooker. Put in the broth. Cover your slow cooker, set it low and let it cook for 5 to 6 hours.

2. Scrape out the vegetables with a slotted spoon when the time is up, and stick them in your blender or any food processor.

3. Add in enough broth to help them quickly process and finely purée them. Put the puréed vegetables back into the slow cooker, using a rubber scraper to clean out any last piece. Now whisk in the heavy cream and sour cream and apply to taste the salt and pepper. If you think it deserves it, thicken the sauce a little with guar or xanthan. Serve asp.

Nutrition: 6 g protein, 5 g carbohydrate, 1 g dietary fiber, 4 usable carbs.

248. Olive Soup

Prep Time: 20 min | **Cook Time:** 1 h | **Serve:** 6-8
- Pepper
- Salt or Vega-Sal
- ¼ cup (60 ml) dry sherry
- ½ teaspoon guar or xanthan
- 1 cup (100 g) minced black olives (You can buy cans of minced black olives.)
- 1 cup (240 ml) heavy cream
- cups (0.9 L) chicken broth, divided

1. Put ½ cup (120 ml) of the chicken broth with the guar gum in the blender and pulse for a few moments. Pour the remainder of the stock and the olives into a saucepan and add the blended mixture.

2. Heat and then whisk in the milk before simmering. Return to a boil, stir in the sherry, then apply salt and pepper to taste.

Nutrition: 3,5 grams of carbohydrates and 1,1 g. of fiber, for a total of 2,5 grams of usable carbs and 2,5 grams of protein.

249. Salmon Soup

Prep Time: 15 min | **Cook Time:** 21 min | **Serve:** 4
- 1 pound salmon fillets
- 1 tablespoon olive oil
- 1 cup carrots, peeled and chopped
- ½ cup celery stalk, chopped ¼ cup yellow onion, chopped 1 cup cauliflower, chopped 3 cups chicken broth

- Salt and ground black pepper, as required ¼ cup fresh parsley, chopped

1. Arrange a steamer trivet in the lower part of the Instant Pot and pour 1 cup of water.
2. Place the salmon fillets on top of trivet in a single layer.
3. Secure the lid and switch to the role of "Seal".
4. Cook on "Manual" with "High Pressure" for about 7-8 minutes.
5. Press "Cancel" and carefully do a "Quick" release.
6. Remove the lid and transfer the salmon onto a plate. Cut the salmon into bite sized pieces.
7. Remove the water and trivet from Instant Pot.
8. Add the oil in Instant Pot and select "Sauté". Then add the carrot, celery and onion and cook for about 5 minutes or until browned completely.
9. Press "Cancel" and stir in the cauliflower and broth.
10. Secure the lid and switch to the role of "Seal".
11. Cook on "Manual" with "High Pressure" for about 8 minutes.
12. Press "Cancel" and do a "Natural" release.
13. Remove the lid and stir in salmon pieces and black pepper until well combined.
14. Serve immediately with the garnishing of parsley.

Nutrition: Calories: 233 | fat: 11.6g | protein: 26.7g | carbs: 6g | net carbs: 4.2g | fiber: 1.8g

250. Cheesy Mushroom Soup

Prep Time: 15 min | **Cook Time:** 15 min | **Serve:** 4

- 2 tablespoons olive oil
- 4 ounces fresh baby Portobello mushroom, sliced
- 4 ounces fresh white button mushrooms, sliced ½ cup yellow onion, chopped
- ½ teaspoon salt
- 1 teaspoon garlic, chopped
- 3 cups low-sodium vegetable broth
- 1 cup low-fat cheddar cheese

1. Heat the oil over normal heat in a medium saucepan and cook the mushrooms and onion with salt for approximately 5-7 minutes, stirring frequently.
2. Add the garlic, and sauté for about 1-2 minutes.
3. Stir in the broth and remove from the heat.
4. With a stick blender, blend the soup until mushrooms are chopped very finely.
5. In the pan, add the heavy cream and stir to combine.
6. Place the pan over medium heat and cook for about 3-5 minutes.
7. Remove from the heat.

MEAT RECIPES

251. Herbed Lemon Chicken

Prep Time: 10 min | **Cook Time:** 20-30 min **Serve:** 4

- 2-3 T fresh chopped herbs (parsley, thyme, rosemary, chives, tarragon, etc.
- 1 T Dash of Desperation Seasoning
- Four teaspoons Luscious Lemon Oil (or oil, fresh lemon juice, and fresh lemon zest)
- 1 1/2 lbs. boneless, skinless chicken breasts (or thighs)

1. Preheat to medium-high heat (about 350) * outdoor grill *
2. In a large-pot, add all the ingredients and toss to cover.
3. Grill each side for 7-12 minutes until the beef is thoroughly cooked (check with the meat thermometer)

252. Char-Grilled Tuscan Chicken Kebabs

- 3 T Apple Cider Vinegar
- 4 tbsp. Roasted Garlic Oil
- 2 T Tuscan Fantasy Seasoning
- 1 C Zucchini cut into ½ inch thick slices
- 1 C Cherry tomatoes*
- 1 C Green bell pepper cut-into 1" pieces
- 1 C Red bell-pepper cut into 1" pieces
- 1½ lb. Boneless chicken breasts cut into 1" pieces

1. Using a big zipper bag to add all the ingredients. Seal the bag and mix the marinade into the vegetables and poultry. Place in the refrigerator for up to one hour overnight. Preheat the outdoor grill to medium-high heat when ready to bake.
2. For best cooking results, thread meat and vegetables onto individual skewers, alternating them. Grill on either side for 5-7 minutes before you hit the target temperature. For better performance, use a meat thermometer.

253. Salmon at Home

Ingredients:

- 1 T Phoenix Sunrise Seasoning
- 1 lb. salmon filet with skin on

Instructions:

1. Preheat a nonstick pan for 1 minute on high flame.
2. Sprinkle seasoning over the salmon during the heating process (NOT on the skin side)
3. Decrease the heat to medium height.
4. Place the fish in the pan and let it cook for 4-6 minutes, seasoning side down depending on the thickness.
5. Lower the heat to medium-low.
6. Flip the fish down to the skin side and cook for 4-6 more minutes. (Less for medium / rare and well finished, more so.)
7. Withdraw from the sun and serve. Fish should slip to the plate right off the skin and on.

254. Simple Chicken Curry

Ingredients:

- Fresh cilantro for garnish if desired.
- 2 C fresh cauliflower, cut into 1" florets (NOT smaller- will overcook)
- 1/2 C water
- 1 tbsp. salt (optional)
- 1 T Garlic Gusto Seasoning
- 1 T Spices of India Seasoning
- 2 C diced tomatoes (fresh or canned)
- 1 C red bell pepper, seeded & chopped into 1" chunks
- 1.25 lbs. boneless-skinless-chicken thighs OR 1.5 lbs. boneless, skinless chicken breasts

1. Put a single layer of chicken on the bottom of a slow cooker.
2. Combine the pepper, onions, cloves, salt, and water in a shallow cup. Throw chicken over it.
3. Comb the chicken with cauliflower florets.
4. Cover and simmer for 6-8 hours, on low heat, until the chicken is fork-tender.
5. Ladle into four bowls and, if needed, garnish with cilantro.

255. Juicy Stuffed Portobellos

- Nonstick cooking spray
- Four large portobello mushrooms, trimmed, stems removed.
- 8 T Cheese- blue, feta, or parmesan (optional)
- 1 T Garlic and Spring Onion Seasoning
- 4 T + 1T Italian Basil Infused Panko
- 1 large egg
- 1 1/4 lb. lean ground beef, chicken, or turkey (85-90% lean)

1. Preheat the oven to 350 ° C. Spray with nonstick cooking spray on a baking sheet.
2. Wash the stems from the mushrooms, cut, and extract them.
3. Take the roots and fine dice them.
4. Apply the stems and steak, bacon, 4 T panko, and Garlic & Spring Onion Seasoning to a large tub.
5. With your hands, combine the ingredients until well combined.
6. Divide the mixture of meat into four equal portions.
7. Pack the meat loosely into the mushroom caps.
8. For the leftover panko and cheese, spread uniformly.
9. Bake until completely baked for 25-30 minutes.

256. Stuffed Bruschetta Chicken

- 4 T Italian Basil Infused Panko Breadcrumbs
- 4 tbsp. Roasted Garlic Oil
- 1 C bruschetta
- Four boneless skinless chicken breasts (about 1 1/2 lbs.)

1. Preheat the oven to 350 ° C.
2. To make a stuffing jar, slice chicken breasts.
3. Place the chicken breast with 1/4 C of bruschetta and place it in a baking dish.
4. Repeat the procedure for and breast of the chicken until they are all stuffed.
5. Drizzle the oil over each chicken breast similarly.
6. Sprinkle the panko with the chicken.
7. Bake for 23-33 minutes, until the chicken is cooked (180 degrees internal temp.)
8. Slicing and cooking!

257. Pork Tenderloins and Mushrooms

Prep Time: 10 min | **Cook Time:** 25 min | **Serve:** 4
- on-stick cooking spray 1 Tablespoon garlic
- 1 Tablespoon marjoram
- 1 Tablespoon basil
- 1 Tablespoon onion
- 1 Tablespoon parsley
- 1 1/2 lbs. pork tenderloin (or beef tenderloin, or chicken breasts) 6 cups portobello mushroom caps, cut into chunks
- 1/2 C low sodium chicken broth
- 1 Tablespoon Stacey Hawkins Garlic Gusto or Garlic & Spring
- Onion Seasoning (or garlic, salt, black pepper, onion, paprika, and parsley)
- fresh parsley for garnish if desired

1. Spray a large skillet with cooking spray.
2. Preheat the stove to medium heat.
3. Place garlic and herbs into the skillet to cook with the cooking spray.
4. Allow the garlic and herbs to cook for 1 minute.
5. Place the pork tenderloin into the pan.

6. Generously season the pork tenderloin with the garlic gusto.
7. Sear the pork for 5 minutes and flip to the other side. Cook the other-side for another 1 minute.
8. Add the mushrooms, broth, and 2 tablespoons of water into the pan.
9. Cover the pan for 20 minutes.
10. Uncover and simmer for an additional 10,5 minutes till tender.
11. Garnish with marjoram. Serve hot.

Nutrition: Energy (calories): 737 kcal Protein: 30.32 g Fat: 62.95 g Carbohydrates: 14.39 g Calcium, Ca40 mg Magnesium, Mg48 mg Phosphorus, P443 mg

258. Garlic Shrimp & Broccoli

Prep Time: 15 min and 30 min marinade | **Cook Time:** 8 minutes | **Serve:** 4
- 1/2 cup honey
- 1/4 cup soy sauce
- 1 teaspoon fresh grated ginger
- 2 tablespoons minced garlic
- 1/4 teaspoon red pepper flakes
- 1/2 teaspoon cornstarch
- 1-pound large shrimp, peeled, deveined, and tails removed if desired
- 2 tablespoon butter
- 2 cups chopped broccoli
- 1 teaspoon olive oil
- salt pepper

1. In a large-bowl, combine honey, soy sauce, ginger, garlic, red pepper flakes, and cornstarch. Add shrimp and toss to combine. Cover and refrigerate for 23 to 33 minutes.
2. Stir-fry in a cast iron pan:
3. In a big-nonstick skillet, heat 1 normal spoon of the butter and olive oil over medium-high heat. Cook and stir broccoli in the hot skillet until crisp-tender, occasionally stirring, 2 to 4 minutes. Remove broccoli from skillet.
4. Add shrimp mixture to hot skillet and stir-fry for 4-5 minutes or until shrimp are done. Stir in broccoli and add salt and pepper to taste.
5. Remove from the heat.
6. Serve with rice; your family will love it!

Nutrition: Energy (calories): 334 kcal Protein: 17.84 g Fat: 11.07 g Carbohydrates: 43.4 g Calcium, Ca100 mg Magnesium, Mg42 mg Phosphorus, P324 mg

259. Chicken with Garlic and Spring Onion Cream

Prep Time: 5 min | **Cook Time:** 15 min | **Serve:** 4
- 6 medium chicken breasts
- 3 spoons butter or 3 espoons margarine 2 spoons all-purpose flour
- One-third cup chopped green onion Three-fourth cup chicken broth One-fourth teaspoon salt
- pepper
- 1 -2 tablespoon Dijon mustard (to taste) 1 cup plain yogurt

1. Heat a large skillet, add 1 tablespoon butter. Add chicken breasts to the pan. Cook for 10 minutes on medium heat, until browned on both sides. Remove and set aside on a plate.
2. Flour a chopping board and cut chicken breasts into thin strips when you're free from extra fat.

3.Melt 2 spoons butter in the same skillet. Stir in flour and cook for 2 minutes, stirring constantly. Gradually add chicken broth, mustard, salt, and pepper. (For a thicker sauce, add 2 tablespoons cornstarch dissolved in 1/2 cup cold water.)

4.Blend in yogurt. Add chicken strips and green onion. Cook until sauce bubbles and thickens, stirring occasionally.

5.Serve with plain white rice or boiled potatoes.

Nutrition: Energy (calories): 1172 kcal Protein: 132.83 g Fat: 63.49 g Carbohydrates: 9.7 g Calcium, Ca162 mg Magnesium, Mg155 mg Phosphorus, P1073 mg

260.Pan-Seared Beef Tips and Mushrooms

Prep Time: 10 min | **Cook Time:** 25 min | **Serve:** 4

- 1 1/2 lbs. lean beef cut into 1 chunk (London broil, filet, strip steak, etc.)
- 1/2 T salt 1/2 T pepper 1/2 T garlic
- nonstick cooking spray
- 4 C mushrooms (either small, whole mushrooms or larger ones cut into quarters)
- 1 C low sodium beef broth 11/2 teaspoons fresh garlic 11/2 teaspoons parsley 11/2 teaspoons onion

1.Sprinkle beef with salt, pepper, and garlic.

2.Coat large skillet with nonstick cooking spray. Heat over medium-high heat and add beef. Cook about 8-10 minutes, stirring frequently or until beef is browned on all sides and no pink remains.

3.Add mushrooms to the skillet. Pour beef broth and boil. Cover and cook over low-heat for 15 minutes.

4.While beef simmers in mushroom sauce, combine garlic, parsley, and onion in a food processor fitted with a steel blade. Pulse a few times until minced.

5.Add garlic mixture to beef and mushrooms and simmer covered for 10 minutes more.

6.Place in the serving bowl and season with parsley. As an alternative, if desired, top with gouda cheese.

Nutrition: Energy (calories): 379 kcal Protein: 42.49 g Fat: 12.44 g Carbohydrates: 25.55 g Calcium, Ca66 mg Magnesium, Mg69 mg

261.Creamy Skillet Chicken and Asparagus

Prep Time: 5 min | **Cook Time:** 20 min | **Serve:** 4

- 1 1/2 tablespoon extra-virgin olive oil
- Salt and fresh-ground pepper to taste, 4 (1 pound) boneless skinless chicken breasts
- 2 spoons Italian Seasoning 1 tablespoon butter
- 1-pound asparagus stalks trimmed and cut into thirds 1 yellow onion sliced
- 1 cup fat-free half & half 1/2 tablespoon all-purpose 1/3 cup grated Parmesan flour
- Lemon slices of salt and fresh ground pepper to taste for garnishing chopped parsley for garnishing freshly rubbed parmesan to garnish

1.Heat a big nonstick omelet pan over medium-high heat. Add olive oil and swirl. Season chicken with salt and pepper and Italian season. Add chicken to the pan and sauté until the tops are brown, about 4 minutes, then flip and cook another 4,3-5,3 minutes, or until golden.

2.Remove chicken from pan and keep warm. Add butter to the pan, asparagus, onion, and sauté until the asparagus is tender, about 4 mins.

3.Season the asparagus. Sprinkle in the flour, constantly stirring, until the mixture is homogenized and bubbly.

Gradually add the 1/2 cup of half and half, constantly stirring, then add parmesan cheese, garlic, lemon juice, salt, and pepper.

4.Cook until sauce thickens, about 2 minutes. Taste and adjust seasoning. Stir in the rest of the half and half. Add chicken back into the pan to reheat and toss together with the sauce.

5.Remove from heat and onto the plates. Serve and garnish with lemon-slices, parsley, and parmesan.

Nutrition: Energy (calories): 703 kcal Protein: 110.07 g Fat: 18.54 g Carbohydrates: 19.52 g Calcium, Ca190 mg Magnesium, Mg171 mg

262.Seared Mahi Mahi with Lemon-Basil Butter

Prep Time: 10 min | **Cook Time:** 20 min | **Serve:** 4-6

- 3 tablespoons unsalted butter
- 1 and one-half teaspoons fresh lemon juice 1 large garlic clove, finely chopped
- One-fourth teaspoon salt, plus additional for seasoning
- One-fourth teaspoon fresh ground black pepper, plus additional for seasoning
- 1 and one-half tablespoons basil leaves, chopped fresh 3 tablespoons olive oil
- 3 mahi-mahi fillet

1.Melt the butter in a small-saucepan over low flame. Add garlic, lemon juice, salt, pepper, and basil. Cook over low heat for 1 minute, regularly stirring the mixture so the butter doesn't burn. Turn off the flame and remove the prepared sauce from the heat. Using a wooden spoon, place the sauce in a bowl, preferably stainless steel, and cool it to room temperature for an even better result. Give it a whisk just before you are ready to use it.

2.Preheat an oven to 450°F. Place a grill-pan over medium flame and add 2 tablespoons olive oil.

3.Season the mahi-mahi fillets with salt and pepper and drizzle 1/4 of the lemon-basil sauce over them. Reserve the remaining sauce for later use.

4.Sear the Mahi mahi on both sides for approximately 2-3 minutes until the fish is opaque and cooked through. Remove the fish-fillet from the grill pan and place them on a baking sheet coated with baking paper.

5.Add the remaaining olive oil to the grill pan you used to cook the fish. Add the fillet to the grill pan and finish cooking the mahi-mahi, searing the top for an additional 1-2 minutes.

6.Serve with any side dish you choose. Eating the fish with a fresh green salad drizzled with lemon-basil sauce is a great combination.

Nutrition: Energy (calories): 222 kcal Protein: 10.19 g Fat: 18.28 g Carbohydrates: 4.76 g Calcium, Ca46 mg Magnesium, Mg12 mg Phosphorus, P198 mg

263.Toasted Sesame Ginger Chicken

Prep Time: 10 min | **Cook Time:** 15 min | **Serve:** 4

- 4 teaspoons olive oil
- 4 teaspoons orange zest
- 1 1/2 lbs. boneless-skinless-chicken breast 1 Tablespoon toasted sesame seeds
- 1 Tablespoon garlic
- 1 Tablespoon onion powder 1 Tablespoon red pepper
- 1 Tablespoon ground ginger 1 Tablespoon salt
- 1 Tablespoon pepper

- 1 Tablespoon lemon

1.Remove the small fillet from each chicken breast, and cut and reserve.
2.Preheat oven to 375 degrees F.
3.Cook sesame seeds over medium heat in oil until they are crisp and turn a little brown.
4.Add chicken and cook for 5,3 minutes on each side, or until it is slightly crispy.
5.Place the chicken-onions, and garlic in a baking dish, and sprinkle with the seasonings. Bake for another 15 minutes, stirring occasionally.
6.Meanwhile, stir together teriyaki sauce and cornstarch in a small saucepan.
7.Bring to a boil, and cook for 1 minute without stirring.
8.Remove the chicken and serve with the glaze.
Nutrition: Energy (calories): 369 kcal Protein: 16.84 g Fat: 15.27 g Carbohydrates: 41.12 g Calcium, Ca58 mg Magnesium, Mg50 mg Phosphorus, P185 mg

264.Tender and Tasty Fish Tacos

Prep Time: 10 min | **Cook Time:** 15 min | **Serve:** 4
- 1 3/4 lbs. cod or haddock (wild-caught)
- 1 capful (1 Tablespoon) Phoenix Sunrise Seasoning or cumin, cilantro, garlic, onion, red pepper, paprika, parsley, salt & pepper (or low sodium taco seasoning)
- 4 little spoons Stacey Hawkins Roasted Garlic Oil or oil of your choice and fresh garlic
- your favorite taco condiments

1.Thaw fish in a separate bowl from other ingredients and heat frying pan at medium (350° - 375° F)
2.Preheat oven at 400° F
3.Line a baking sheet with parchment paper
4.Cut fish into cubes evenly about 1/2"x1/2". Prepare the oil mixture with the chopping knife by adding the Stacey Hawkins Roasted Garlic Oil or Olive Oil to the oiling bowl and fresh garlic cloves with the skins still on. Extra garlic makes food taste good.
5.Preheat a clean frying pan on medium to high heat
6.Add fish to the frying pan and allow it to cook for 2-4 minutes, or until it becomes opaque. With your cooking tweezers or fork, flip the fish to cook the other side for an additional 2-4 minutes. Keep fish-warm in the oven while preparing tortillas.
7.To prepare the tortillas, heat the frying pan at medium heat, add tortilla to the pan, and heat on each side for 20 seconds (you might need to add a small amount of oil). To keep the tortillas warm, put the tortillas in the oven at 400° F and close the door.
8.Remove tortillas from the oven and immediately add fish and other ingredients and fold it all together.
Nutrition: Energy (calories): 202 kcal Protein: 32.59 g Fat: 6.08 g Carbohydrates: 2.02 g Calcium, Ca25 mg Magnesium, Mg44 mg Phosphorus, P458 mg

265.Sausage Stuffed Mushrooms - an LB. D LG Recipe

Prep Time: 5 min | **Cook Time:** 25 min | **Serve:** 4
- 4 large portobello mushrooms (caps and stems) 1 1/2 pounds lean Italian sausage (85-94% lean) 1 capful (1 Tablespoon) chopped garlic
- 1 capful (1 Tablespoon) chopped chives
- 1 capful (1 Tablespoon) garlic powder

- 1 capful (1 Tablespoon) onion powder
- 1 capful (1 Tablespoon) salt and pepper to taste

1.Preheat the oven to 425 degrees F.
2.Sauté the sausage with the garlic and onion/garlic powders in a skillet without coloring it. Place the mushroom caps on a plate.
3.Mix the salt and pepper with the bread crumbs and stuff it inside the mushroom caps. Stuff the sausage mixture in the mushroom caps.
4.Spoon about a teaspoon of oil over the cap and place it stem side up on a cookie sheet.
5.Bake the caps for about 23 minutes or until the stuffing is fully cooked. Garnish with chives.
Nutrition: Energy (calories): 645 kcal Protein: 29.16 g Fat: 54.06 g Carbohydrates: 11.38 g Calcium, Ca49 mg Magnesium, Mg47 mg Phosphorus, P429 mg

266.Smoky Chipotle Shrimp and Tomatoes

- 2 T fresh cilantro, chopped (optional)
- 1/2 large lime, juiced (optional)
- 1 T (one capful) Cinnamon Chipotle Seasoning
- 1 C diced tomatoes (unflavored, no sugar added)
- 1 1/2 lbs. wild-caught shrimp, shelled, deveined, and tails removed
- 1 C scallions (whites and greens) or chopped onion
- 4 tbsp. Roasted Garlic Oil

1.Heat oil over medium-high-heat in a medium-sized frying pan.
2.Put the onion and cook until translucent, for 2 minutes. Add shrimp and cook on each-side for 1 minute. Connect the chipotle tomatoes and cinnamon seasoning.
3.Cook for an extra 2-3 minutes until the tomatoes and shrimp are heated and opaque.
4.Drizzle and substitute the cilantro with the lemon juice. Serve it hot.

267.Simply Scrumptious Bruschetta

- 4 tbsp. Balsamic Mosto Cot to
- 1 T Garlic Gusto Seasoning
- 1 tbsp. Viva Italian Blend
- 2 C fresh tomatoes, diced (you can use unseasoned, no sugar added canned tomatoes as well)

1.Place all the ingredients in a small-bowl and cover them with a toss.
2.Let it rest for 20 minutes, and then enjoy it.
3.It can be placed in an airtight-container and kept refrigerated for one week.

268.Rosemary Pulled Pork

- 1 tbsp. Dash of Desperation Seasoning
- 1 1/2 T Rosemary Versatility Seasoning
- 1 C water
- 3 lbs. pork loin, excess fat removed

1.Place all the ingredients in order in the crockpot. Place the lid on and let it cook on low for 8-10 hours. The average size of the meat can depend on timing and tenderness.
2.It will take a little less time for smaller, longer parts, and it will take a little longer for narrower, stockier cuts (or those with bones).

3.Remove the lid when ready, and remove any bones carefully. Shred the meat using two big forks and throw it to cover in the juices in the crockpot.

4.Serve warm over salads or cauliflower rice as an entree. Superbly chilled over vegetables or on zero carb rolls as a sandwich.

269.Zesty Chicken with Artichokes and Garlic

- 1/4 C green onions (scalions) tops only for garnish 1 T Skinny Scampi Seasoning 1 T Garlic Gusto Seasoning
- One 12-15oz. jar artichoke-hearts IN WATER NOT OIL drained well & chopped.
- 1½ lb. boneless-chicken-breasts, cut into 1" cubes 4 tbsp. Roasted Garlic Oil

1.Heat the Roasted-Garlic Oil in a pan in a large skillet over medium-high heat.

2.Include the chicken and cook on either side for 5-7 minutes, until the chicken is painted and solid.

3.Attach seasonings and artichokes. Turn the heat-to-low and simmer until the artichokes are sufficiently heated, and the chicken is completely cooked for an additional 5 minutes.

270.Crispy Baked Scampi Chicken

- 4 T Lemon Pepper Infused Panko Bread Crumbs
- 1 T Skinny Scampi Seasoning
- 2 lbs. boneless, skinless chicken thighs, all visible fat removed

1.Preheat the oven to 350 ° C.

2.Place the chicken in one layer of a roasting oven.

3.Using Skinny Scampi Seasoning to sprinkle chicken.

4.Sprinkle the Lemon Pepper Panko with the chicken.

5.Bake until thoroughly fried, 30-40 minutes.

6.Take out froom the oven, leave to rest for about 5,3 minutes, and serve.

271.No Carb Garlic "Rolls"

- 1 T Garlic & Spring Onion Seasoning
- 1 T cream cheese
- 1 T grated Parmesan cheese
- 1/8 tbsp. cream of tartar
- Three large eggs, separated

1.Preheat the oven to 300 ° F.

2.Separate the white and egg yolks into two wide cups.

3.Apply the tartar cream to a cup with the whites. Beat on high, using an electric-mixer, until very rigid peaks develop. And put aside.

4.Apply the remaining ingredients and the yolks to the dish. Beat together on high, using an electric mixer until all ingredients are combined.

5.Pour over the whites of the egg yolks and fold them softly until fully mixed.

6.Line 2 cookie sheets OR GENEROUSLY brush with nonstick cooking spray or silicone baking mats. Use a large spoon to put a dollop of egg mixture on the mat and spread it on a scale. DO NOT make them too thin, or they're going to roast and crisp. For better results, keep the egg mixture about 1/3 "deep. "Repeat the process to produce 12" rolls.

7.Take out from the oven and bake for 30 minutes. While still mildly warm, extract from your oven and place to cool aside.

8.The bread will be crispy in texture as it comes right out of the oven.

9.Place it in a zipper-type bag until cooled, and it will turn into fluffy, pliable bread that is delicious overnight!

272.Pan-Seared Lemon Tarragon Cod

Prep Time: 5 min | **Cook Time:** 15 min | **Serve:** 4

- 1 3/4 lbs. cod fillets- fresh or frozen and thawed
- 4 tbsp. Luscious Lemon Oil
- 1 Tablespoon Rockin' Ranch Seasoning (or garlic, lemon, tarragon, pepper, onion, salt, and pepper)

1.Using a large frying pan to add oil, and cook over medium-high heat. Cut cod into 2″ chunks while the oil is heating.

2.Heat oil over medium-high-heat in a wide frying pan.

3.Break the cod into 2" chunks when boiling the oil.

4.Add fish to the pan while the oil is hot and cook on either side for 2-3 minutes, browning slightly. To be fully cooked and ready to eat, fish can take between 6-8 minutes.

5.It's done until the fish is translucent and flaky. Serve instantly.

273.Citrus Kissed Shrimp and Spinach

- 6 cups baby spinach greens, arugula greens, beet greens, or a combination
- 2 T Simply Brilliant Seasoning
- 1 1/2 lbs. wild-caught, raw shrimp, cleaned and tails removed
- 4 tbsp. Luscious Lemon Oil

1.Heat oil over medium-high-heat in a wide frying pan. Sprinkle with seasoning and put shrimp. Stir to cover and cook for about 3-4 minutes.

2.Switch the shrimp over once using tongs and cook for one minute. To the pan, add the vegetables. Toss it to coat it. Let the greens cook until wilted, for 1-2 minutes. Serve it warm.

274.Zesty Turkey and Kale Chili

- 2 C chopped vegetables* (eggplant, zucchini, mushroom, etc.)
- 2 C chopped kale
- 2 T Zesty White Chili Seasoning
- 1 lb. ground turkey
- 2 C diced tomatoes
- 4 tbsp. Roasted Garlic Oil

1.In a medium-sized kettle, apply oil and fire over low heat.

2.Sprinkle with seasoning and substitute ground turkey.

3.Cook, stirring regularly, for 4,3-5,3 minutes, until the turkey is opaque.

4.Add the remaining ingredients, blend well, and reduce heat to mild.

5.Cover the pot and cook for 10,5 minutes, until the vegetables are tender.

6.Offer over some cauliflower rice.

275.Muscle Meatballs

Prep Time: 15 min | **Cook Time:** 20 min | **Serve:** 3

- 1 1/2 lb. extra-lean ground turkey breast 2 egg whites
- 1/2 cup of toasted wheat-germ 1/4 cup fast-cooking oats
- 1 tbsp. of whole linseed seeds
- 1 tbsp. of grated parmesan cheese One-half tsp. All-purpose seasoning 1/4 tsp. ground black pepper

1.Preheat the furnace to 400° F. Use cooking spray to cover a large baking dish.

2.In a container, mix all the ingredients.

3.Make and place 16 meatballs in the baking dish.

4.Bake the meatballs for 7 minutes and turn them around. Bake for 8–13 minutes longer, or until the center is no longer pink.

Nutrition: Energy (calories): 460 kcal Protein: 77.65 g Fat: 9.13 g Carbohydrates: 16.9 g Calcium, Ca78 mg Magnesium, Mg151 mg

276.Orange Chicken

Prep Time: 15 min | **Cook Time:** 30 min | **Serve:** 4
- 1 lb. of skinless, boneless-chicken, cut into bite-sized pieces 1/2 tsp. Crystal Light Orange Drink
- 1 tsp. of powdered garlic 1/2 tsp. Dried ground ginger 1/4 tsp. Red flakes of pepper 1/8 tsp. pepper
- 2 tsp. of olive oil
- 2 tbsp. Of rice vinegar 2 tbsp. water
- 1/2 tsp. of sesame oil
- 1 tsp. of medium soy sauce
- 1/2 tbsp. of minced dried onion 1/4–1/2 tsp. of dried orange peel

1.Preheat the oven to 350° C.

2.Put the chicken in a 13x9 inches baking dish.

3.In a small bowl, mix the remaining ingredients. Pour over the chicken. Bake until done, for 25–30 minutes.

Nutrition: Energy (calories): 171 kcal Protein: 25.78 g Fat: 6.06 g Carbohydrates: 1.42 g Calcium, Ca11 mg Magnesium, Mg35 mg

277.Salma Lime Chicken

Prep Time: 10 min | **Cook Time:** 45 min | **Serve:** 5
- 5 boneless, skinless breasts of chicken 4 tbsp. of lime juice
- 1 1/4 tbsp. of chili powder 1 1/4 cup of fresh salsa

1.Preheat the oven to 350° C.

2.Line the foil with a 13x9 inches baking dish. Spray with non-stick cooking spray.

3.Put the chicken in your baking dish. Sprinkle the chili powder. Add lime juice and salsa.

4.Bake until done, for 40–45 minutes.

Nutrition: Energy (calories): 817 kcal Protein: 43.37 g Fat: 26.21 g Carbohydrates: 101.14 g Calcium, Ca132 mg Magnesium, Mg104 mg Phosphorus, P433 mg

278.Scandinavian Chicken

Prep Time: 10 min | **Cook Time:** 45 min | **Serve:** 6
- 1 lb. boneless chicken breasts without skin 1 tbsp. Mrs. Dash Seasoning Original Blend 1/2 tsp. dried ground ginger
- 1/4 tsp. pepper
- 1/4 tsp. Ground cinnamon 1/4 tsp. ground nutmeg
- 1 tbsp. of olive oil
- 3 tbsp. of wine vinegar
- 1/2 tbsp. Worcestershire sauce
- 1 1/2 tbsp. Brown sugar substitute 1/2 tbsp. dried minced onion
- 1 garlic clove, hacked

1.Make a fire in the oven to 350° C.

2.Put the chicken in a baking dish that is 13x9 inches.

3.In a small cup, mix up the remaining ingredients. Pour the chicken over. For 45 minutes, cook.

Nutrition: Energy (calories): 169 kcal Protein: 20.71 g Fat: 7.87 g Carbohydrates: 2.11 g Calcium, Ca18 mg Magnesium, Mg18 mg

279.Spinach and Mushroom Stuffed Chicken

Prep Time: 20 min | **Cook Time:** 30 min | **Serve:** 4
- 4 boneless skinless halves of chicken breast
- 4 softened laughing cow light cheese wedges (any flavor) 1 cup of chopped spinach
- 1 cup of white mushrooms, sliced or chopped Italian seasoning
- Parmesan cheese

1.Heat the oven to 350° C.

2.Fillet chicken breasts by cutting a "pocket" horizontally into the middle of the meat around ¾ of the way down, being careful not to cut through to the other side. To absorb some water within the breast, add a paper towel.

3.Place one wedge of laughing cow cheese in the middle of each breast. Cover with 1 tbsp. Of mushrooms and about 2 tbsp. Of spinach. Close them very well. If needed, secure it with a toothpick. Season with Italian seasonings (or any seasoning of your choice) and a little Parmesan cheese outside the chicken.

4.Bake for 32 minutes or until the chicken isn't pink anymore.

Nutrition: Energy (calories): 847 kcal Protein: 113.9 g Fat: 26.44 g Carbohydrates: 30.96 g Calcium, Ca252 mg Magnesium, Mg152 mg

280.Rosemary Chicken

Prep Time: 20 min | **Cook Time:** 45 min | **Serve:** 4
- 4–5 (4–6 oz.) boneless chicken breasts without skin 1/2 cup white cooking wine (or chicken broth)
- 1 tbsp. of lemon juice
- 1 1/2 tsp. Balsamic vinegar 1 tsp. Of powdered garlic 1/2 tsp. Dried rosemary 1/4 tsp. salt (optional)
- 1/8 tsp. pepper

Instructions:

1.Prepare the cooking machine to 350° C.

2.In a cookie sheet that is 13x9 inches, bring the chicken in.

3.In a small cup, mash up the best ingredients. Drop the chicken over. Cook until done, about 40-45 minutes.

Nutrition: Energy (calories): 327 kcal Protein: 47.78 g Fat: 12.92 g Carbohydrates: 2.03 g Calcium, Ca26 mg Magnesium, Mg42 mg

281.Stuffed Chicken Breasts with Tomato Salad

Prep Time: 20 min | **Cook Time:** 15 min | **Serve:** 4
- 1 6.5-oz pot drained and chopped artichoke hearts 2 tbsp. grated parmesan
- 2 spoonsful of new thyme leaves
- 4 6-oz boneless, skinless breasts of chicken 2 tbsp. + 1 tsp. extra-virgin olive oil Pepper and kosher salt
- 2 beefsteak tomatoes, sliced into bite-sized bits 1 shallot, sliced thinly
- 1 tablespoon red wine vinegar
- 8 toasted baguette slices (optional)

1.In a small cup, combine the artichokes, parmesan, and 1 tablespoon of thyme.

2.Cut a 2-inch pocket into each chicken breast's thickest section. Use a quarter of the artichoke mixture to stuff each bag.

3.With 1 teaspoon of oil, rub the chicken breasts and season with a three-fourth teaspoon of salt and one-fourth teaspoon of pepper.

4.Heat the grill or barbecue pan to medium. Grill the chicken for 7 minutes, turning once, until cooked through.In a wide bowl, mix the tomatoes, shallot, vinegar, one-fourth teaspoon of salt and pepper, and the remaining oil and thyme.

5.If needed, slice the chicken and, if desired, serve with the tomato salad and baguette slices.

Nutrition: Energy (calories): 1818 kcal Protein: 63.07 g Fat: 134.17 g Carbohydrates: 114.55 g Calcium, Ca425 mg Magnesium, Mg960 mg Phosphorus, P2234 mg

282.Super-fast Chicken Salad Sandwich

Prep Time: 20 min | **Cook Time:** 0 min | **Serve:** 2
- 2 cans of chicken (3 oz. each), rinsed and drained twice 1 celery stick, finely chopped
- 1 tbsp. Onion, finely chopped 1 tbsp. of pine nuts
- 1 tsp. of spicy brown mustard
- 1 heaping tsp. of sour cream free of fat 1 heaping tsp. of plain yogurt free of fat Ground black pepper pinch
- 4 whole-grain bread slices 2 lettuce leaves

1.Combine the celery, onion, pine nuts, vinegar, sour cream, yogurt, and pepper in a dish. Mix the chicken in.

2.On a slice of bread, spread out half of the mixture. Place a lettuce leaf on top and then another slice of bread on top.

3.To make a second sandwich, repeat with the remainder of the mixture.

Nutrition: Energy (calories): 764 kcal Protein: 34.8 g Fat: 50.96 g Carbohydrates: 40.18 g Calcium, Ca131 mg Magnesium, Mg94 mg

283.Quick and Easy Protein Salad

Prep Time: 20 min | **Cook Time:** 0 min | **Serve:** 2
- 2 cups of baby spring mix 2 chopped scallions
- ½ cucumber, cut in half and sliced 4 spores, halved and cut
- 1/4 of a medium avocado, diced
- 1/2 cup of cottage cheese free of fat 1 hardboiled egg, diced
- 1 lemon juice
- 1 garlic clove, minced
- 3 tbsp. low-fat buttermilk
- Salt and ground black pepper, to taste

1.In a medium-sized mixing bowl, add the spring mix, scallions, cucumber, mushrooms, avocado, cottage cheese, hardboiled egg, and toss. Switch to a wide tray.

2.In a little-mixing bowl, add the lemon juice, garlic, buttermilk, salt, pepper, and incorporate well.

3.Work over the salad with the sauce.

Nutrition: Energy (calories): 628 kcal Protein: 60.98 g Fat: 27.46 g Carbohydrates: 33.82 g Calcium, Ca355 mg Magnesium, Mg102 mg

284.Feta Chicken with Zucchini

Prep Time: 20 min | **Cook Time:** 20 min | **Serve:** 2
- 2 tbsp. olive oil 1 lemon

- 4 boneless, skinless-chicken breasts (about 1 1/2 lb.) One-fourth tsp. kosher salt
- 2 mid-sized zucchinis
- One-fourth cup fresh, chopped flat-leaf parsley leaves 13 tsp. of black pepper
- One-third cup of crumbled Feta (about 2 oz.)

1.Heat the furnace to 400° F. In a roasting pan, drizzle one-half tablespoon of the oil. In thin stripes, remove the skin from the lemon; set aside. Slice the lemon thinly. In the pan, place half the slices.

2.On top of the lemon slices, place the chicken and season with 1/8 of a teaspoon of salt.

3.Lengthwise, split each zucchini in half, then split each half into one-fourth inch-thick half-moons. Combine the zucchini, parsley, pepper, the remaining oil, slices of lemon, salt in a bowl; toss.

4.Spread the mixture over the chicken and sprinkle it over the top with the Feta.

5.Roast for 16 to 21 minutes until the chicken is fully cooked. Switch it to a cutting board and cut it into thirds for each piece.

6.Divide the chicken, zucchini mixture, and lemons between individual plates, and sprinkle with the zest.

Nutrition: Energy (calories): 2176 kcal Protein: 111.16 g Fat: 88.45 g Carbohydrates: 236.31 g Calcium, Ca819 mg Magnesium, Mg343 mg

285.Cinnamon Chicken

Prep Time: 20 min | **Cook Time:** 20 min | **Serve:** 2
- 4 or 5 (4-6 oz.) boneless chicken breasts without skin 2 tbsp. Italian Dressing Low-Calorie
- 1 tsp. of cinnamon
- 1 1/2 tsp. Powdered garlic 1/4 tsp. salt (optional)
- 1/4 tsp. pepper

1.Heat the oven the 350 ° C oven.

2.In a 13x9 baking dish, bring the chicken in. Pour the Italian sauce over it.

3.Blend the remaining ingredients in a small bowl. Sprinkle chicken over it. Bake for 40–45 minutes.

Nutrition: Protein: 94.9 g Fat: 26.29 g Carbohydrates: 6.69 g Calcium, Ca66 mg Magnesium, Mg79 mg Phosphorus, P552 mg

286.Chinese Five Spice Chicken

Prep Time: 20 min | **Cook Time:** 20 min | **Serve:** 2
- 2 entire chicken breasts bone-in, with skin 2 tsp. of five-spice Chinese powder
- 1 tsp. Of powdered garlic, Salt and pepper, for taste 1 tbsp. olive oil

1.Rinse the breasts and pat the chicken dry. Sprinkle with garlic powder, five-spice powder, salt, and pepper. Cover securely in aluminum foil and cool for at least 2 hours to marinate.

2.Bring to fire your oven to 175° C (350° F).

3.Remove the wrapping from the chicken breasts and put them in a 9x13 inches baking dish that is lightly greased.

4.Drizzle with olive oil and bake for 46 minutes at 350° F (175° C), or until the juices are cooked through and clear.

Nutrition: Energy (calories): 572 kcal Protein: 61.02 g Fat: 33.68 g Carbohydrates: 3.01 g Calcium, Ca45 mg Magnesium, Mg81 mg

287.Chicken with Acorn Squash and Tomatoes

Prep Time: 20 min | **Cook Time:** 20 min | **Serve:** 2

- 1 little-acorn squash (about 1 1/2 lb.), 1/4 inch thick, halved, seeded, and sliced
- 1 pint of grape tomatoes, halved 4 garlic cloves, cut
- 3 tbsp. olive oil
- Black pepper and kosher salt
- 4 6-oz boneless, skinless breasts of chicken One-half tsp. ground cilantro
- 2 tbsp. of fresh oregano, chopped

1.Heat the furnace to 425° F.
2.Toss the squash, tomatoes, and garlic with 2 little spoons of oil, one-half teaspoon of salt, and one-fourth teaspoon of pepper on a broad-rimmed baking sheet.
3.Roast the vegetables for 21 to 25 minutes until the squash is tender.
4.Meanwhile, over medium heat, heat the remaining tablespoon of oil in a large skillet.
5.Season the coriander, one-half teaspoon salt, and one-fourth teaspoon pepper with the poultry. Cook, 6 to 7 minutes per hand, until golden brown and cooked through.
6.Serve the squash and tomatoes with the chicken and sprinkle with the oregano.

Nutrition: Energy (calories): 877 kcal Protein: 34.11 g Fat: 39.9 g Carbohydrates: 98.08 g Calcium, Ca165 mg Magnesium, Mg144 mg

288.Chicken Cordon Blue

Prep Time: 15 min | **Cook Time:** 20 min | **Serve:** 2

- 2 4-oz boneless chicken breasts, skinless,
- 2 large leaves of spinach, washed, stems removed 2 wedges laughing cow light cheese
- 1 oz. of reduced-ham without nitrate sodium Paprika, to taste
- 1 garlic clove, minced
- 1 tsp. of extra-virgin olive oil
- 1 cup Baby Bella mushrooms, sliced 1/8 tsp. ground black pepper
- 2 tsp. yogurt sauce
- 1/2 cup Greek nonfat yogurt 1 tbsp. Dijon mustard
- 1/2 tsp. buttermilk
- 2 tbsp. chives, chopped

1.Set up the oven to 400° F.
2.Pound the chicken with a mallet till it is 1/4-inch thick. Take care not to rip a breast apart.
3.On top of each breast lay 1 spinach leaf. Spread a slice of cheese to cover the spinach. Top with 1/2 slice of ham and fold the ham over to match the breast as desired.
4.Roll each breast up gently and protect it with a toothpick. Sprinkle with paprika on the outer side of the breast. Bake for 20 minutes in the oven until the chicken is completely cooked.
5. Sauté the garlic in the oil in a non-adhesive skillet over medium-high heat for 1 minute while the chicken is cooking. Add pepper and mushrooms. Stir regularly until soft for 10 minutes. Withdraw from the sun. Cover and set aside.
6.Whisk together the yogurt, mustard, and buttermilk for sauce preparation. Mix the chives in.
7.Divide the mushrooms evenly, about 1/4 cup each, between 2 plates. Then put the chicken on the mushroom bed and drizzle the top with 1/4 cup of yogurt sauce.

Nutrition: Energy (calories): 180 kcal Protein: 29.41 g Fat: 5.35 g Carbohydrates: 1.95 g Calcium, Ca21 mg Magnesium, Mg42 mg

289.Chicken Kampala

Prep Time: 15 min | **Cook Time:** 1 and 1/2 h | **Serve:** 4-5

- 3 lbs. chicken parts
- 2 tbsp. butter
- 2 tbsp. olive oil
- 2 med. Onions, chopped two cloves garlic, minced 1 c. canned tomatoes
- 3 oz. tomato paste
- 2 sticks cinnamon
- 1/4 tsp. Ground allspice 1/4 tsp. sugar
- 1/4 c. red wine

1.Heat 2 tbsp. Butter, and 1 tbsp. Olive-oil in a skillet and add the chicken—Cook chicken over medium heat for about 15 minutes, often stirring to keep chicken from burning. Take it out of the skillet once the chicken is browned and apply the remaining butter and oil to the pan.
2.Ensure the skillet is still hot before adding the onions and cooking for about 5 minutes over medium heat. Stir in the garlic and tomatoes, cooking for another 5 minutes. Stir in the tomato paste, cinnamon, allspice, sugar, red wine, and chicken, including juices.
3.Bring to a boil and cover tightly (you can use foil and cover with foil). Reduce heat and simmer, occasionally stirring, for 1 and 1/2 hours.
4.Serve with white rice.

Nutrition: Energy (calories): 421 kcal Protein: 56.41 g Fat: 17.51 g Carbohydrates: 6.43 g Calcium, Ca46 mg Magnesium, Mg73 mg

290.Garlic and Citrus Turkey with Mixed Greens

Prep Time: 5 min | **Cook Time:** 15 min | **Serve:** 4

- 4 teaspoons (or oil of your choice and fresh chopped garlic) 1 C scallion greens, thinly sliced
- 1 3/4 pounds lean ground turkey
- 1 Tablespoon (or lemon, pepper, garlic, onion, parsley, salt & pepper)
- 8 cups mixed green lettuce
- 1 lemon cut into wedges for garnish

1.Heat a large non-stick skillet with oil and sauté the garlic over medium-high heat for 1 minute, stirring.Add scallion greens, green onions, ground turkey, and seasonings. Stir and cook for 16 minutes, or until meat is thoroughly cooked.
2.Divide greens between 4 plates and top each plate with 1/4 of the meat mixture.
3.Serve with lemon wedges.

Nutrition: Energy (calories): 355 kcal Protein: 38.71 g Fat: 21.33 g Carbohydrates: 3.54 g Calcium, Ca81 mg Magnesium, Mg57 mg Phosphorus, P421 mg

291.Greek Chicken with Yogurt

Prep Time: 10 min | **Cook Time:** 20 min | **Serve:** 4

- oil spray
- 5 oz. plain Greek yogurt 2 tbsp mayonnaise
- 1/2 cup grated parmesan-cheese 1 tsp garlic powder
- 1/4 tsp salt
- 1/4 tsp black-pepper
- 1.5 lb. chicken-tenders (whole) or chicken-breasts (cut in quarters) Parsley (chopped, for garnish)

1.Fire up the oven to 480 degrees F.

2.Line a baking sheet with parchment paper. Spray oil on parchment, then place chicken on top (the oil will help prevent the chicken from sticking to the parchment paper).

3.In a little-mixing bowl, whisk together the yogurt, mayo, parmesan, garlic powder, salt, and pepper. Toss the chicken tenders or breasts with the yogurt mixture and place them on the baking sheet.

4.Repeat with the remaining chicken and yogurt/spices mixture.

5.For 20 minutes, bake. Garnish with extra parsley and immediately serve sprinkled on top with extra Greek yogurt, mayo, and grated parmesan.

Nutrition: Energy (calories): 325 kcal Protein: 42.78 g Fat: 14.13 g Carbohydrates: 4.87 g Calcium, Ca189 mg Magnesium, Mg60 mg

292.Sliced Steak with Canadian Crust

Prep Time: 10 min | **Cook Time:** 20 min | **Serve:** 5

- 10-ounce steaks good for grilling (ask your butcher for suggestions) about 1 and one-half thick
- 1 Tablespoon (1 Capful) (or other dry steak seasonings)

1.Preheat broiler

2.Sprinkle on both sides of steak dry steak seasonings seasoning

3.Place steak under pre-heated broiler

4.Broil each side to taste (approx. 5 minutes per side for medium-rare)

5.Slice steak in thin, 3/4" slices against the grain.

6.Arrange slices on a serving platter and top with a generous amount of butter.

Nutrition: Energy (calories): 51 kcal Protein: 6.58 g Fat: 2.02 g Carbohydrates: 1.03 g Calcium, Ca7 mg Magnesium, Mg8 mg

293.BBQ Chicken with Sesame Ginger "Rice"

Prep Time: 10 min and refrigerate for 3 h up to overnight. | **Cook Time:** 12 min | **Serve:** 4

- 4 (4 to 6 ounces each) boneless (skinless-chicken breasts) For the Marinade:
- 1/2 cup soy-sauce
- 3 garlic cloves (peeled and crushed) 1/4 cup seasoned rice wine vinegar 2 normal spoons honey
- 1 normal spoon fresh ginger root (peeled and grated) 4 medium green onions (chopped)
- 2 normal spoons toasted sesame oil 1 little spoon toasted sesame seeds
- Garnish: 2 normal spoons whole fresh cilantro leaves

1.Using a mallet, pound the chicken until 1/2 inch thick. Cut into 1- inch strips.

Preparation:

2.Place the chicken in a resealable bag.

3.In a 9x13x2 baking pan, mix the soy sauce, garlic, Rice Vinegar, honey, and ginger. Add the chicken-breasts and turn to coat. Seal with a non-reactive covering. Refrigerate for 3 hours up to overnight.

4.Preheat a gas grill to medium-high heat. Discard the marinade and remove the chicken

5.Arrange the chicken strips on the grill pan with tongs to cook for 8 to 12 minutes until the chicken is thoroughly cooked. DO NOT overcook. The chicken is done when the juices-run clear. Transfer the chicken to a platter. Cover with foil and set aside (if finishing later).

6.In a medium casserole dish, add the ¼ cup water and bring to a boil. Stir in the sesame oil, sesame seeds, and the rice vinegar and salt.

7.While the rice is cooking, prepare the barbecue-cooked chicken.

8.To serve, divide the chicken strips among 4 servings.

Nutrition: Energy (calories): 268 kcal Protein: 8.75 g Fat: 13.55 g Carbohydrates: 28.93 g Calcium, Ca43 mg Magnesium, Mg39 mg Cholesterol14 mg

294.Fork Tender Beef Goulash with Peppercorn & Sage

Prep Time: 15 min | **Cook Time:** 35 min | **Serve:** 4

- 2 Tbsp Olive oil
- 2 Onions, chopped roughly 4 garlic cloves, crushed
- 2 Celery stalks, sliced
- 800 g Beef rump steaks, or use stewing steak, cut into 3cm cubes 1 Tbsp Paprika
- ½ bottle Red wine
- 1 tin Chopped tomato, approx. 420g 1 Tbsp Balsamic vinegar
- 1/2 Peppercorn
- 2 tsp Brown sugar
- 1 stalk Sage, leaves only 1 pinch Chili flakes
- 1 pottle Sour cream, for serving

1.In a heavy saucepan, sauté the onion, celery, and garlic till soft. Add the meat and brown well.

2.Set aside a small amount of the meat, sliced thinly, and return the rest to the pan along with the paprika, wine, chopped tomatoes, balsamic vinegar, and sugar.

3.Preheat the oven to 160°C.

4.Gently simmer for 20–30 minutes, adding the whole peppercorn and sage bundle. With a sharp knife, remove the peppercorn and sage.

5.Increase the heat and simmer vigorously for another 10 minutes.

6.Serve garnished with the reserved meat slices, sour cream, and chili flakes.

Nutrition: Energy (calories): 417 kcal Protein: 44.36 g Fat: 18.21 g Carbohydrates: 17.78 g Calcium, Ca58 mg Magnesium, Mg73 mg Phosphorus, P507 mg

295.Simple Sonoma Skillet

Prep Time: 15 min | **Cook Time:** 30 min | **Serve:** 4

- 4 teaspoons of your choice of oil
- 1 cup scallions (or onions if permitted in your program) 1 cup red-bell-pepper, thinly sliced
- 1 cup of yellow-bell pepper, thinly sliced
- Thinly cut 20 ounces-chicken or steak (can be cooked leftovers or uncooked)
- Stacey Hawkins Phoenix Sunrise Seasoning 1 normal-spoon (one capful)

1.Put a big-skillet on medium heat and let it heat up.

2.Add the extra virgin olive oil and the scallion or onion, and thinly sliced bell peppers.

3.Sauté them for about 5 minutes until they start to soften.

4.Add the meat and let it cook for 6 minutes or so until it's no longer pink.

5.Add the Phoenix Sunrise Seasoning.

6.Cook for a few more minutes, and it is ready to serve.

Nutrition: Energy (calories): 307 kcal Protein: 38.65 g Fat: 12.37 g Carbohydrates: 8.49 g Calcium, Ca43 mg Magnesium, Mg42 mg Phosphorus, P360 mg

296. Italian Chicken with White Wine, Peppers, and Anchovy

Prep Time: 10 min | **Cook Time:** 25 min | **Serve:** 4

FOR THE CHICKEN
- 1 normal spoon olive oil
- 4 boneless-skinless chicken breasts salt and fresh ground pepper to taste 1 little spoon garlic powder
- 1 tablespoon anchovy

FOR THE SMOOTH SAUCE OF WHITE WINE
- 1 regular spoon of unsalted butter 1 diced large-yellow onion 3 minced garlic cloves
- Salt and fresh ground pepper, 1 cup of dry white wine to taste
- 1 dried thyme small-spoon
- New chopped parsley
- 1/2 cup half-and-half/heavy cream/evaporated milk

1. Pan Heat the olive oil in a heavy large skillet over medium-high heat. Season the chicken with salt, pepper garlic powder and combine it with the anchovy flakes. Ad the chicken to the pan and cook on both sides until it is golden brown. Ensure that you are sauteing in the pan, lower the heat to keep from burning.

2. Magnetic Mixer Dispersion Whip the wine, thyme, garlic, pepper, and salt in a glass bowl. Add the cream, mix in the cubes of butter. Keep mixing for a few minutes, and then add the peppers. Keep mixing and cook the fusion.

3. Mixer-ext. Ended Hand Cut the chicken into strips (or very small pieces if desired. The pieces are easier to eat). Combine the chicken with the mixture—Cook the fusion for 10 minutes. Serve with pasta or on warm pieces of French bread.

Nutrition: Energy (calories): 742 kcal Protein: 110.07 g Fat: 26.87 g Carbohydrates: 9.25 g Calcium, Ca262 mg Magnesium, Mg150 mg Phosphorus, P1171 mg

297. Tagine of Chicken and Olives

Prep Time: 10 min and marinate for 3-4 h **Cook Time:** 45 minutes | **Serve:** 4

- 5 cloves garlic, finely chopped
- One-fourth teaspoon saffron threads, pulverized One-half teaspoon ground ginger
- 1 teaspoon sweet paprika
- Half a little-spoon of ground cumin, half a teaspoon of turmeric
- 1 chicken, salt and freshly ground black pepper, cut into 8 to 10 pieces.
- 3 medium onions, sliced thin, 2 tablespoons extra virgin olive oil
- 1 cinnamon stick
- 8 pitted and halved kalamata olives
- 8 cracked green, pitted and halved olives
- 1 big or 3 small lemons preserved (sold in specialty food shops) 1 cup of stock of chicken
- 1/2 lemon juice
- 1 tablespoon of flat-leaf parsley chopped

1. In a big-plastic food bag, combine the garlic, saffron, ginger, parsley, paprika, cumin, turmeric, salt, and pepper. To coat the spices with the chicken, add the chicken and shake the bag. Set it aside for 1 hour to 3 hours to marinate.

2. Transfer the chicken to a large pot and add the remaining ingredients. If there isn't any liquid in the bag, add enough water to cover the pot's ingredients. Cover and cook for 36 to 46 minutes, until the chicken is tender and the liquid is reduced. 3. Serve garnished with lemon juice and parsley.

Nutrition: Energy (calories): 1090 kcal Protein: 115.01 g Fat: 64.59 g Carbohydrates: 6.08 g Calcium, Ca111 mg Magnesium, Mg137 mg

298. Citrus Chicken

Prep Time: 10 min | **Cook Time:** 3-4 h | **Serve:** 3

- 6 bone-in chicken breast halves, 1 tea separated from the flesh.
- 1/2 teas seasoned salt 1/4 teas pepper
- 2 Tbsp olive oil 1/4 cup water
- 3 Tbsp lemon juice
- 2 garlic cloves, minced
- 1 teas chicken bouillon granule 2 teas minced fresh parsley

1. Rinse chicken; pat dry. Place chicken in a 4-qt. Slow cooker.

2. Combine the oregano, seasoned salt, pepper, oil, water, lemon juice, garlic, bouillon, and parsley; pour over the chicken.

3. Cover and cook until tender, for 3-4 hours or until the chicken is tender.

Nutrition: Energy (calories): 1379 kcal Protein: 151.74 g Fat: 80.84 g Carbohydrates: 1.75 g Calcium, Ca86 mg Magnesium, Mg140 mg

299. Chunky Chicken Pie

Prep Time: 10 min | **Cook Time:** 30 min | **Serve:** 3

- 3 boneless skinless chicken breasts 2 tablespoons sunflower oil
- 300 ml of milk
- 200 ml chicken stock (it's okay from a cube) 2 tablespoons of flour
- Fifty g of butter
- 1 clove of garlic, hacked
- 1 tablespoon of chopped freshly grated nutmeg parsley
- About salt
- 1 Shortcrust pastry ready to roll, rolled eggs moderately thinly pounded, glazed

1. Pounding with a rolling pin on the chicken breasts with until they are about three to eight thick and set aside. Cook the garlic in the oil in a saucepan until it is pale yellow.

2. Precisely Mix the flour and everything, add to the oil and cook for 5 minutes over low heat, stirring at first, until the flour turns clear and the dish is thick. Add the nutmeg and season with salt, mix well. Take the pan from the heat and let it cool slightly. Add this to the chicken breasts to obtain a heavy pin.

3. Shape into a square by covering them with wax paper and pounding them with a rolling pin. Spread the chicken mixture evenly over the pastry. Roll the pastry's edges over the outsides of the chicken mixture to form a rim and bake in a preheated hot oven 220 ° C. until golden brown, about 20 minutes. Serve hot with fresh vegetables.

Nutrition: Energy (calories): 10597 kcal Protein: 614.33 g Fat: 511.1 g Carbohydrates: 867.92 g Calcium, Ca14044 mg Magnesium, Mg1576 mg

300. Tender Rosemary Pork Chops

Prep Time: 15 min | **Cook Time:** 20 min | **Serve:** 4
- 4 pork loin chops kosher salt
- Freshly ground black pepper
- 1 tbsp. freshly minced rosemary 2 cloves garlic, minced
- 1/2 c. (1 stick) butter melted 1 tbsp. extra-virgin olive oil

1. Preheat grill or broiler with 1/2 inch of oil in the pan.
2. With paper towels, pat the chops dry, and season with salt and pepper to taste.
3. Brush the chops with the melted butter and sprinkle the rosemary and garlic over them on both sides.
4. Grill the chops for 20 minutes or until tenderness comes
5. Serve with a simple carrot and red bell pepper medley.

Nutrition: Energy (calories): 547 kcal Protein: 40.57 g Fat: 41.81 g Carbohydrates: 0.6 g Calcium, Ca49 mg Magnesium, Mg41 mg Phosphorus, P355 mg

301. Low Carb Shakshuka

Prep Time: 15 min | **Cook Time:** 40 min | **Serve:** 4
- 2 tablespoons EVOO- extra virgin olive oil 4 teaspoons crushed garlic
- 1 red pepper seeds and pith removed, diced 1 onion finely chopped
- 2 teaspoons turmeric
- 1 little spoon ground coriander 1 teaspoon ground cumin
- 5 teaspoon ground cinnamon
- 3 tablespoons Harissa homemade or store-bought 2 medium tomatoes chopped
- 400 grams /14 oz diced tomatoes no added sugar 8 eggs
- 200 grams /7 oz diced feta cheese salt and pepper to taste fresh coriander to garnish

1. In a big sauté pan, heat 2 tablespoons olive oil and sauté the onion for a few minutes.
2. Add the garlic, turmeric, coriander, cumin, cinnamon, and harissa and sauté for another minute.
3. Add the red pepper and the diced tomatoes and simmer for 20 minutes until the sauce thickens.
4. Make 8 little wells in the sauce, crack the eggs into the well, and season with salt and pepper.
5. Put a lid on the pan and cook for a bit gently for 8-10 minutes, or until the eggs are just set.
6. Place one egg on each serving plate and sprinkle with feta.
7. Spoon over the sauce and garnish with fresh coriander.

Nutrition: Energy (calories): 7621 kcal Protein: 252.86 g Fat: 331.54 g Carbohydrates: 1007.48 g Calcium, Ca7721 mg Magnesium, Mg861 mg Phosphorus, P6091 mg

302. Thai Cashew Chicken

Prep Time: 10 min | **Cook Time:** 15 min | **Serve:** 4
- 200 grams of chicken breast, 1 tbsp., cut into bite-sized bits. Flour cassava or all-purpose flour
- 1/3 cup cooking oil with a natural flavour (I used sunflower oil for frying everything)
- For 1 tbsp. Crushed and sliced garlic (I used about 4 cloves)
- 1/2 cup of yellow onions, cut into wedges (1 small onion I used) 1/3 cup of dry red chilies from Thai birds' eye, deep-fried
- 1/2 cup raw unsalted cashew nuts
- 1/3 cup of fresh, thinly julienned, long red chili peppers (I used red spur chilies)
- 1/3 cup of fresh chili peppers from the banana, cut into thin strips
- Seasoning sauce: 1/3 cup green onions (spring onions), cut into 2.5 cm bits.
- For 1 tbsp. 1/2 tbsp. mild soy sauce. 1/2 tbsp. dark soy sauce. Sauce of oysters
- Tsp. 1/4. White ground pepper with a pinch of salt
- The sugar pinch
- Oh. 3 tbsp. Water or stock

1. In a large bowl, add in chicken. Add in seasonings (1 tbsp. light soy sauce, 1/2 tbsp. dark soy sauce, 1/2 tbsp. oyster sauce, ground white pepper, ground black pepper, and a pinch of salt and sugar). Toss to coat evenly. Set aside.
2. In another non-stick pan, heat oil on medium-high heat. Pan-fry the chicken until cooked through but still tender and juicy. Set aside. Pan-fry garlic, ginger, and onions until fragrant and onions are translucent. Do not burn. Set aside.
3. Pour-in the leftover oil. Pan-fry cashew nuts, chilies, and chicken. Toss till fragrant.

Nutrition: Energy (calories): 412 kcal Protein: 15.69 g Fat: 33.8 g Carbohydrates: 15.56 g Calcium, Ca62 mg Magnesium, Mg81 mg Phosphorus, P227 mg

303. Cheesy Pepper Taco Bake

Prep Time: 10 min | **Cook Time:** 30 min | **Serve:** 4
- 1 lb. 95-97% lean ground beef (chicken or turkey)
- 1T garlic, cumin, paprika, cayenne, salt, black pepper, onion, and parsley
- 1C no sugar added, fresh vegetable salsa plus 4 additional Tablespoons for garnish
- 1 1/2 lbs. fresh peppers (green, red, poblano, your choice) stems removed, cut in half lengthwise, and seeded.
- 1/2 C shredded low-fat-cheddar cheese 4 T Sour Cream

1. Preheat oven to 375 degrees.
2. In a large skillet – brown meat, garlic, spices, and parsley for about 4 min. Over medium heat. Add Fresh salsa and cook for 5 more minutes.
3. Carefully spoon 1/2 cup mixture in each pepper half going up the open side. The goal is to fill up the pepper in an orderly fashion.
4. Pour 1 C of salsa over the stuffed pepper halves in a small baking pan, cover the pepper mixture with the cheese.
5. Bake for about 10-15 min, or until cheese is completely melted.
6. To serve, divide equally into 4 bowls, and pour 1/2 T of sour cream on top of each.

Nutrition: Energy (calories): 362 kcal Protein: 35.6 g Fat: 14.66 g Carbohydrates: 23.03 g Calcium, Ca122 mg Magnesium, Mg84 mg Phosphorus, P397 mg

304. Summer Shrimp Primavera

Prep Time: 10 min | **Cook Time:** 10 min | **Serve:** 4
- 4 ounces of uncooked angel pasta for hair
- 8 shrimp jumbo, peeled and deveined

- 6 fresh asparagus spears, cut into 1/4 cup of olive oil and cut into 2-inch pieces.
- 2 cloves of garlic, minced
- 1/2 cup of fresh sliced mushrooms, 1/2 cup of chicken broth
- 1 tiny, peeled, seeded, and diced plum tomato, 1/4 teaspoon of salt
- 1/8 teaspoon of crushed flakes of red pepper
- 1 tablespoon of fresh basil, oregano, thyme and parsley each, 1/4 cup of grated Parmesan cheese

1. In a big-saucepan, cook pasta according to package directions for al-dente pasta; drain.
2. Preheat broiler. Spray a broiler-proof baking dish with nonstick spray. Sprinkle shrimp with salt and pepper. Arrange on a metal baking pan coated with nonstick spray. Broil for two minutes, 4 inches from the sun. Turn shrimp and broil for 2 minutes longer or until done.
3. Cook the pasta until tender in boiling water (1 to 2 minutes). Run under cold water, drain well, and keep warm.
4. In a big/large non-stick skillet, heat the olive oil over a medium-high heat. Add the garlic, asparagus, mushrooms, tomato and chicken broth; heat through. Stir in the pasta and shrimp; cook until it is completely cooked. Season with salt and pepper flakes. Stir herbs into shrimp mixture. Sprinkle with cheese. Serve immediately.

Nutrition: Energy (calories): 291 kcal Protein: 20.7 g Fat: 17.84 g Carbohydrates: 12.43 g Calcium, Ca100 mg Magnesium, Mg39 mg Phosphorus, P229 mg

305. Pan-Seared Pork Loin and Balsamic Caramelized Onions

Prep Time: 5 min | **Cook Time:** 25 min | **Serve:** 4
- on stick cooking spray 1 teaspoon garlic
- 1 teaspoons salt
- 1 teaspoon black pepper 1 teaspoon onion
- 1 teaspoons parsley
- 1 1/2 lbs. pork tenderloin (or beef tenderloin, or chicken breasts)

1. Preheat oven to 350 degrees. Lightly spray a shallow baking PanSprinkle salt and pepper with the steaks and put them in a baking pan.
2. Bake until the meat and internal temperature are tender and reaches 150 degrees, approximately 15 to 20 minutes.
3. While meat is cooking, prepare your gravy. In a large skillet, sauté onion and garlic in olive oil for 3 to 4 minutes. Add sugar to the pan and let cook until caramelized. Once onions are caramelized, add balsamic vinegar and butter. Allow this to simmer until onions are very soft. Thickens as it simmers.
4. Brush top of pork loin with olive oil. Place the pan under the broiler for around 1-2 minutes, until the top layer is caramelized.
5. Remove/Take it from the oven and let it rest for 15 minutes.
6. Slice into medallions and top with gravy. Serve.

Nutrition: Energy (calories): 688 kcal Protein: 23.91 g Fat: 61.78 g Carbohydrates: 7.89 g Calcium, Ca29 mg Magnesium, Mg25 mg

306. Citrus Shrimp & Spinach

Prep Time: 5 min | **Cook Time:** 10 min | **Serve:** 4
- on stick cooking spray 1 teaspoon garlic
- 1 teaspoons salt
- 1 teaspoon black pepper 1 teaspoon onion

- 1 teaspoons parsley
- 1 1/2 lbs. wild-caught, raw shrimp, cleaned and tails removed
- 6 cups baby spinach greens, arugula greens, beet greens, or a combination

1. Pour the olive oil into a big-skillet over medium heat (you may want to spray your pan with a non-stick cooking spray).
2. In a small bowl, combine the garlic, salt, pepper, onion powder, and parsley. Then sprinkle over the shrimp and leave to rest while you heat.
3. Add one normal spoon of the olive oil; heat for about 1 minute until hot but not scorching. Add shrimp to the pan. Cook, occasionally stirring, until the shrimp are pink and opaque. Remove from the pan to a plate and serve over a greens bed with additional olive oil and balsamic vinegar.

Nutrition: Energy (calories): 815 kcal Protein: 37.58 g Fat: 4.03 g Carbohydrates: 164.19 g Calcium, Ca118 mg Magnesium, Mg357 mg

307. Mediterranean Roasted Chicken with Lemon Dill Radishes

Prep Time: 5 min | **Cook Time:** 30 min | **Serve:** 4
- 2 lbs. chicken thighs (remove skin)
- Pinch Stacey Hawkins Dash of Desperation Seasoning (or garlic, salt, black pepper, onion, and parsley)
- 1 Tablespoon garlic
- 1 Tablespoon marjoram
- 1 Tablespoon basil
- 1 Tablespoon rosemary
- 1 Tablespoon onion

1. Preheat the oven to 350 degrees.
2. Dice onion.
3. Put the chicken in a deep baking dish.
4. Chop the vegetables. Then put them with some oil on the baking dish.
5. Pour all the seasoning.
6. Bake for 30 minutes, then put the radishes.
7. The radishes cook with the chicken.
8. Serve at room temperature.

Nutrition: Energy (calories): 507 kcal Protein: 37.72 g Fat: 37.74 g Carbohydrates: 1.88 g Calcium, Ca31 mg Magnesium, Mg44 mg Phosphorus, P362 mg

308. Pan-Seared Balsamic Chicken and Vegetables

Prep Time: 10 min | **Cook Time:** 13 min | **Serve:** 4
- 1/4 cup + 2 tablespoons of Italian salad dressing (I recommend using Kraft light Italian; this is the best quality, and it's what I've used) 3 tablespoons of balsamic vinegar
- Honey 1 1/2 tbsp
- 1/8 tsp (more or less to taste) crushed red pepper flakes 1 1/4 lbs. Tenderloins with chicken breast
- 2 Teaspoons of olive oil
- Salt and black pepper freshly ground
- With 1 lb. New asparagus, cut with tough ends, cut into two-inch sections (look for thinner stalks. Green beans are another good option)
- 1 1/2 cups of matchstick-carrots, 1 cup of grape tomatoes, half the grape tomatoes

1. Combine 1/4 cup of the Italian dressing, 2 Tbsp balsamic vinegar, honey, 1/8 tsp red pepper flakes in a bowl. Put the

chicken from the tenderloin package into a big zip-top baggie and pour the marinade over the top.

2.Preheat the oven to 400 degrees.

3.Heat the oil in a pan. Preheat the broilerBegin to add the asparagus to the pan once the oil is hot.

4.Season with salt & pepper and cook only until barely tender, about 3 mins. Remove from skillet and set aside. Add the tomatoes, carrots, and chicken to the pan and continue sautéing for an additional 5-6 mins. (Or until most chicken pieces are lightly browned on both sides)

5. Remove/take the pan (from the heat), and pour over the chicken mixture with the second tablespoon of balsamic vinegar. Cover and place with a lid in the 400-degree oven for an additional 5 mins or until the chicken is completely cooked through.

6.Add the cooked asparagus and the remaining tablespoons of dressing right before serving.

Nutrition: Energy (calories): 439 kcal Protein: 32.85 g Fat: 23.26 g Carbohydrates: 25.5 g Calcium, Ca66 mg Magnesium, Mg61 mg Phosphorus, P332 mg

309.Tex-Mex Seared Salmon

Prep Time: 5 min | **Cook Time:** 15 min | **Serve:** 4

- 1 1/2 pounds wild-caught salmon filet (will cook best if you have it at room temp)
- 1 Tablespoon salt
- 1 Tablespoon pepper
- 1Tablespoon garlic
- 1 Tablespoon cumin
- 1 Tablespoon paprika
- 1 Tablespoon cayenne
- 1 Tablespoon onion to taste

1.Wash your salmon filet, then cut a 6-inch slit across the middle of the fillet (I use a sandwich knife to make the slit)

2.In a bowl, mix-all the ingredients, then rub your mixture in the filet, let it sit for 10-15min

3.HEAT OIL TO MEDIUM HIGH

4.Sautéed your filet on both sides till it has a nice dark sear; best to use tongs, be careful it is hot!

Nutrition: Energy (calories): 279 kcal Protein: 44.26 g Fat: 9.09 g Carbohydrates: 6.47 g Calcium, Ca46 mg Magnesium, Mg73 mg Phosphorus, P513 mg

310.Charred Sirloin with Creamy Horseradish Sauce

Prep Time: 5 min | **Cook Time:** 15 min | **Serve:** 4

- 1 1/2 pounds sirloin steaks, trimmed & visible fat removed 1/2 Tablespoon salt
- 1/2 Tablespoon pepper
- 1/2 Tablespoon garlic and onion to taste 6 Tablespoons low-fat sour cream
- 1-3 T horseradish (from the jar)

1.Preheat oven to high broil

2.Season your steaks with salt, pepper, garlic, and onion, and then place on a cookie sheet lined with foil.

3.Place your sheet on the top rack of your oven and broil until the steaks are charred to your desired doneness. The steaks will also continue to cook once they are removed from the oven.

4.Remove steaks from the oven and let them rest for a few minutes.

5.Warm-up your horseradish sauce in the microwave and set aside.

6.Meanwhile, in a medium saucepan over medium-high heat, warm up the cream, horseradish, and Worcestershire sauce. Whisk constantly until it is warm and remove from heat.

7.Spoon your horseradish sauce over top of your steak.

Nutrition: Energy (calories): 218 kcal Protein: 35.2 g Fat: 6.38 g Carbohydrates: 2.77 g Calcium, Ca50 mg Magnesium, Mg50 mg Phosphorus, P392 mg

311.Rosemary Beef Tips and Creamy Fauxtatoes

Prep Time: 5 min | **Cook Time:** 30 min | **Serve:** 4

- 1 1/2 lbs. top sirloin steak, cubed into 1 chunk 1 T (one capful) fresh rosemary
- 1 T (one capful) sage
- 1 T (one capful) black pepper
- 1 T (one capful) onion and garlic 2 1/2 C low sodium beef broth
- 4 C sliced baby portobello mushrooms 1 T fresh minced garlic,
- 1 T (one capful) scallions 1 teaspoon salt and pepper
- 1/2 tsp guar gum & 1/4 C water 2 C hot cauliflower mashed potatoes

1.Note: To speed up the preparation, all ingredients except steak, mushrooms, and a hint of olive oil for searing/cooking can be pre-chopped and stored in baggies ahead of time.

2.In a big-pot, cook beef over medium to high heat. Add onion, garlic, and mushrooms. Stir occasionally. Add oregano, thyme, parsley, salt, and pepper. Stir.

3.Add chopped rosemary, sage, black pepper, and garlic powder. Stir. Add beef broth. Bring to boil. Lower the heat to simmer.

4.Add half the cooked mushrooms into the pot on top and alongside the beef.

5.When beef is cooked to medium-rare, remove from pan and keep warm. Strain broth into a measuring cup to get 4 1/2 cups of broth. Pour broth into a large mixing bowl.

6.Discard solids. Add cornstarch and salt to hot broth and whisk. Add guar gum (or other thickeners) and water and whisk.

7.Bring the water to a boil.

8.Add additional mushrooms and cooked beef to the gravy. Mix. 9.Add chopped garlic and green onions. Mix. Serve sauce alongside beef.

Nutrition: Energy (calories): 492 kcal Protein: 47.47 g Fat: 23.56 g Carbohydrates: 26.14 g Calcium, Ca106 mg Magnesium, Mg70 mg Phosphorus, P606 mg

312.Balsamic-Glazed Chicken Thighs with Broccoli

Prep Time: 5 min | **Cook Time:** 20 min | **Serve:** 4

- 4 (~6 ounces) boneless, skinless chicken thighs
- 2 teaspoons (one capful) salt and pepper, garlic, onion, and parsley
- 4 Tablespoons balsamic reduction
- 1/4 C low sodium chicken broth
- 4 C broccoli florets, lightly steamed (crisp-tender) nonstick cooking spray

Instructions:

1.Mix the chicken thighs to coat with salt, pepper, garlic, onion, and parsley, in a medium bowl. Spray a nonstick skillet loosely with cooking spray to reduce the amount of fat absorbed into the thighs. Heat the skillet to medium-high.

2. Cook and add the thighs to the skillet, uncovered, for about 6 minutes on each side until browned and no longer pink inside.

3. Add the balsamic reduction to deglaze the pan, and cook for one minute. Put the chicken and balsamic reduction into the slow cooker.

4. Turn the slow-cooker to high and add the chicken broth. Cook for 15 minutes or until the chicken is tender enough to pull apart with a fork. Stir in the broccoli florets and cook with the chicken for extra 5 minutes or until the broccoli is cooked through but still crisp.

5. Serve hot with a side of wild rice and chopped green onion.

Nutrition: Energy (calories): 823 kcal Protein: 44.87 g Fat: 26.37 g Carbohydrates: 100.81 g Calcium, Ca172 mg Magnesium, Mg121 mg Phosphorus, P476 mg

313. Chicken with Lemon Caper Butter Sauce (Instant Pot Lean and Green Recipe)

Prep Time: 10 min | **Cook Time:** 5 min | **Serve:** 4

- 2 Chicken breasts
- low sodium pink Himalayan salt Black pepper
- 2 normal spoon extra-virgin olive oil 1 teaspoon minced garlic
- 1/2 cup unsalted chicken broth or stock 1/3 cup dry white wine
- 1/4 cup low sodium capers, rinsed and drained Juice from one lemon
- Lemon slices for garnish
- 2 Tablespoon parsley, for garnish

1. Set aside and season the chicken breast with salt and pepper.

2. Heat olive oil for 10 seconds in an instant pot in sauté mode. Add garlic and sauté for 10 seconds.

3. Add chicken broth or stock, white wine, capers, and lemon juice. Press cancel and close lid with a vent in sealing position. Cook on manual mode for 5 minutes.

4. When the instant pot beeps, do a 5-minute natural pressure release.

5. Drain chicken and place it on the cutting board. Use two forks to shred chicken into chunks.

6. Gently stir in the pan sauce and return to the instant pot. Add 1/2 cup of water or chicken bone broth.

7. Press sauté mode and bring to a boil for 2 minutes, stirring occasionally. Add lemon slices and parsley and serve.

Nutrition: Energy (calories): 326 kcal Protein: 32.76 g Fat: 18.52 g Carbohydrates: 6.42 g Calcium, Ca78 mg Magnesium, Mg43 mg Phosphorus, P301 mg

314. Tender Taco Chicken

Prep Time: 5 min | **Cook Time:** 10 min | **Serve:** 4

- 1 1/2 pounds boneless, skinless-chicken breast 1 Tablespoon, low salt Tex-Mex seasoning
- 1/2 C fresh chopped tomatoes or low carb, no sugar added salsa 1 tsp Stacey Hawkins Dash of Desperation Seasoning
- Your favorite on-program taco condiments

1. Cutting the chicken into 1/2-inch strips and sprinkle with the Tex Mex and dash of desperation seasoning.

2. In a large pan, heat the over medium and sauté the chicken for about 10 minutes, until cooked through and no longer pink.

3. Remove to a bowl and add tomatoes or salsa and toss to combine.

Nutrition: Energy (calories): 325 kcal Protein: 16.43 g Fat: 10.65 g Carbohydrates: 40.05 g Calcium, Ca47 mg Magnesium, Mg41 mg Phosphorus, P169 mg

315. Garlic Crusted Baby Back Ribs

Prep Time: 15 min | **Cook Time:** 1-h | **Serve:** 2

- 11 and 3/4 rack baby back ribs
- 2 tablespoon extra-virgin olive oil Kosher salt and freshly ground pepper 6 clove garlic
- 12 sprig thyme
- 8 sage leaves with stems 2 sprig rosemary

1. For the ribs, trim the excess fat and slice down the middle into one and a half-inch sections. Add olive-oil and season with salt and pepper.

2. Lay the food grilling rack over a gas or charcoal grill and grill for 1-hour basting with extra-virgin olive oil and coating each side.

3. And then line it in the middle of the grill for 8 minutes.

4. In the meantime, place the garlic and herbs on a large sheet of foil and wrap it tightly.

5. Transfer the ribs and ragout to a platter and drizzle with juices, and top with the foil's garlic and herbs.

Nutrition: Energy (calories): 19328 kcal Protein: 1710.36 g Fat: 1364.22 g Carbohydrates: 76.49 g Calcium, Ca1726 mg Magnesium, Mg2093 mg

316. Blistered Tomatoes with Balsamic and Goat Cheese

Prep Time: 5 min | **Cook Time:** 10 min | **Serve:** 12

- 9 oz. Mission Organics® Blue Corn Tortilla Chips 16 oz. Cream Cheese
- 8 oz. Goat Cheese
- 1 Clove Garlic, Minced
- ¼ Cup Chives – Fresh, Chopped
- 2 Tbsp. Scallions – Greens Chopped 1 ½ Cups Cherry Tomatoes, Chopped 2 Tbsp. Olive Oil
- 2 Tbsp. Balsamic Vinegar
- Salt and Black Pepper to Taste

1. Preheat the oven to 350°. Lightly grease a 2 ¼ cup ramekin with non-stick canola oil spray. Place 1/3 cup of the chip bag into the ramekin.

2. Preheat oven to 350°. Using an electric-mixer on medium-high speed, combine the cream cheese, 2 oz of the goat cheese, 2 tbsp. Of the chives, garlic, and scallions. Season with salt and black pepper.

3. Place the ramekin in the oven and cook for about 10 minutes until the mixture starts to bubble. Remove and allow for 5 minutes to cool. Stir in the tomatoes, drizzle with the oil and vinegar, and sprinkle with the remaining goat cheese and chives.

4. Serve with the remaining chips.

Nutrition: Energy (calories): 656 kcal Protein: 20.01 g Fat: 49.1 g Carbohydrates: 34.47 g Calcium, Ca443 mg Magnesium, Mg65 mg Phosphorus, P451 mg

317. Mediterranean Style Grilled Lamb Burgers

Prep Time: 20 min | **Cook Time:** 10 min | **Serve:** 8

- 2 lb. ground-lamb or a combination of lamb and beef (see cook's tip #1)
- 1 small-red-onion, grated 2 garlic cloves, minced
- 1 cup chopped fresh-parsley 10 mint leaves, chopped
- 2 and one-half tsp dry oregano 2 tsp ground cumin
- One-half tsp paprika
- One-half tsp cayenne-pepper, optional Kosher salt, and black pepper
- Extra virgin-olive-oil (I used Private Reserve Greek extra virgin olive oil)
- To Serve:
- Warm Greek pita bread or buns Homemade Tzatziki sauce Sliced tomatoes
- Sliced Green bell pepper Sliced cucumbers
- Sliced red onions
- Pitted Kalamata olives, sliced Crumbled feta

1.Combine the ground meat, the onion, the garlic, herbs, and spices in a large mixing bowl and lightly mix with your hands until combined. Do not over mix.
2.Form 8 patties approximately three-fourths inch thick.
3. Brush the olive oil on the outside of the patties and season all sides with salt and pepper.
4.Preheat the grill on medium-high.
5.Cook the patties for 5-6 minutes per side for medium-rare. Well done, burgers can be drier and a bit tougher.
6.Spread 2 Tbsp of Tzatziki sauce on both sides of the pita bread or buns.
7.Place the patties on the pita-bread and top with the sliced kalamata olives, sliced cucumbers, sliced red onions, sliced tomatoes, and grated feta cheese.
8.Wrap the pita bread or buns around the patties and serve.
Nutrition: Energy (calories): 336 kcal Protein: 36.43 g Fat: 17.36 g W Carbohydrates: 8.31 g Calcium, Ca186 mg Magnesium, Mg78 mg Phosphorus, P333 mg

318.Basil Chicken Sausage & Zucchini Spaghetti

Prep Time: 10 min | **Cook Time:** 10 min | **Serve:** 4
- 1 normal spoon extra-virgin olive oil, or more as needed 4 chicken sausage links, sliced
- 2 tablespoons minced garlic 1 large tomato, chopped
- 4 zucchinis, spiralized using the 3mm blade and trimmed 1/4 cup chopped fresh basil
- salt and ground black pepper to taste
- 1 pinch-red-pepper flakes, or more to taste 1/4 cup grated Parmesan cheese, or to taste

1.Heat-oil in a large-skillet over medium heat. Add chicken sausage and cook for about 4 minutes, or until lightly browned.
2.Add garlic, tomato, and zucchini noodles and cook until the zucchinis get tender and begin to soften.
3.Stir in basil. Add salt, pepper, and chili.
4.Move the mixture to a bowl and top with parmesan cheese before serving.
Nutrition: Energy (calories): 232 kcal Protein: 18.95 g Fat: 11.75 g Carbohydrates: 14.81 g Calcium, Ca125 mg Magnesium, Mg61 mg Phosphorus, P232 mg

319.Cheat Kebabs

Prep Time: 10 min | **Cook Time:** 25-35 min | **Serve:** 4

- 4 C mixed veggies (peppers, zucchini, mushrooms, yellow squash, etc.) chopped into 1 piece
- 1 1/2 pounds (24 oz) chicken breast meat cut into 1" chunks
- 1-2 Tablespoons Garlic Gusto Seasoning or Tuscan Fantasy Seasoning (or lemon, pepper, garlic, onion, parsley, salt & pepper) 4 teaspoons Stacey Hawkins Roasted Garlic Oil (or lemon, pepper, garlic, onion, parsley, salt & pepper)
- 1/4 C apple cider vinegar

1.Preheat the grill to medium-high. {Note: For temps, see grill manufacturer's instructions}. Spray grill with non-stick cooking spray.
2.Cut the veggies into 1 piece.
3.Pat the chicken-dry and season with the Gusto or Tuscan Fantasy or other favorite seasonings. {Note: Try and keep it simple. Salt, pepper, and onion powder work wonderfully}.
4.Pour the vinegar into a shallow bowl.
5.Dip the chicken pieces in the vinegar and then coat with the Gusto or Tuscan Fantasy.
6.Dip the vegetables into the vinegar and then place them on the chicken.
{Note: It is fine if the pieces overlap. We are creating a packet that will deliver wonderful flavors as it cooks. We'll account for the remaining vinegar in the marinade}.
7.Press the veggies and chicken into the Gusto or Tuscan fantasy and really press down hard! Stuff should be touching all surfaces of the chicken.
8.When your grill is smoking, but the kebabs on the grill and over medium-high heat, close the lid and cook for 10-15 minutes and then check to see if the chicken is done.
9.To have the chicken to be a little crispy after it is cooked, place the finished kebabs onto a hot grill for 1 minute just before you serve.
10.Serve with fresh pita and various toppings and the remaining marinade.
Nutrition: Energy (calories): 363 kcal Protein: 38.97 g Fat: 18.84 g Carbohydrates: 8.15 g Calcium, Ca46 mg Magnesium, Mg71 mg Phosphorus, P342 mg

320.Lemony Roasted Beets

Prep Time: 10 min | **Cook Time:** 20 min | **Serve:** 6
- 6 Cups red beets cut into three-fourth chunks 1 Tablespoon olive oil
- 1 Tablespoon salt
- 1 Tablespoon pepper
- 1 Tablespoon onion and garlic 1 Tablespoon fresh lemon juice 1/2 cup crumbled feta cheese

1.Preheat oven to 400 degrees F.
2.Sauté the onions, garlic, and lemon juice in the olive oil with salt and pepper for about 3 minutes.
3.After sautéing the onions and lemon juice, spread the beets evenly in a lightly oiled baking dish.
4.Sprinkle the crumbled feta cheese over the beets.
5.Pour the sautéed onions mixture over the beets.
6.Bake the lemony roasted beets for 20 minutes, and serve.
Nutrition: Energy (calories): 206 kcal Protein: 3.84 g Fat: 5.12 g Carbohydrates: 38.82 g Calcium, Ca91 mg Magnesium, Mg39 mg Phosphorus, P87 mg

321.Creamy Paprika Pork

Prep Time: 10 min | **Cook Time:** 15 min | **Serve:** 4

- 1 pork-tenderloin (1 pound), cut into 1-inch cubes 1 little spoon all-purpose flour
- 4 little spoons paprika 3/4 teaspoon salt 1/4 teaspoon pepper 1 little spoon butter
- ¾ cup heavy-whipping cream Hot-cooked egg-noodles or rice Minced fresh parsley, optional

1.Preheat oven to 355 F. Coat a large baking dish with vegetable cooking spray. In a bowl, toss pork with flour, paprika, salt, and pepper until coated. Heat butter in a large skillet over medium-high heat until it starts to sizzle.

2.Add pork, sauté for 3 minutes. Add cream; cover and bring to a boil, reduce heat, simmer for 15 minutes.

3.Serve over hot cooked noodles or rice. Sprinkle with parsley if desired.

Nutrition: Energy (calories): 308 kcal Protein: 32.86 g Fat: 17.9 g Carbohydrates: 2.89 g Calcium, Ca40 mg Magnesium, Mg42 mg

322.Tender & Tangy BBQ Ribs

Prep Time: 15 min | **Cook Time:** 45 min | **Serve:** 6

- 1/4 C apple-ider-vinegar 1/4 C water
- 2 lbs. boneless-pork ribs, all visible fat trimmed off & discarded 1-2 normal spoons SH Cinnamon Chipotle
- Sugar-Free BBQ Sauce – Mesquite Style (or your favorite)

1.Preheat oven to 350 degrees.

2. Mix the apple cider vinegar with water in a small tub. Place the ribs in a large plastic bag that can be resealed. Pour the apple cider vinegar mixture and the ribs into a plastic jar. Seal the bag and put it for a minimum of 15 minutes in the refrigerator.

3. On a rimmed-baking mat, put the ribs and with a brush, generously coat both sides of the ribs with barbecue sauce. Sprinkle cinnamon chipotle sugar-free syrup on both sides of the ribs.

4.Cook ribs in the preheated 350-degree oven for 45 minutes. Take out and brush with more BBQ sauce. Then place back in the oven for another 5 to 10 minutes.

5.Let it cool for a minute, then serve.

Nutrition: Energy (calories): 221 kcal Protein: 31.49 g Fat: 8.57 g Carbohydrates: 2.75 g Calcium, Ca53 mg Magnesium, Mg37 mg Phosphorus, P310 mg

323.Tender Beef Stew with Rosemary

Prep Time: 20 min | **Cook Time:** 2 h | **Serve:** 8

- 4 slices-cut bacon into thin strips
- After trimming, 4 pounds beef chuck roast bits - cut into 1 1/2 - 2- inch pieces
- 1/2 small spoon of kosher salt I use 1/2 small spoon of black pepper with Morton coarse kosher salt
- 1 1/2 cups chopped onion
- 2 cups of fresh (peeled) or frozen pearl onions
- 2 1/2 cups of peeled carrot pieces and cut into 1 - 1 1/2-inch of 1 tablespoon of oil if necessary3-4 cloves garlic
- 2 sprigs of rosemary
- 4 sprigs of thyme
- 2 bay leaves dried
- Two cups of low-sodium beef broth, two tablespoons of soy sauce
- 2-3 tablespoons of butter, 2-3 tablespoons of flour, softened

- If required, 1/2 teaspoon kosher salt
- 2 tablespoons of chopped fresh flat-leaf parsley – Optional

1.Place the meat in a large mixing bowl. Sprinkle with salt and pepper.

2.In a medium-sized sauté pan put the 2 tablespoons of oil, add the bacon strips. Cook for about 2-3 minutes.

3.Add the onion, carrot, pearl onions (fresh or frozen), garlic cloves, and rosemary springs. Until the vegetables begin to soften, cook for 5-6 minutes.

4.Add the vegetables and bacon to the meat mixture.

5.Add the thyme, bay leaves, and broth.

6.Refrigerate until ready to cook the stew. This can be done a day ahead.

7.After refrigerating the stew, let the stew come to room temperature.

8.Heat the oven to 350 °F.

9.Grease a large baking pan (if needed) and put the meat and vegetables into it.

10.With the gravy, cover the meat and vegetables. Cook for about 90-120 minutes until the meat starts to get tender.

11.Take the meat out of the baking pan and place it on a platter or in a large bowl using 2 forks to shred the pot's meat.

12.Place the meat back in the potting mixture. Add the soy sauce and the butter and stir it.

13.Reduce the heat to medium-low. If the stew starts to get very thick and dry, add a little more broth and stir.

14.Mix the 2 tablespoons of flour with 1/2 cup of water until very thin paste forms. Stir into the stew while whisking regularly. Add a little-extra-water if needed if the stew gets too dry. Add the salt and mustard and mix well at the end.

15.Add the parsley to the stew at the end.

Nutrition: Energy (calories): 474 kcal Protein: 51.48 g Fat: 22.46 g Carbohydrates: 18.46 g Calcium, Ca85 mg Magnesium, Mg64 mg Phosphorus, P520 mg

324.Glazed Ginger Chicken and Green

Prep Time: 5 min | **Cook Time:** 20-35 min | **Serve:** 4

- 1 Tablespoon Toasted Sesame Ginger Seasoning
- 1 1/2 pounds boneless-skinless-chicken (breasts or thighs) nonstick cooking spray
- ¼ cup low-sodium soy sauce ½ cup water
- 4 cups fresh green beans, ends snipped

1.Preheat oven to 350F.

2.In a medium bowl, add the chicken, ginger seasoning, and soy sauce. Toss to combine. Marinate at room temperature.

3.Spray a large baking sheet; add the chicken mixture and spread evenly.

4. Place the sheet in the oven on the center rack and roast it for 20 minutes. If desired, baste the chicken with the liquid from the bowl (2- 4 tablespoons) three times while roasting.

5.Remove the baking sheet from the oven.

6.Add the green beans (in the bowl) and water; cover the pan with aluminum foil and bake for 10 to 15 more minutes.

7.Remove the pan and stir the beans. Bake for a further five to seven minutes, or until the beans are fluffy.

8.Serve and sprinkle with some fresh ground pepper.

Nutrition: Energy (calories): 259 kcal Protein: 41.77 g Fat: 6.23 g Carbohydrates: 8.04 g Calcium, Ca77 mg Magnesium, Mg86 mg Phosphorus, P435 mg

325.Zucchini Pappardelle with Sausage

Prep Time: 5 min | **Cook Time:** 15 min | **Serve:** 4

- • 1 ½ lbs. Lean turkey or chicken sausage, seasoned in Italy (your choice is hot or sweet) 2 C chopped tomatoes
- Stacey Hawkins Garlic and Spring Onion Seasoning 1 Tablespoon (1 capful)
- • 4 cups of fresh zucchini noodles (about 3 cups) zucchinis, 8 long)
- 4 teaspoons Olive Oil
- A little bit of Stacey Hawkins Dash of Desperation Seasoning

1.Wash and gently dry zucchini. Cut it lengthwise into spaghetti sized strips; using a vegetable peeler, peel zucchini into thin shreds. Transfer zucchini to a salad spinner. Sprinkle with 1 teaspoon of the olive oil and a Dash of Desperation Seasoning. Toss gently to coat with oil and seasoning.

2.In a skillet, brown sausage; drain fat and transfer sausage to a large pot. Add 2 teaspoons olive oil, chopped tomatoes, and Stacey Hawkins Garlic and Spring Onion Seasoning. Cook over high heat until tomatoes are softened, about 5 minutes.

3.Fill a large pot with generously salted water. Bring water to boil and cook zucchini pasta for 7 minutes. While you are cooking zucchini, add sausage, tomato, and seasoning combination to the zucchini pasta and cook together on medium heat.

4.Use tongs to submerge zucchini noodles one at a time into a large pot of boiling water with 1 teaspoon olive oil stirred in. Once done, strain it along with other ingredients.

5.Preheat oven to 350 degrees. Transfer all ingredients to a large casserole or baking dish and mix thoroughly. Top dish with fresh grated Parmesan cheese. Bake for about 15 minutes in the preheated oven, until the cheese is bubbly and golden brown.6.This dish is equally delicious served either hot or cold. Serve in a bowl and stir in a little bit of pasta water.

Nutrition: Energy (calories): 801 kcal Protein: 33.31 g Fat: 51.13 g Carbohydrates: 49.95 g Calcium, Ca58 mg Magnesium, Mg41 mg Phosphorus, P321 mg

326.Garlic Crusted Flank Steak with Roasted Tomato Relish

Prep Time: 5 min and 1 h refrigerate | **Cook Time:** 25 min | **Serve:** 6

- Steak
- 2 tablespoons chopped fresh thyme
- 2 normal spoons chopped fresh rosemary 1 tablespoon chopped fresh tarragon
- 2 garlic cloves, minced 2 teaspoons salt.
- 1 ½ little spoons ground black-pepper 2 1 ½ pound flank steaks
- 1 tablespoon olive oil Tomatoes
- 2 cups halved cherry tomatoes
- 1 cup chopped fresh Italian parsley
- 1/4 cup of Kalamata pitted olives coarsely chopped or other black olives brine-cured
- ¼ cup coarsely-chopped pitted green olives with brine-cured
- 1/4 cup chopped new basil
- 1/4 cup of extra virgin olive oil
- 2 tablespoons Sherry wine vinegar

1.Preheat oven to 375 degrees F.

2. Process the tomatoes in a food processor until smooth. Pulse the beef herbs into the sprigs, along with the garlic, salt, and pepper, until the mixture is finely chopped and the herbs are gone. Drizzle in the olive oil with the engine running. The relish can be made, covered, and refrigerated a day in advance.

3.On a work surface, lay the steaks out side by side. Spoon a third of the relish over the steaks, spread it over the meat with a spatula, and be careful not to tear it. Sprinkle with the herb-garlic mixture and roll up the steaks lengthwise. Place them and drizzle them with olive oil in a baking dish. Let stand at room temperature for 30 minutes.

4.Roast the steaks for 10 minutes. Turn them and continue roasting until medium-rare (135 degrees F) or medium (140 degrees F), about 10 minutes more. The steaks can rest up to 10 minutes before slicing.

5.In a bowl, to make the tomatoes, toss together the tomatoes, herbs, olives, and basil with the vinegar and oil; season to taste with salt and pepper.

6.Cut the steak rolls crosswise on the diagonal into 1 1/2-inch-thick slice. Serve the steak between the tomato slices

Nutrition: Energy (calories): 2236 kcal Protein: 334.68 g Fat: 84.92 g Carbohydrates: 10.36 g Calcium, Ca372 mg Magnesium, Mg359 mg Phosphorus, P3165 mg

327.Seafood & Scallions Creole

Prep Time: 10 min | **Cook Time:** 30 min | **Serve:** 5

- 4 regular butter spoons 1 big onion, diced 1 celery rib, diced
- 1 green bell pepper, 2 cloves of garlic, 1/2 teaspoon of thyme salt, 1/2 teaspoon of thyme salt
- One-half teaspoon black pepper
- ½ teaspoon cayenne pepper 1 Tablespoon flour
- 1/3 cup dry white wine (optional)
- 1 15 oz of tomatoes or around 1 ¼ cups of fresh tomatoes peeled and diced
- 1 cup stock of chicken, 2 bay leaves
- 2 lb of spicy pepper sauce, such as Tabasco, to taste. Oh, huge uncooked shrimp (about 32)
- For serving, 6-8 cups of hot cooked rice
- 2 green onions for garnish, sliced,

1.In a big saucepan or Dutch oven, heat 2 tablespoons of the butter over medium-high. Add the onion, celery, bell pepper, and garlic and cook stirring, until softened, about 3 minutes.

2.Ad the shrimp and cook, stirring, until they just turn pink, about 2 minutes. Stir in the salt, thyme, black pepper, and cayenne.

3.Stir in the remaining 2 normal spoons of butter and melt. Stir in the flour and cook, stirring, for 1 minute, until it is cooked.

4.Stir in the wine, tomatoes, stock, bay leaves, and hot pepper sauce. Reduce heat to medium-low and simmer for 16 minutes, periodically stirring.

5.Remove bay leaves. Using a spoon, push the shrimp mixture to one side of the pot. Pour the eggs into the opposite side, and begin to scramble. Stir the eggs into the shrimp mixture and again push to one side. Pour the rice into the pot and mix it in. Cover the pot, reduce the heat to low, and cook for 5 minutes longer to heat through.

6.Sprinkle with green onions when serving

Nutrition: Energy (calories): 1017 kcal Protein: 89.27 g Fat: 52.71 g Carbohydrates: 95.46 g Calcium, Ca322 mg Magnesium, Mg1400 mg Phosphorus, P3672 mg

328. Sweet & Smoky Pulled Chicken

Prep Time: 10 min | **Cook Time:** 20 min | **Serve:** 6

- 750 g skinless and boneless chicken breasts (1.65 lb.) 400 ml unsweetened passata tomato (sauce) (13.5 fl oz) 100 ml apple cider vinegar (3.5 fl oz)
- 3 tbsp Erythritol or Swerve (30 g/ 1.1 oz)
- Optional: 1 tbsp of molasses (20 g/0.7 oz) - see note 1 tsp of sea salt above
- 1 black pepper tablespoon
- 1 TL garlic powder
- 1/4 tsp of Cayenne-pepper or 1 tbsp of smoked paprika to taste 3 tbsp of amino coconut (45 ml)
- 1/4 Cup of Virgin Olive Oil Extra (60 ml)
- Optional: 1 cup of sour cream, full-fat yogurt, or fresh cream for serving.

1. In a large bowl, place the chicken breasts and cover with the tomato passata. To that, add the ground or whole peppercorns, salt, black pepper, and garlic powder. Toss to combine and transfer to the crockpot. Toss again to coat and let it cook on low for 5 hours.
2. Cook the rice according to the direction of the box and move it to a big bowl. Add the sour cream, coconut cream, and Swerve. Whisk until combined.
3. Finely mince the fresh parsley. Mix the parsley and the smoked paprika with the rice. To serve, pile the rice onto the chicken and top with the sour cream or yogurt or creme fraiche.

Nutrition: Energy (calories): 2924 kcal Protein: 85.2 g Fat: 27.19 g Carbohydrates: 515.51 g Calcium, Ca578 mg Magnesium, Mg347 mg Phosphorus, P1475 mg

329. Garlic Crusted BBQ Baby Back Ribs

Prep Time: 15 min | **Cook Time:** 1-h | **Serve:** 2

- 11 and three-fourth rack baby back ribs 2 tablespoons extra-virgin olive oil Kosher salt and freshly ground pepper 6 clove garlic
- 12 sprig thyme
- 8 sage leaves with stems 2 sprig rosemary

1. To 350F, preheat the oven. With salt and pepper, season the ribs and poke them all over with a fork. Rub both sides with olive oil and put them over a baking sheet in a roasting rack package.
2. Sprinkle garlic over the meat, and place 4 sage leaves, 4 sage leaves with stems, and 4 rosemary leaves on top of the meat.
3. Bake the ribs for 30 minutes. Reduce the oven temperature to 310F and bake the ribs for 25 minutes. Place 4 more sage leaves, 4 sage leaves with stems, another 30 all the and brush
4. And 4 rosemary leaves on top of the meat. Bake for minutes.
5. Place 1 cup of barbecue sauce in a bowl. Scrape
6. Sauce from the roaster. Return the ribs to the pan the meat with the sauce. Bake for 15 additional minutes.
7. Scrape the sauce again from the roaster and spread it over the meat. More sauce.
8. Remove the meat from the oven and serve with

Nutrition: Energy (calories): 19863 kcal Protein: 1754.29 g Fat: 1401.07 g Carbohydrates: 82.05 g Calcium, Ca1903 mg Magnesium, Mg2170 mg Phosphorus, P12527 mg

330. Juicy Rosemary Pulled Pork

Prep Time: 10 min | **Cook Time:** 35 min | **Serve:** 4

- 1 tbsp olive-oil 1 tsp sea salt
- 1/2 tsp ground black-pepper
- 4 boneless center-cut pork chops
- 6-8 cloves garlic, peeled and whole

1. Combine olive-oil, salt, and pepper in a small bowl. Rub into the pork chops. Refrigerate for 30 minutes.
2. Rub 2 cloves of garlic into the pork chops 2. Rub 2 cloves of garlic into the pork chops3. Preheat the grill. Grill pork chops 6-8 minutes on each side or until done.
3. Chop the remaining cloves of garlic. Add to a bowl with the rosemary, onion, and barbeque sauce. Mix to blend.
4. Preheat the oven to 325-degree F / 160 C.
5. Thinly slice the red-onion and place in a bowl. Add enough balsamic vinegar to cover and let marinate for 10 minutes.
6. In the same bowl, add the tomato halves. Sprinkle with garlic salt and olive oil. Stir to coat everything evenly.
7. In a baking dish, put the onions at the bottom of the dish. Place the pork chops on top and pour over any leftover marinade.
8. Cook covered for 30-35 minutes.
9. To make the sauce, place all the ingredients into a blender and blend until smooth.
10. Serve pork with sauce and lime wedges on the side.

Nutrition: Energy (calories): 265 kcal Protein: 39.52 g Fat: 10.02 g Carbohydrates: 1.98 g Calcium, Ca44 mg Magnesium, Mg48 mg Phosphorus, P400 mg

331. Slow-Cooked Chicken with Fire Roasted Tomatoes

Prep Time: 10 min | **Cook Time:** 3 10 min | **Serve:** 4

- 1 1/2 lbs. boneless, skinless chicken breast
- 1 15oz can fire-roasted tomatoes (any variety- BUT make sure no extra added sugar)
- 2 T salt
- 2 T ground black pepper 2 T oil
- 2 T (one capful) sage
- 2 T (one capful) black pepper
- 2 T (one capful) onion and garlic

1. Add oil and chicken breasts to the slow cooker.
2. Pour a bottle of spices over the chicken and cover.
3. Cook on high for 3 hours.
4. Add fire-roasted tomatoes and cook for additional 10 minutes
5. Using a handheld blender or an upright blender, blend 6 tbsp of the liquid into the chicken.
6. Remove chicken and place on a plate.
7. Shred chicken into smaller pieces using two forks.
8. Serve over white or brown rice.

Nutrition: Energy (calories): 400 kcal Protein: 17.7 g Fat: 17.12 g Carbohydrates: 45.65 g Calcium, Ca131 mg Magnesium, Mg62 mg Phosphorus, P188 mg

332. Finger Licking BBQ Crock Pot Chicken

Prep Time: 10 min | **Cook Time:** 6 h | **Serve:** 4

- 1.5 lbs. – Boneless-Skinless-Chicken (thigh or breasts) 1 T – Stacey Hawkins Honey BBQ Seasoning
- 1 T – Stacey Hawkins Garlic & Spring Onion Seasoning 1 T – Phoenix Sunrise Seasoning

1. In a slow cooker, mix all of the seasonings.
2. Remove from the chicken any fat and skin and cut into equally-sized pieces.

3.Add chicken pieces to the seasonings in the slow cooker.

4.Drizzle 2T honey BBQ over the chicken pieces. Mix.

5.Cook for 5 ½ hours on a low setting.

6.Before serving, add one-fourth cup BBQ sauce to the chicken in the crockpot.

7.Mix thoroughly and cook for 6 minutes on high to let the BBQ sauce cook into the chicken.

Nutrition: Energy (calories): 400 kcal Protein: 17.7 g Fat: 17.12 g Carbohydrates: 45.65 g Calcium, Ca131 mg Magnesium, Mg62 mg Phosphorus, P188 mg

333.Big Mac in a Bowl

Prep Time: 10 min | **Cook Time:** 10 min | **Serve:** 4
- 1 lb lean ground beef lean beef
- 1 tbsp of onion powder
- 1 Tbsp garlic Powder
- 2 or 3 dashes Worcestershire sauce
- 8 cups of roman lettuce
- 16 Pickle slices
- Fat cheddar reduced in 4 oz
- 8 tbsps of red, diced onion
- 2 diced Tomato Roma
- 8 Lite Thousand Island Dressing Spoons

1. Cook the ground beef in a nonstick skillet over medium-high heat. Drain any excess fat when the beef is brown and no longer pink in the middle. Add the ground onion, garlic powder, and Worcestershire sauce. Only set aside.

2. Attach the top of the lettuce with 2 cups of sliced romaine lettuce, pickles, tomatoes, onions, cheese, and ground beef.

3. Put 2 tbsps of Thousand Island dressing on top of the salad.

Nutrition: 1; Calories: 390; Sugar: 7.4g; Fat: 20.7; Carbohydrates: 15.4g;Fiber: 4.5g; Protein: 34.9g

334.Coconut Flour Chicken Nuggets

- Thighs of 1 pound of skinless chicken
- 3/4 cup mayo
- ⅓ cup of flour with arrowroot
- ¼ cup of flour for coconut
- ½ Tbsp powdered onion
- ½ Tbsp powdered garlic
- ¼ tbsp of turmeric
- ½ tbsp of basil dried
- ½ tbsp oregano
- ¼ tbsp Smoked Paprika
- ¼ tsp of cayenne
- ¼ tbsp of salt
- ⅛ tbsp of black pepper

1. Preheat to 450 ° F in the oven.

2. Put the parchment paper into a large baking sheet.

3. Combine the arrowroot starch, coconut meal, and spices in a dish.

4. Dip every piece of chicken into the mayo (or wash the eggs), then dip into the mixture of coconut flour. On the baking sheet, put the chicken and repeat for the remaining pieces of chicken.

5. Bake for twenty minutes at 450 ° F or until the juices from the chicken are clear.

335.Skinny Chicken Salad

Prep Time: 25 min | **Cook Time:** 15 min | **Serve:** 5
- Boneless 1.5 lbs, skinless breast of chicken, fried ani finely shredded

- 2 chopped green onions
- 2 halved and chopped celery stalks
- 1/3 cup of congrats parsley
- ½ cup of paleo mayo
- 1/2 C Greek yogurt
- Juice from 1 lemon
- Salt and pepper

1. Chicken's generous season with salt and pepper and cook in a crockpot, instant pot, or cooked poach and no longer pink.

2. Move the cooked chicken to your stand mixer or cutting board to finely shred. Use the paddle connector and turn it to medium speed while using a stand mixer and let it be shredded to your taste.

3. Place shredded chicken in a medium side mixing bowl to all other ingredients. Whisk to combine.

4. Serve over greens, on crostini's, etc., in a wrap, as a dip.

5. In an airtight jar in the fridge for 5 days.

336.Chicken Marsala

Prep Time: 15 min | **Cook Time:** 20 min | **Serve:** 4
- 1 1/4 cups of dry marsala wine
- 1 1/4 cups of unsalted chicken broth
- 2 (10 - 11 oz) pounded, boneless skinless chicken breasts Salt and freshly ground black pepper 1/3 cup of all purpose flour
- 2 Tbsp of unsalted butter
- 2 Tbsp of olive oil
- 8 oz. of sliced cremini mushrooms
- 3 1 Tbsp minced garlic cloves
- 1 tsp of minced fresh thyme
- 1 tsp of minced fresh oregano
- 1 1/2 tsp of cornstarch whisked with 1 Tbsp chicken broth (well combined)
- 1/3 cup of heavy cream
- 1 Tbsp of minced fresh parsley

1. To a medium saucepan, add marsala wine and chicken broth. Heat over medium-high-heat, bring to a boil, reduce to medium heat, and cook gently until it is reduced to 1 cup, about 15 min.

2. With salt and pepper, season the chicken on both sides.

3. Dredge in the flour mixture on either side.

4. In a 12-inch skillet over medium-high heat, melt 1 Tbsp of butter with 1 Tbsp of olive oil. Add pieces of chicken and let it sear until it is cooked through (165 in the center), turning around 10-12 minutes once halfway through.

5. Move your chicken to an oven. Tent on the foil.

6. Reduce burner to medium flame. Melt the remaining 1 tbsp of butter and 1 tbsp of olive oil, then add the mushrooms.

7. Stir in mushrooms, tossing just periodically (and growing the burner temp slightly as required to promote browning), until the mushrooms have shrunk and are golden brown, around 8 min. During last one minute of sautéing, add garlic.

8. Then pour in marsala reduction, thyme and oregano, remove the pan from fire.

9. Return to flame, bring to a simmer and scrape brown bits from the rim, then whisk in a mixture of cornstarch chicken broth. Delete to thickened.

10. Stir off heat in heavy cream, and season with salt and pepper to taste. Put the chicken breasts back in the pan, then spoon the sauce over the top.

11. Sprinkle and serve immediately with parsley.

Nutrition: Calories 448, Fat 24 g; Cholesterol 133 mg; Sodium 200 mg; Potassium 944 mg; Carbo. 11 g; Fiber 1 g; Sugar 3 g; Protein 33 g; Calcium 45 mg; Iron 2 mg

337. Turkey Meatloaf

Active Time: 30 min | **Total Time:** 1 1/2 h

- 1 1/2 cups of onion finely chopped
- 1 tbsp of minced garlic
- 1 tsp of olive oil
- 1 medium of carrot
- 3/4 pound trimmed and very finely chopped cremini mushrooms 1 tsp of salt
- 1/2 tsp of black pepper
- 1 1/2 tsps of Worcestershire sauce
- fresh parsley, finely chopped (1/3 cup)
- 1/4 cup of plus 1 tbsp ketchup
- Fine fresh bread crumbs (1 cup)
- 1/3 cup of milk
- 1 whole of a lightly beaten large egg
- 1 large lightly beaten egg white
- 1 1/4 pound of ground turkey Accompaniment: roasted red pepper tomato sauce

1. Preheat the oven to 204.444°C.
2. In a 11-inch nonstick skillet, cook the onion and garlic in oil over moderate heat, stirring, until the onion is tender, around 2 minutes. Add carrot and cook, stirring for about 3 minutes, until softened. Add mushrooms, 1/2 tsp of salt, and 1/4 tsp of pepper and cook, occasionally stirring, until liquid mushrooms are evaporated and very tender, 10 to 15 minutes. Stir in Worcestershire sauce, parsley, and ketchup for 3 tsps, then switch vegetables to a large bowl and cool down.
3. In a small cup, mix together the bread crumbs and milk and let stand for 5 minutes. Stir in the white egg and egg, and add to the vegetables. Apply the turkey and remaining 1/2 tsp salt and 1/4 tsp pepper to the mixture of vegetables and blend well with hands. (The mixture was going to be very humid.)
4. In a lightly oiled 13- by 9- by 2-inch metal baking pan, shape a 9- by 5-inch oval loaf and brush meatloaf evenly with the remaining 2 tablespoons ketchup. Bake in the center of the oven until 170 ° F, 50 to 55 minutes of thermometer inserted into meatloaf registers.
5. Let meatloaf to stand five minutes before serving.

338. Chicken Piccata

- ½ cup of reduced-sodium chicken broth 2 tsp of cornstarch
- 2 (8 ounces) skinless, boneless chicken breast halved ¼ cup of all-purpose flour ½ tsp of kosher salt
- black pepper freshly ground (1 tsp)
- 4 tsp of olive oil
- 4 lemon slices
- 2 tsp of butter
- 3 large minced cloves garlic
- ¼ cup of dry white wine
- 2 tbsp of lemon juice
- 1 ½ tbsp. of drained capers
- 1 ½ tsp of snipped fresh thyme

1. Stir together the broth and the cornstarch in a small bowl; set aside. Flatten the chicken between two sheets of plastic wrap until 1/2 inch thick using the flat side of a meat mallet.

Stir together rice, salt, and pepper in a shallow dish. Sprinkle the chicken into a mixture of flour, turning to cover.
2. Hot oil over medium-high heat in a 12-inch nonstick skillet. Add chicken; cook 8 to 9 minutes, turning once. Withdraw from the skillet; keep warm. Add lemon slices to skillet if necessary. Cook for 30 to 60 seconds or, turning once, until brown. Take off the skillet.
3. For the sauce, melt butter over medium in skillet. Add the garlic for 30 seconds, cook and stir. Put the wine in carefully. Cook for one to two minutes or until slightly thick, stirring up crusty brown bits to scrape. Stir in a mixture of cornstarch. Take to boil; minimize heat. Simmer for 1 minute, or until dense. Incorporate lemon juice, capers, and thyme.
4. Drizzle the chicken with the sauce and top with the slices of lemon and extra thyme.

Nutrition: 249 calories; total fat 9.6g 15% DV; saturated fat 2.5g; cholesterol 88mg 29% DV; sodium 354mg 14% DV; potassium 461mg 13% DV; carbohydrates 9.7g 3% DV; fiber 0.6g 2% DV; sugarg; protein 27.2g 54% DV; exchange other carbs 1; vitamin a iu 274IU; vitamin c 7mg; folate 39mcg; calcium 23mg; iron 1mg; magnesium 39mg.

339. Chicken, Bell Pepper & Carrot Curry

Prep Time: 15 min | **Cook Time:** 12 min | **Serve:** 4

- 1 (14-ounce) can unsweetened coconut milk
- 2 tablespoons Thai red curry paste
- 1 pound of boneless-chicken breast cut into thin pieces
- 1 cup carrots, peeled and sliced
- 1½ cups green bell pepper, seeded and cubed
- ½ cup onion, sliced ¼ cup chicken broth
- 2 tablespoon fish sauce
- 1 tablespoon fresh lime juice
- 12 fresh basil leaves, chopped
- Salt and ground black pepper, as required.

1. Add the oil to Instant Pot and select "Sauté." Then add half of coconut milk and curry paste and cook for about 1-2 minutes.
2. Press "Cancel" and stir in remaining coconut milk, chicken, carrot, bell pepper, onion, and broth.
3. Secure the lid and switch to the location of the "Seal".
4. Cook on "Manual" with "High Pressure" for about 5 minutes.
5. Press "Cancel" and carefully do a "Quick" release.
6. Remove the lid and select "Sauté".
7. For the rest of the ingredients, stir in and cook for 4-5 minutes or so.
8. Stir in the salt and black pepper and press "Cancel".

Nutrition: Calories: 282 | fat: 24.0g | protein: 10.1g | carbs: 6.9g | net carbs: 2.8g | fiber: 4.1g

340. Chicken Chili

Prep Time: 15 min | **Cook Time:** 20 min | **Serve:** 4

- 3 (5-ounce) chicken breasts
- 1 carrot, peeled and chopped
- 1 celery stalk, chopped
- 1 medium yellow onion, chopped
- 2 garlic cloves, chopped
- 1 teaspoon dried oregano
- 1 teaspoon ground cumin
- Salt and ground black pepper, as required
- ½ cup unsweetened coconut milk
- 1 cup chicken broth

1.Ad all the ingredients to the Instant Pot pot and mix to blend.
2.Secure the lid and switch to the location of the "Seal".
3.Select "Poultry" and just use the default time of 20 minutes.
4.Press "Cancel" and do a "Natural" release.
5.Remove the lid and, with a slotted spoon, transfer the chicken breasts into a bowl.
6.With 2 forks, shred chicken breasts and then return into the pot.

Nutrition: Calories: 306 | fat: 15.6g | protein: 33.4g | carbs: 7.1g | net carbs: 5.2g | fiber: 1.9g

341.*Beef and Kale Casserole*
Prep Time: 15 min | **Cook Time:** 29 min | **Serve:** 4
- 2 tablespoons olive oil
- 2 cups fresh kale, trimmed and chopped
- 1 1/3 cups scallion, sliced
- 8 egg, beaten
- 1½ cups cooked beef, shredded
- Salt and ground black pepper, as required

1. In the Instant Pot, add oil and pick "Sauté". Then add the kale and scallion and cook for about 3-4 minutes.
2. Press "Cancel" and transfer the kale mixture into a bowl.
3. Add eggs and beef and mix well.
4. Move the mixture into a baking dish that is lightly greased.
5. Arrange a steamer trivet in the lower part of the Instant Pot and pour 1½ cups of water.
6. Place the baking dish on top of the trivet.
7. Secure the lid and turn to the "Seal" position.
8. Cook on "Manual" with "High Pressure" for about 25 minutes.
9. Press "Cancel" and carefully do a "Quick" release.
10. Remove the lid and serve immediately.

Nutrition: calories: 345 | fat: 20.2g | protein: 34.2g | carbs: 6.6g | net carbs: 5.2g | fiber: 1.4g

342.*Beef and Mushroom Soup*
Prep Time: 15 min | **Cook Time:** 15 min | **Serve:** 4
- 2 teaspoons olive oil
- 1 pound sirloin steak, trimmed and cubed
- 1 small carrot, peeled and chopped
- 1 bell pepper, seeded and chopped
- 1 celery stalk, chopped
- 1 onion, chopped
- 8 ounces fresh mushrooms, sliced
- 2 cups beef broth
- 1½ cups water
- 1 cup tomatoes, crushed
- 1½ tablespoons fresh oregano chopped 1 bay leaf
- 2 teaspoon garlic powder
- Salt and ground black pepper, as required

1. Add the oil in an Instant Pot Mini and select "Sauté". Now, add the steak and cook for about 4-5 minutes or until browned.
2. Add the carrots, bell pepper, celery, and onion and cook for about 2-3 minutes.
3. Attach the mushrooms, then cook for 4-5 minutes or so.
4. Push and stir in the remaining ingredients with "Cancel".
5. Secure the lid and turn to the "Seal" position.
6. Select "Soup" and just use the default time of 15 minutes.
7. Press "Cancel" and do a "Quick" release.
8. Remove the lid and serve hot.

Nutrition: Calories: 298 | fat: 10.6g | protein: 39.9g | carbs: 10g | net carbs: 6.7g | fiber: 3.3g

343.*Beef & Veggies Stew*
Prep Time: 15 min | **Cook Time:** 45 min | **Serve:** 4
- 1¼ pounds beef stew meat, cubed
- 2 small zucchinis, chopped
- ½ pound small broccoli florets
- 2 garlic cloves, minced
- ½ cup chicken broth
- 1 tablespoon curry powder
- 1 teaspoon ground cumin
- Salt and ground black pepper, as required 7 ounces unsweetened coconut milk 2 tablespoons fresh cilantro, chopped.

1. In the pot of Instant Pot, place all ingredients except coconut milk and cilantro and stir to combine.
2. Secure the lid and turn to the "Seal" position.
3. For about 45 minutes cook on "Manual" with "High Pressure".
4. Click "Cancel" and perform a "Natural" release carefully for about 10 minutes. Then do a "Quick" release.
5. Stir in the coconut milk and remove the cap.
6. Serve immediately with the garnishing of cilantro.

Nutrition: Calories: 389 | fat: 17.9g | protein: 46.7g | carbs: 10g | net carbs: 7g | fiber: 3g

344.*Beef & Carrot Chili*
Prep Time: 15 min | **Cook Time:** 40 min | **Serve:** 4
- 1 tablespoon olive oil
- 1 pound ground beef
- ½ green bell pepper, seeded and chopped
- 1 small onion, chopped
- 1 medium carrot, peeled and chopped
- 2 tomatoes, chopped finely
- 1 jalapeño pepper, chopped
- Salt and ground black-pepper, as required 1 tablespoon fresh parsley, chopped
- 1 tablespoon Worcestershire sauce
- 4 teaspoons red chili powder
- 1 teaspoon paprika
- 1 teaspoon ground cumin

1. Add the Instant Pot oil and pick 'Sauté.' Then add the beef and cook for
approximately 5 minutes or until fully browned.
2. Push and stir in the remaining ingredients with 'Cancel'.
3. Secure the lid and turn to the "Seal" position.
4. Choose 'Soup' and use the default time of 35 minutes only.
5. Press "Cancel" and do a "Natural" release.
6. Remove the lid and serve hot.

Nutrition: Calories: 287 | fat: 11.4g | protein: 36g | carbs: 9g | net carbs: 6g | fiber: 3g

345.*Beef & Carrot Curry*
Prep Time: 15 min | **Cook Time:** 33 min | **Serve:** 4
- 2 tablespoons olive oil
- 1¼ pounds of stew meat with beef, cut into 1-inch sections Salt and ground black pepper, as required 1 cup onion, chopped
- 1 tablespoon fresh ginger, minced
- 2 teaspoons garlic, minced
- 1 jalapeño pepper, chopped finely

- 1 tablespoon curry powder
- 1 teaspoon red chili powder
- 1 teaspoon ground cumin
- 2 cups beef broth
- 1½ cups carrots, peeled and cut into 1-inch pieces 1 cup unsweetened coconut milk
- ¼ cup fresh cilantro, chopped

1. Add the oil in an Instant Pot Mini and select "Sauté". Now, add the beef, salt, and black pepper and cook for about 4-5 minutes or until browned completely.
2. Move the beef into a bowl with a slotted spoon.
3. In the pot, add the onion, ginger, garlic, and jalapeño pepper and cook for about 4-5 minutes.
4. Press "Cancel" and stir in the beef, spices, and broth.
5. Secure the lid and turn to the "Seal" position.
6. For about 15 minutes cook on "Manual" with "High Pressure".
7. Press "Cancel" and do a "Quick" release.
8. Remove the lid and mix in the carrots.
9. Secure the lid and turn to the "Seal" position.
10. For about 5 minutes cook on "Manual" with "High Pressure".
11. Press "Cancel" and do a "Natural" release for about 10 minutes. Then do a "Quick" release.
12. Remove the lid and mix in the coconut milk.
13. Now, select "Sauté" and cook for about 2-3 minutes.
14. Press "Cancel" and stir in the cilantro.

Nutrition: Calories: 399 | fat: 18.1g | protein: 46.7g | carbs: 10g | net carbs: 7g | fiber: 3g

346.Pork Lettuce Wraps

Prep Time: 15 min | **Cook Time:** 25 min | **Serve:** 4

For Pork
- 1 garlic clove, minced finely
- 1 teaspoon dried rosemary
- 1 tablespoon olive oil
- Salt and ground black pepper, to taste
- 1½ pounds pork tenderloin, trimmed and cubed 4 tablespoons water
- 2 tablespoon fresh lemon juice

For Wraps
- ½ cup tomato, chopped finely
- ½ cup cucumber, chopped
- ½ cup onion, chopped
- 2 tablespoons fresh parsley, chopped
- 8 butter lettuce leaves

1. For the pork: Add the garlic, rosemary, oil, salt and black pepper in a wide bowl and mix well.
2. Add the pork and coat with the garlic mixture generously. Set aside for about 15-20 minutes.
3. Place the pork, water, and lemon juice and stir to combine in the pot of Instant Pot.
4. Secure the lid and turn to the "Seal" position.
5. Cook with "High Pressure" on "Manual" for about 25 minutes.
6. Press "Cancel" and do a "Natural" release.
7. Remove the lid and pour the pork into a large bowl with a slotted spoon.
8. With 2 forks, shred the meat.
9. In a bowl, mix together tomato, cucumber, onion, and parsley.
10. Arrange the lettuce leaves onto serving plates.
11. Divide the shredded pork over lettuce leaves evenly and top with tomato mixture.

Nutrition: Calories: 291 | fat: 19.7g | protein: 45.2g | carbs: 3.7g | net carbs: 2.7g | fiber: 1g

347.Chicken Alfredo Pesto Pasta

Prep Time: 10 min | **Cook Time:** 30 min | **Serve:** 2
- ½ pound angel hair pasta, uncooked
- 2 teaspoons oil
- Half kg boneless skinless chicken breasts, cut into bite-size pieces
- 2 cups of milk
- ½ cup PHILADELPHIA Cream Cheese Spread
- 1 large-red-pepper, cut into strips
- ¼ cup KRAFT Grated Parmesan Cheese 2 tablespoons pesto

Cook the pasta omitting salt. Over medium heat, heat oil in a big nonstick skillet. Put chicken and then cook and stir until done or for 7 minutes.
Mix in cream cheese spread and milk. Cook until sauce is well blended and cream cheese is completely melted or for 3 minutes. Put pesto, parmesan and peppers, then stir. Cook until heated through or for 3 minutes, stirring occasionally.
Drain the pasta and place it in the sauce with cream cheese. Coat by tossing it.
Nutrition: Calories 309, Fat 16, Carbs 26, Protein 33, Sodium 755

348.Chicken Pesto Paninis

Prep Time: 10 min | **Cook Time:** 15 min | **Serve:** 2
- 1 focaccia bread, quartered
- 1/2 cup prepared basil pesto
- 1 cup diced cooked chicken
- 1/2 cup diced green bell pepper
- 1/4 cup diced red onion
- 1 cup shredded Monterey Jack cheese

Start preheating a panini grill.
Horizontally cut each quarter of the focaccia bread in half. Spread pesto on each half. Layer equal portions of the chicken, the bell pepper, the onion, and the cheese onto the bottom halves. Place the rest of the focaccia halves on top to have 4 sandwiches.
Place paninis in the prepared grill and grill until cheese is melted and focaccia bread turns golden brown, about 5 minutes.
Nutrition: Calories 350, Fat 12, Carbs 7, Protein 26, Sodium 309

349.Chicken With Ginger Pesto

Prep Time: 10 min | **Cook Time:** 30 min | **Serve:** 2
- 2 pounds skinless, boneless chicken breast halves
- 1/2 cup dry white wine
- 1/4 cup vegetable oil
- 2 little spoons grated fresh ginger root
- 2 cloves garlic_-minced
- 1 littlespoon salt
- 1 littlespoon white sugar
- 1 bunch green onions, cut into 1/4-inch-pieces

1.Combine lightly salted water and wine in a saucepan, place the chicken breasts into the pan. Lower the heat to simmer, bring to a boil, for 8 to 10 minutes until chicken is white and cooked through. Take the chicken out of the sun and let it sit until it cools in the broth. Remove chicken from the broth, set aside.

2.A skillet is placed over medium-low heat, heat vegetable oil, stir in sugar, salt, garlic, and ginger. Cook for about 20 minutes until the garlic is tender and browned and the oil is flavored; remember to stir occasionally when cooking. Stir in green onions, and cook for additional 10 minutes until the onions' white parts are tender; remember to stir occasionally while cooking.

3.Cut poached chicken breasts on the bias into 1 inch wide slices, place decoratively on a plate. Place green onion mixture on top of chicken breasts. Serve.

Nutrition: Calories 584, Fat 21, Carbs 26, Protein 18, Sodium 532

350.Creamy PHILLY Pesto Chicken

Prep Time: 10 min | **Cook Time:** 30 min | **Serve:** 2

- 1 teaspoon oil
- 4 small boneless skinless chicken breasts
- 1/4 cup PHILADELPHIA Cream Cheese Spread 1/3 cup 25%- less-sodium chicken broth 2 tablespoons pesto

In a big nonstick frying pan, heat oil over medium heat. Put in chicken, cook until done (170°F), or for about 6-8 minutes per side. Remove to a dish; put a cover on to keep warm.

Add cream cheese spread to the frying pan, cook over medium heat until melted, or for about 5 minutes, whisking continually. Mix in pesto and broth, stir and cook until the sauce fully combines and thickens, or for about 2-3 minutes. Add onto the chicken.

Nutrition: Calories 328, Fat 12, Carbs 26, Protein 12, Sodium 459

FISH AND SEAFOOD RECIPES

351.Keto Lobster Roll But With Crab

Prep Time: 20 min | **Cook Time:** 11 min

BUN:

- 1 cup of (100g) almond flour
- 1 scoop (30g) unflavoured whey isolate
- 1.5 tsp of baking powder
- 1 tsp of xanthan gum
- 1/4 cup of melted (50g) butter
- 1/4 cup of (60ml) water
- salt & pepper

"LOBSTER" (crab) SALAD:

- 250g chopped real crab or lobster meat
- 1-2 chopped sticks of celery
- 2-3 chopped green onions
- 1/4 cup of (80g) chopped onions
- 1 tsp of dill
- 1 tsp of minced garlic
- 1/2 cup of (100g) mayonnaise
- Juice from 1/2 a lemon
- A few leaves of lettuce

1. For the buns-combine, all the ingredients in a mixing bowl together until a thick batter forms.
2. Scoop the batter (I used parchment paper to line mine) into greased hot dog bun molds.
3. Wet your hands to make the surface of the dough smooth.
4. Bake for 10-12 minutes at 350 ° F / 175 ° C.
5. Stir all the ingredients for the lobster/crab salad together in a mixing bowl as your buns cook.
6. When the buns are done, let them cool for a few minutes.

7. Like a hot dog bun, slice them open and put a few lettuce leaves in the crack.
8. Fill the lobster/crab salad with it.

352.Salmon with Veggies

Prep Time: 15 min | **Cook Time:** 6 min | **Serve:** 4

- 1 pound skin-on salmon fillets
- Salt and ground black pepper, as required
- 1 fresh parsley sprig
- 1 fresh dill sprig
- 3 teaspoons coconut oil, melted and divided ½ lemon, sliced thinly
- 1 carrot, peeled and julienned
- 1 zucchini, peeled and julienned
- 1 red bell pepper, seeded and julienned

1. The salmon fillets are similarly seasoned with salt and black pepper.
2. Arrange a steamer trivet and put herb sprigs and 1 cup of water at the bottom of the Instant Pot.
3. Place the salmon fillets, skin side down on top of the trivet.
4. Drizzle salmon fillets with 2 teaspoons of coconut oil and top with lemon slices.
5. Secure the lid and turn to the "Seal" position.
6. Choose 'Steam' and use the default time of 3 minutes only.
7. Press "Cancel" and do a "Natural" release.
8. Meanwhile, for the sauce: in a bowl, add remaining ingredients and mix until well combined.
9. Remove the lid and transfer the salmon fillets onto a platter.
10. Remove the steamer trivet, herbs, and cooking water from the pot. With paper towels, pat dries the pot.
11. Place the remaining coconut oil in the Instant Pot and select "Sauté". Then add the veggies and cook for about 2-3 minutes.
12. Press "Cancel" and transfer the veggies onto a platter with salmon.

Nutrition: Calories: 204 | fat: 10.6g | protein: 23.1g | carbs: 5.7g | net carbs: 4.3g | fiber: 1.4g

353.Baked cod with tomatoes and feta

Total time: 30 min | **Serve:** 4

- 2½ tbsp. olive oil
- 2 garlic cloves
- 2½ cups chopped tomatoes (preferably canned tomatoes with the juice)
- 4 scallions (chopped and separate the white parts from the green parts)
- ¼ tsp. dried oregano
- 12 oz. zucchini
- ½ tsp. salt
- ½ tsp. black pepper
- 1¾ lbs. cod fillet (sliced into 12 pieces)
- 1/3 cup feta cheese
- 1 cup basil (chopped)

1.Take a pan and cook the garlic and the scallions (the white parts) in 1 tbsp. of olive oil until fragrant.
2.Now, add the tomatoes and the oregano and cook them for about 20 minutes, until the tomato sauce gets thicker.
3. In the meantime, the zucchini should be sliced into 1/8-inch thick slices (lengthwise) and, then, put them on the side.
4.When the tomato sauce is thick and ready, remove from heat, put the green parts of the scallions, and stir everything.
5.Preheat the oven to 425°F.

6.Take a tray, arrange the slices of zucchini, and then place the cod on top. Season the cod with ¼ tsp. of black pepper, ½ tsp. of salt, and drizzle with remaining olive oil.

7.Cover the sliced cod with the tomato sauce and the feta cheese. Bake for about 23 minutes, until the cod reaches the temperature of 145°F. When ready, season everything with the chopped basil and the remaining black pepper.

354.Salmon with cucumbers, tomatoes, and dill salad

Total time: 30 min | **Serve:** 4
- 1-pint cherry tomatoes (cut in half)
- 4 cups cucumber (sliced)
- ¼ cup cider vinegar
- ¼ cup dill (chopped)
- ¼ tsp. salt
- ¼ tsp. black pepper
- 1½ lbs. salmon (skinless)
- 1 tbsp. Za'atar
- 4 lemon wedges

1.Preheat the oven to 350°F.

2.In the meantime, prepare the salad. Take a bowl and put the sliced cucumbers, the cherry tomatoes, the cider vinegar, and the chopped dill. Toss everything until thoroughly combined.

3.Now, take the salmon and season it with Za'atar on both sides, and place them on a tray. Roast the salmon until it reaches the temperature of 145°F.

4.When ready, serve the salmon with the salad and lemon wedges.

355.Salmon burgers with cucumber salad

Total time: 25 min | **Serve:** 2
- 1 egg (slightly beaten)
- 1½ tbsp. light mayo
- ½ tsp. lemon juice
- 1 tbsp. onion (diced)
- ¼ tsp. dried parsley
- dash of pepper
- 1,5 oz. salmon (skinless, boneless, and can drain)
- 1 packet of multigrain crackers (crushed)
- cooking spray
- 1,5 oz. low-fat Greek yogurt
- 2 tbsp. apple cider vinegar
- 1 tbsp. dill
- dash of salt
- 3 cups cucumber (peeled and thinly sliced)

1.Take a bowl and whisk together the egg, mayo, lemon juice, onion, parsley, and pepper. Gently fold in salmon and crushed crackers. Break the mixture, then form it into two patties. Cook on a lightly greased pan over medium-high heat until golden brown on both sides (about 5 minutes per side).

2.Meanwhile, whisk together the Greek yogurt, apple cider vinegar, dill, salt, and pepper. Pour over cucumber slices, and stir to mix in Chill until ready to serve.

356. Roasted red pepper sauce scallops and zucchini noodles

Total time: 30 min | **Serve:** 2
- 6 oz. jarred roasted red peppers (drained)
- ½ cup unsweetened almond or cashew milk
- 2 oz. avocado

- 2 tsp. lemon juice
- 1 clove garlic
- ¼ tsp. red pepper (crushed)
- ¼ tsp + 1/8 tsp salt
- 2 small zucchini (cut into spaghetti-like strands)
- ½ tbsp. butter
- 1 lbs. raw scallops

1. Place the roasted red peppers, milk, avocado, lemon juice, garlic, crushed red pepper and ¼ tsp. in a blender.

2.Heat roasted red-pepper sauce in a pan over medium heat, occasionally stirring, for about 3-5 minutes. Then, add zucchini noodles, stir to incorporate, and continue cooking until cooked to your liking (about 3-5 minutes).

3. Meanwhile, in a broad skillet over medium-high heat, melt-butter. With the remaining salt, season the scallops. Cook the scallops until golden brown on each side and translucent in the centre (about 1-2 minutes per side).

4.Serve zucchini noodles with scallops on top.

357.Stir-fried winter melon with shrimp

Total Time: 30 min | **Serve:** 4
- 4 tsp. olive oil
- 1 tbsp. ginger root (peeled and minced)
- 1 scallion (trimmed and minced)
- 30 oz. raw shrimp (peeled and deveined)
- ½ tsp. salt (divided)
- 4 tsp. canola oil
- 6 cups winter melon (trimmed and sliced)
- ½ cup water
- ½ tsp. black pepper
- 2 tsp. fresh chili paste
- ¼ cup coriander (chopped)

1.Heat the mustard oil in a non-stick wok or skillet and gently cook the ginger and scallion until fragrant.

2.Add the shrimp to the wok and continue to stir fry until pink. Add half the salt.

3.Once the shrimp are cookeed, remove them from the wok or skillet and set aside.

4.In the same wook or skillet, heat the canola oil. Add the sliced winter melon, and stir-fry over medium heat until they become tender (about 5-8 minutes). Add the water as needed and cover with a lid. Adjust seasoning with the remaining salt and add the pepper.

5.Return the shrimp into the same wok or skillet, heat through. Add the chili paste and green coriander.

358.Roasted lemon pepper salmon and garlic Parmesan asparagus

Total time: 35 min | **Serve:** 4
- 1½ lbs. salmon (skin on)
- 2½ tbsp. olive oil
- 1 tsp. lemon zest
- 1 tbsp. fresh lemon juice
- 4 cloves garlic (minced)
- 1 tsp. Dijon mustard
- ¾ tsp. onion powder
- ½ tsp. each salt and black pepper (plus more for asparagus)
- ½ lemon (thinly sliced)
- 1½ – 2 lbs. asparagus (ends trimmed)
- ½ cup parmesan (finely shredded)

1.Preheat oven to 400°F. Place salmon in the ceenter of the pan. In a mixing bowl, whisk together 1½ tbsp of olive oil, the lemon zest, lemon juice, 2 cloves of garlic, Dijon mustard, and onion powder. Brush evenly over the top of the salmon, and then sprinkle ½ tsp. of salt and black pepper. Arrange lemon slices on top.

2.Toss asparagus with 1 tbsp. Of olive oil, 2 cloves of garlic and season with salt, then place around salmon. Bake in a preheated oven (about 10 minutes).

3.Remove from oven, toss asparagus, then sprinkle asparagus with Parmesan. After sprinkling the Parmesan, put it into the oven and bake it until salmon has cooked through (about 5 – 10 minutes). Cut salmon into portions and serve it warm.

359.Avocado lime shrimp salad

Total time: 15 min | **Serve:** 2
- 14 oz. jumbo cooked shrimp (peeled and deveined, chopped)
- 1½ cup tomato (diced)
- 4½ oz. avocado (diced)
- ¼ cup jalapeño (seeds removed, finely diced)
- ¼ cup green onion (chopped)
- 2 tbsp. lime juice
- 1 tsp. olive oil
- 1 tbsp. coriander (chopped)
- 1/8 tsp. salt
- ¼ tsp. black pepper

1.Take a bowl and combine green onion, lime juice, olive oil, a pinch of salt, and pepper. Let them marinate to soften the onion (at least 5 minutes).

2.In a bowl, mix in chopped shrimp, avocado, tomato, jalapeño. Combine all the ingredients, add coriander, and gently toss. Adjust salt and pepper to taste.

360.Steamed Seafood Pot

Total Time: 1 h 15 min | **Serve:** 4
- 14 oz. winter melon (peeled, seeded, and thinly sliced)
- 7 oz. Oriental radish (peeled and thinly sliced)
- 17 oz. Chinese cabbage (wash, drain, and sliced)
- 21 oz. firm tofu (drain and sliced)
- 11 oz. fresh prawns with shells (washed and drained)
- 32 oz. fresh clams with shell (cover with water and 1 tsp. of salt for 1 hour to remove the sands, washed and drained)
- 4 blue crabs with shells (about 35 oz., washed and drained)
- 1 cup water
- ½ cup fresh coriander
- 1 scallion (trimmed and chopped)
- 2 fresh red hot chilies (cut into half and remove seeds)
- 2 tbsp. soy sauce
- 4 tsp. sesame oil

1.Layer the winter melon, Oriental radish, and cabbage at the bottom of the pot.

2.Layer tofu slices on top of the vegetables.

3.Spread prawns, clams, and crabs on top.

4. Place the water on the side of the bowl. Cover the lid and cook until all the ingredients are well cooked (about 15 minutes).

5.Garnish with coriander and scallions. Serve with chili, soy sauce, and sesame oil.

361.Avocado lime tuna salad

Total time: 15 min | **Serve:** 4
- 3 cans of tuna water (drained)
- 1 cup cucumber (quartered and sliced)
- 1 avocado (seeded, peeled, and diced)
- 2 tbsp. onion (thinly sliced)
- ¼ cup coriander (chopped)
- 2 tbsp. lime juice
- ¼ cup olive oil
- ½ tsp. chili powder
- ¼ tsp. cumin
- salt and black pepper to taste

1.take a bowl and place the tuna, cucumber, avocado, onion, and coriander.

2.In another bowl, whisk together the lime juice, olive oil, chili powder, cumin, salt, and black pepper.

3.Over the tuna mixture, add the dressing; toss gently to cover.

362.Low-carb lobster roll

Total Time: 15 min | **Serve:** 2
- 2 small heads of romaine lettuce
- 1 tbsp. butter (melted)
- 1/3 cup Greek yogurt (low-fat)
- 2 tbsp. mayonnaise
- 1 small stalk celery (finely diced)
- 2 tsp. lemon juice
- 1 tbsp. chives (chopped)
- ¼ tsp. paprika
- ¼ tsp. salt
- ¼ tsp. pepper
- 12 oz. cooked lobster meat

1.Preheat grill.

2.Slice romaine hearts in half lengthwise. Remove one or two of the inner leaves from each half to create a boat-like shape for the lobster filling. Lightly coat the inner parts and edges of each "boat" with butter, and grill cut-side-down to get a slight char and bring out the lettuce's flavors (about 2-3 minutes).

3.Take a bowl and mix the remaining ingredients except for the lobster meat. Once ingredients are well mixed, fold in the lobster meat until completely coated.

4.Arrange the lobster mixture evenly among the boats.

363.Tom Yum noodle soup

Total Time: 45 min | **Serve:** 4
- 8 oz. Celtuce ("spiralized" into noodle-like strands)
- 4 cups of water
- 3 oz. lemongrass sticks (mashed and cut into 2 inches long)
- 4 shallots (peeled and sliced)
- 0.3 oz. Thai lime leaves
- 2.4 oz. blue ginger (sliced)
- 2 pieces fresh red hot chili (cut in half, seeds and membranes removed)
- 2 medium tomatoes (cut each tomato into 6 wedges)
- 14 oz. firm tofu (cut into ½inch x ½inch cubes)
- 2 cups oyster mushrooms (sliced)
- 10 oz. frozen shrimps (defrost, washed, and drained)

- 10 oz. frozen scallops (defrost, washed, and drained)
- 2 tbsp. fish sauce
- ½ cup coconut milk
- 2 tbsp. lime juice
- ½ cup fresh coriander (slightly chopped)

1. Take a pot, pour waater into it, and bring it to a boil. Add the Celtuce "noodles" and cook for 2 minutes. Drain the noodlees, put them in a bowl on the side.
2. Take a pot, pour water into it. When the water is boiling, add lemongrass, shallots, Thai lime leaves, blue ginger, chili, tomatoes, tofu, and mushrooms. Cook for about 3 minutes.
3. Add shrimp and scallops and cook for 3,3 minutes.
4. Turn off the heat, add fish sauce, coconut milk, and lime juice. Stir to combine well.
5. Carefully remove the lemongrass sticks, shallot slices, Thai lime leaves, and blue ginger with a slotted spoon.
6. Pour the soup over the Celtuce "noodles." Garnish with coriander leaves.

364. Steamed white fish street tacos

Total Time: 20 min | **Serve:** 2

- 16 oz. raw cod fillets
- ½ tsp. garlic powder
- ½ tsp. salt, divided
- ½ cup tomato (diced)
- 2 tbsp. onion (chopped)
- ½ jalapeño pepper (seeds and membranes removed, chopped)
- 2 tbsp. cilantro (chopped)
- 1 tbsp. lime juice
- 6 large romaine lettuce leaves
- 1 avocado (about 6 oz., sliced)

1. Season cod with garlic powder and ¼ tsp. of salt. Steam fish until cooked through (about 5-10 minutes). Flake the fish, using a fork, removing any bones.
2. Meanwhile, prepare pico de gallo. Take a bowl and combine tomato, onion, jalapeño pepper, cilantro, lime juice, and the remaining salt.
3. To prepare tacos: Top each romaine lettuce leaf with fish, avocado, and pico de gallo.

365. Stir-fry shrimps with champignon mushroom and broccoli

Total time: 25 min | **Serve:** 4

- 1 lb. shrimps
- 2 garlic cloves
- 1 onion (chopped)
- 1 crown broccoli (chopped)
- ¼ lb. champignon mushroom
- 1 tbsp. + 2 tsp. corn starch
- 2 tbsp. soy sauce
- 1 tsp. rice vinegar
- ½ tbsp. brown sugar
- ½ cup chicken broth
- 2 tbsp. canola oil
- ½ tbsp. lemon juice

1. Take the shrimps and mix them with 1 tbsp. Of corn starch, then ass salt and pepper to taste.
2. Take the soy sauce and mix it with vinegar, brown sugar, chicken broth, and 2 tsp. Corn starch.
3. Now take the wok and put it over medium-high heat. Add 1 tbsp. Of canola oil, heat it, and then add the shrimps to it.

Cooked the shrimps until they will get a golden color. Then remove the shrimps from the pan and set aside.
4. Once you removed the shrimps from the pan, put it over medium-high heat, and add the remaining canola oil. Now, add the garlic cloves and then the chopped onions with a dash of salt. Cooked the onions until they become soft (about 2 minutes).
5. Add broccoli and season them with a bit of salt. Stir-fry for about 2 minutes, add sliced champignon mushrooms, and season them with a salt dash.
6. Now, add the shrimps back in. Push all the ingredients to the pan's side to form a circle in the middle. Then, put the sauce mixture into the pan's center (in case the corn starch has sunk to the bottom, stir it).
7. Cook until shrimps are ready. Then, remove the pan from heat and add1/2 tbs. of lemon juice. Add salt and pepper to taste.

366. Steamed stuffed mushrooms (with pork)

Total Time: 30 min | **Serve:** 2

- 6 oz. raw pork tenderloin (minced into bite-sized pieces)
- 7 oz. cooked shrimp (peeled, deveined, and minced into bite-sized pieces)
- 7 oz. fresh white mushrooms (stems removed)
- 2 tbsp. soy sauce
- 1 tbsp. rice wine vinegar
- 2 tsp. sesame oil
- ¼ tsp. black pepper
- 1 spring onion (trimmed and minced)
- ½ tsp. chili oil

1. Combine minced pork and shrimp with soy sauce, vinegar, oil, and pepper. Marinate for at least one hour. Drain liquid when finished.
2. When ready to serve, stuff each mushroom cap with the pork and shrimp mixture and place on a steamer plate (if needed, put any extra meat and shrimp alongside the mushrooms on the plate). Steam on the stovetop until the meat and shrimp are fully cooked (about 15 minutes).
3. Garnish with spring onions and chili oil.

367. Sheet pan shrimp scampi

Total Time: 15 min | **Serve:** 2

- 12 oz. zucchini (ends removed)
- 16 oz. raw shrimp (peeled and deveined)
- 2 tbsp. grated Parmesan cheese
- Juice of half a lemon
- 1 tbsp. butter (unsalted, melted)
- 2 tsp. olive oil
- 1 clove garlic (minced)
- ¼ tsp. salt

1. Preheat oven to 400°F.
2. Using a vegetable peeler, cut zucchini into thin strips.
3. Then, take a re-sealable plastic bag and combine zucchini strips and the remaining ingredients. Seal the bag and toss it to evenly coat zucchini and shrimp.
4. Distribute the mixture in an even layer onto a foil-lined baking sheet. Bake until shrimp are cooked through (about 8 minutes).

368. Sambal Kang Kong with bay scallops

Total Time: 30 min | **Serve:** 4

- 6 scallions (trimmed and chopped)
- 2 garlic cloves (chopped)
- 1 tbsp. lemongrass (minced)
- 2 tsp. ginger root (peeled and minced)
- 1 tbsp. chili paste
- 2 fresh Thai bird chilies (seeds and membranes removed)
- 1 tbsp. shrimp paste
- 4 tsp. lime juice
- 2 tbsp. + 2 tsp. canola oil
- 25 oz. bay scallops
- 25 oz. water spinach
- 1 tbsp. fish sauce

1.Combine the scallions, garlic, lemongrass, ginger, chili paste, Thai bird chilies, shrimp paste, and lime juice in a blender and puree fine paste, adding water as needed to facilitate blending. Alternatively, you can use a pestle and a mortar. Set the paste aside when done.

2.Heat 2 tsp. Oil in a wok or pan-and add the scallops, and stir-fry until almost cooked through (about 3-5 minutes). Remove from the wok, put them on the side, and keep warm.

3.Heat the remaining 2 tbsp. Of oil in the same wook or skillet and cook the spice paste over moderate heat until almost dry (about 5 to 6 minutes).

4.Add the water spinach, fish sauce, and cook quickly until the spinach is wilted (about 3-5 minutes).

5.Arrange the water spinach on a platter and top with the scallops.

369.Crab and asparagus frittata

Total Time: 30 min | **Serve:** 4
- 2½ tbsp. extra virgin olive oil
- 2 lbs. asparagus
- 1 tsp. salt
- ½ tsp black pepper
- 2 tsp sweet paprika
- 1 lb. lump crabmeat
- 1 tbsp. chives (finely cut)
- ¼ cup basil (chopped)
- 4 cups liquid egg substitute

1.Remove the ends of the asparaagus and cut it into small pieces.

2.Pre-heat an oven to 375°F.

3.In a 12-inch to 14-inch tray, heat the olive oil and gently sweat the asparagus until tender; then, season them with salt, pepper, and paprika.

4.In a bowl, add the chives, basil, and crab meat. Pour in the eggbeaters and gently mix until combined.

5.Carefully pour the crab and egg mixture into the tray with the cooked asparagus, and gently stir to combine. Cook over low to meedium heat until the egg beaters start bubbling.

6.Placee the tray in the oven and bake until the egg beaters are fully cooked and golden brown (about 15-20 minutes).

370.Shrimp and cauliflower grits

Total Time: 20 min | **Serve:** 2
- 1 lb. shrimp (raw and peeled)
- ½ tbsp. Cajun seasoning
- cooking spray
- 1 tbsp. lemon juice
- ¼ cup chicken broth
- 1 tbsp. butter
- 2 ½ cups cauliflower (finely riced)
- ½ almond or cashew milk (unsweetened)
- ¼ cup sour cream
- ¼ tsp. salt
- 1/3 cup cheddar cheese (low-fat)
- ¼ cup scallions (thinly sliced)

1.In a big, re-sealable plastic bag, placed the shrimp and Cajun seasoning. Close the bag and toss in the seasoning to coat the shrimp evenly.

2. Use cooking spray to spray a pan and heat over medium heat. Cook the shrimp (about 2,3-3,3 minutes on each side) until yellow. Then add the chicken broth and lemon juice, boil for 1 minute, and then place it on the side.

3. Heat the butteer in a separate pan over medium heat. Connect the cauliflower 'riced' and cook (about 5 minutes). Add the milk and salt, then cook for an extra 5 minutes.

4.Remove pan from heat, and stir in sour cream and cheese until melted.

5.Serve shrimps atop cauliflower grits, and top with scallions.

371.Zucchini sheet with shrimp and scampi

Total Time: 15 min | **Serve:** 2
- 3 small zucchini (ends removed)
- 1 lb. raw shrimp (peeled and deveined)
- 2 tbsp. grated Parmesan cheese
- juice of half a lemon
- 1 tbsp. butter (unsalted, melted)
- 2 tsp. olive oil
- 1 clove garlic (minced)
- ¼ tsp. salt

1.Preheat oven to 400 °F.

2.Peel the zucchini into thin-ribbons using a vegetable peeler.

3. Combine the zucchini ribbons and residual ingredients in a large resealable plastic container. Seal the bag and toss well to mix all the ingredients together.

4. Spread the mixture onto a tray in an even layer and place it in the oven. Bake until the shrimp is cooked (about 8 minutes).

372.Crab zucchini sushi rolls

Total Time: 15 min | **Serve:** 4
- 3 cups lump crab meat
- 1 cup of Greek yogurt (low-fat)
- 2 tbsp. Sriracha sauce
- 1 medium avocado (peeled and sliced)
- 4 medium zucchini (remove ends)
- 1 small cucumber (chopped into matchstick-sized pieces)
- ¼ cup of soy sauce

1.Take a bowl and combine the crab meat with the Greek yogurt and the Sriracha sauce.

2.Take the zucchini and use a vegetable peeler or mandolin slicer to peel them into long, thin strips (8 per zucchini).

3.Lay the zucchini strips flat vertically and spread a spoonful (about 1-2 tbsp. of mixture per strip) of crab mixture on each one. On each strip, place a few matchsticks of cucumber and a slice of avocado horizontally.

4. Roll up the strips of zucchini, secure them with toothpicks, and serve.

373.Oyster omelet

Total Time: 30 min | **Serve:** 4

- 10 eggs
- 10 oz. oysters (chopped)
- 1 tbsp. soy sauce
- 1 tsp. canola oil
- 3 garlic cloves (minced)
- 1 tbsp. ginger root (peeled and minced)
- 1 scallion (trimmed and diced)
- 2 medium red bell peppers (8 oz., deseeded, deveined, and diced)
- 8 cups baby spinach

1.Take a bowl and combine eggs, oysters, light soy sauce, and beat with a fork. Put it on the side.
2.Take a pan and heat oil over medium-high heat. Add garlic, ginger, scallions, and red bell peppers. Sauté until aromatic.
3.Pour the beeaten egg mixture into the pan and gently push the cooked portion from the center's edges.
4.Keep cooking, tilting the pan, and moving the cooked portions gently as required.
5.When the top surface of eggs is set, and no visible liquid egg remains, place spinach on top and cover with a lid to wilt. The omelet is folded in half and moved to a tray. Serve hot or room temperature.

374.Spicy crab stuffed avocado

Total time: 10 min | **Serve:** 1

- 2 tbsp. light mayo
- 2 tsp. sriracha (plus more for drizzling)
- 1 tsp. chives (chopped)
- 4 oz. lump crab meat
- ¼ cup cucumber (peeled and diced)
- 1 small avocado (4 oz., pitted and peeled)
- ½ tsp. furikake
- 2 tsp. soy sauce

1.Take a bowl and combine mayo, sriracha, and chives.
2.Add crab meat and cucumber and gently toss.
3.Cut the avocado open, remove the pit, peel the skin, or spoon the avocado.
4.Fill the avocado halves with crab salad in the same way.

375.Blackened shrimp lettuce wraps

Total time: 20 min | **Serve:** 4

- 2 lb. raw shrimp, peeled and deveined
- 1 tbsp. blackened seasoning
- 4 tsp. olive oil (divided)
- 1 cup of Greek yogurt (low-fat)
- 6 oz. avocado
- 2 tbsp. lime juice (divided)
- 1 ½ cups diced tomato
- ¼ cup green bell pepper (diced)
- ¼ cup onion (chopped)
- ¼ cup coriander (chopped)
- 1 jalapeño (chopped and deseeded)
- 12 large romaine lettuce leaves

1.In a re-sealable plastic bag, put the shrimp and blackened seasoning (you will need to split the shrimp into two batches). Shake the contents of the sack to uniformly disperse the seasoning.
2.Heat two teaspoons. In a saucepan, add olive oil and half the shrimp in a single layer. Cook until the shrimp is pink and fried. (approximately 2 to 3 minutes per side). Repeat with remaining shrimp and olive oil.

3.For the avocado salsa: combine Greek yogurt, avocado, and one tbsp. In a food proceessor, add lime juice and blend until smooth.
4.For the tomato salsa: take a bowl and stir the tomatoes, green bell pepper, onion, coriander, jalapeño, and remaining tbsp of lime juice.
5.Prepare lettuce wraps by dividing the shrimp, avocado salsa, and tomato salsa evenly among the lettuce leaves.

376.Shrimp cucumber bites

Total time: 60 min | **Serve:** 6

- 1/3 cup olive oil
- ¼ cup lime juice
- 2 tbsp. honey
- 2 cloves garlic (minced)
- 1 tsp. Cajun seasoning
- ½ tsp. salt (divided)
- 1 lb. shrimp (peeled, deveined, and tails discarded)
- 2 avocados
- 2 tbsp. lime juice
- ½ onion (finely minced)
- 1 jalapeño (finely chopped)
- 2 tbsp. coriander (chopped, plus more for garnish)
- 2 cucumbers (sliced ½ inch thick)

1.Combine the oil, lime juice, sugar, garlic, and the Cajun seasoning in a dish. With salt, season. Attach the shrimp and toss until thoroughly coated, then cover and leave for 30 minutes or up to an hour to rest in the fridge.
2.Take a pan and place it over medium heat, cook shrimp until pink (about 2 minutes per side). Remove from heat.
3.Meanwhile, in a bowl, mash avocados, add lime juice, red onion, jalapeño, coriander, and stir to combine. Season with the remaining salt.
4.On each cucumber slice, put a tablespoon-sized amount of guacamole.

377.Savory coriander salmon

Total time: 110 min | **Serve:** 4

- 4 cups coriander (divided)
- 2 tbsp. lemon/lime juice
- 2 tbsp. hot red pepper sauce
- 1 tsp. cumin
- ½ tsp. salt (divided)
- ½ cup of water
- 4, 7 oz. salmon filets (raw)
- 2 cups yellow bell pepper (sliced)
- 2 cups green bell pepper (sliced)
- ½ tsp. black pepper
- cooking spray

1.In a food processor, put half of the coriander, lemon or lime juice, hot red pepper sauce, cumin, salt, and water, and blend until smooth. Transfer the marinade to a resealable plastic bag.
2.Add salmon to marinade. Seal the bag by squeezing out the air; turn it to coat the salmon. Let it rest in the fridge for 65 minutes, turning the bag now and then.
3.Meanwhile, preheat the oven to 410°F. Arrange pepper-slices in a single layer in a lightly-greased baking tray, and sprinkle with black pepper and the remaining salt. Bake for 23 minutes, turning pepper slices once.
4.Drain salmon, and discard the marinade. Crust tops of salmon with the remaining fresh coriander. Place salmoon

on top of pepper slices, and bake until fish flakes easily when tested with a fork (about 12-14 minutes).

378.Grilled shrimp skewers
Total time: 35 min | **Serve:** 1
- ¾ lb laarge shrimp (raw)
- green pepper (cut into thick chunks)
- 1 cup whole mushrooms
- ½ tsp Old Bay seasoning
- tbsp. roasted red pepper vinaigrette

1.Marinate the shrimp in the roasted red pepper vinaigrette for 30 minutes (discard dressing).
2.Alternate shrimp, peppers, and mushrooms on a skewer.
3.Grill skewers on foil, turning once.
4.Sprinkle shrimp with Old Bay seasoning.

379.Salmon and asparagus with peppers puree
Total time: 40 min | **Serve:** 1
- 6 oz. raw salmon
- 1 cup fresh asparagus
- ¼ cup red bell peppers (diced)
- ¼ cup raw tomatoes (diced)
- 1/8 tsp. salt
- ½ cup water
- 2 tbsp. red wine vinegar
- cooking spray
- ¼ tsp. pepper

1.Preheat oven to 350° F.
2.Dice the tomatoes and peppers; spray lightly with some cooking spray on a cookie sheet.
3. Season both sides of the salmoon lightly with salt and pepper. Place the salmon in a baking dish and add water to the baking tray.
4.Bake for about 22-24,5 minutes with the salmon and vegetables.
5. For asparagus, boil water. As it heats up, it finishes with clean and trim asparagus. Leave or cut in half as whole stalks. Place in boiling water and cook (about 10 minutes) until soft-crisp.6. After removing peppers and tomatoes from the oven, let them cool down (about 2-3 minutes). Place in a bleender, add vinegar and blend until the consistency of applesauce.
7.On a plate with salmon on top, arrange the asparagus.
8.Add salt and pepper to taste.

380.Tuna Nicoise salad
Total time: 10 min | **Serve:** 4
- 4tsp. olive oil
- 3 tbsp. balsamic-vinegar
- 2 garlic-cloves (minced)
- 6 cups-mixed greens
- 2 cups string-beans (steamed until just tender)
- 1 cup grape-tomatoes (halved)
- 6 hardboiled eggs (sliced)
- 2, 7 oz. cans-of-tuna

1.Whisk together olive oil, garlic, and vinegar.
2.Prepare a bed of mixed greens. Layer with string beans, tomatoes, egg slices, and tuna. Drizzle with oil mixture.

381.Ancho tilapia on cauliflower rice
Total time: 30 min | **Serve:** 4

- 2 lb. tilapia
- 1 tsp. lime juice
- 1tsp. salt
- 1 tbsp. ground ancho pepper (or 1 tbsp. of curry powder)
- 1 tsp. cumin
- 1½ olive oil
- ¼ cup toasted pumpkin seeds
- 6 cups cauliflower rice
- 1 cup fresh coriander (chopped)

1.Preheat oven to 450°F.
2.Take the tilapia and season it with lime juice, and then set on the side.
3.Take a bowl and combine salt, ancho pepper, and cumin. Season the tilapia with the spice mixture.
4.On a baking sheet, arrange the tilapia and bake for 7 minutes.
5.Meanwhile, take a pan and sweat the cauliflower rice in olive oil until tender (about 2 minutes).
6.Mix in the pumpkin seeds and the coriander into the cauliflower rice. Remove from heat, and serve with tilapia.

382.Salmon Florentine
Total time: 35 min | **Serve:** 4
- ½ cup green onions (chopped)
- 1 tsp. olive oil
- 2 garlic cloves (minced)
- 1, 12 oz. frozen chopped spinach (thawed and patted dry)
- 1½ cups cherry tomatoes (chopped)
- ¼ tsp. red pepper flakes (crushed)
- ¼ tsp. salt
- ¼ tsp. black pepper
- ½ cup ricotta cheese (part-skim)
- 4, 5½ oz. salmon fillets
- cooking spray

1.Preheat oven to 350°F.
2.Take a pan, cook green onions in olive oil until they begin to soften (about 2 minutes). Add garlic and cook 1 minute more. Add the spinach, tomatoes, red pepper flakes, salt, and pepper. Cook, stirring for 2 minutes. Take it from heat and let it cool for 10 minutes. Then, mix in the ricotta cheese.
3.Then, take the salmon fillets and place a quarter of the spinach mixture on top of them. On a lightly greased sheet, arrange the salmon fillets and bake until salmon is cooked through (about 15 minutes).

383.Light tuna casserole
Total time: 45 min | **Serve:** 2
- 1 cup almond milk (unsweetened)
- 4 wedges of garlic and herb cheese (low-fat)
- 1 cup shredded cheddar cheese (low-fat)
- 1 tbsp. chives
- ¼ tsp. cayenne pepper
- 1, 5 oz. can drained tuna packed in water
- 2 cups cooked spaghetti squash
- salt to taste
- black pepper to taste

1.Preheat oven to 350°F.
2.Take a pan and heat almond milk, then add cheese and stir until they melt and the sauce thickens up. Add the rest of the ingredients, leaving some of the cheddar cheese to sprinkle on top.

3.Spread everything in a casserole dish, sprinkle cheese on top and bake for about 30 minutes.

384.Curry crusted salmon with chili braised cabbage

Total time: 30 min | **Serve:** 4
- 4, 6 oz. salmon fillets (raw, skinless)
- ¼ tsp. salt
- 1½ tbsp. curry powder
- 1¼ lb. cabbage (trimmed and chopped into bite-sized pieces)
- 2 tsp. fresh ginger root (minced)
- 1 cup chicken broth
- ¼ tsp. red pepper flakes
- 2 green onions (minced)

1.Preheat oven to 425°F.
2.Take the salmon fillets and rub the salt over them until dissolved. Let the fillets sit for 5 minutes
3.Take a plate, spread the curry powder, and then roll each salmon fillet in the curry powder until evenly coated.
4.Place salmon on a baaking sheet and bake for about 8-10 minutes.
5.Meanwhile, cut the cabbage into bite-sized pieces and put it on the side.
6.Take a pan, combine the chicken broth and ginger, and bring to a boil. Add the red pepper flakes and cabbage, cover, and bring to a boil. Reduce heat and simmer until-cabbage is tender (about 3,3-5,3 minutes).
7.Mix the green onions in with the cabbage. Serve salmon on a bed of cabbage.

385.Shrimp ceviche

Total time: 70 min | **Serve:** 4
- 2 lb. shrimp (raw, peeled, and deveined)
- ¼ cup lemon juice
- ¼ cup lime juice
- ½ cup fresh tomatoes (diced)
- ½ cup cucumbers (diced)
- 1 jalapeño (seeds removed, diced)
- 1 large red bell pepper (diced)
- ¼ cup green onion (diced)
- ½ cup fresh coriander (chopped)
- 1 avocado
- 4 cups mixed greens-hot sauce

1.Make a big pot of water boil. Immerse the shrimp in boiling water and cook for a period of one to two minutes (depending on the size of the shrimp). Remove it with a slotted spoon from the bath.
2.Place the shrimp in a ceramic or glass tub. Add lemon and lime juice to the mixture. Cover for at least 30 minutes and refrigerate.
3. Combine the shrimp with the onions, cucumbers and peppers. Refrigerate until ready to serve or for at least 33 minutes.
4. Combine the bits of green onion, coriander, and avocado.
5.Serve over a bed of mixed greens. Top with green hot sauce, if desired.

386.Cajun shrimp sausage and vegetable skillet

Total time: 10 min | **Serve:** 6
- 28 oz. cooked shrimp
- 12 oz. turkey sausage
- 3 cups zucchini (sliced)
- 3 cups yellow squash
- 1 cup asparagus
- 2 cups red bell pepper
- ¼ tsp. salt
- ½ tsp. black pepper
- 2 tbsp. olive oil
- 2 tbsp. Cajun seasoning

1. Take a bowl and mix in the shrimp, zucchini, sausage, yellow squash, bell pepper, asparagus, and salt and pepper. Add olive oil and cajun-seasoning and toss until well coated.
2. Add to a pan and put on medium heat; cook until the shrimp is pink and the vegetables are tender (about 5-7 minutes).

387.Parmesan garlic shrimp zucchini noodles

Total time: 20 min | **Serve:** 4
- 16 oz. frozen uncooked shrimp
- 1 cup cherry tomatoes (halved)
- 8 cups zucchini noodles (3 medium zucchini)
- 3 tbsp. olive oil (divided)
- 2 tbsp. garlic (minced, divided)
- ½ cup grated Parmesan cheese
- 1 tsp. dried oregano
- ½ tsp. chili powder
- ½ tsp. salt
- ½ tsp. black pepper

1.Preheat the oven to 400 degrees. Line a large sheet pan with foil.
2.In a colander, position the frozen shrimp and run cool water over them to thaw (approximately 5 minutes).
3. Toss the parmesan cheese, oregano, chili powder, salt and pepper together.
4. Using a paper towel, drain the shrimp and pat them dry. Put a bowl in it. Uh, pour 1 tbsp. Petroleum, and 1 tbsp. Shrimp with garlic and stir to cover.
5.Sprinkle ½ the cheese mixture on the shrimp and stir to coat. Sprinkle on top with the remaining cheese and keep stirring. Put the shrimp onto the pan and spread out, so they are lying flat. Place in the oven for about 8-10 minutes.
6.Pour the remaining oil and garlic into a large pan, heat for 1 minute, and then stir in the zucchini noodles and tomatoes. Toss to coat. Keep stirring and tossing the noodles as they saute for about 6-8 minutes.
7.Serve the hot veggies and shrimp right away. Sprinkle with extra parmesan cheese, if desired.

388.Garlic and herb squash stir fry

Total time: 10 min | **Serve:** 1
- ¾ cup zucchini (sliced)
- ¾ cup yellow squash (sliced)
- 7 oz. cooked shrimp
- 1 tbsp. butter (low-fat)
- 2 tbsp. water
- ½ tsp Mrs. garlic and herb seasoning
- 1 tbsp. grated parmesan cheese (low-fat)
- dash of salt or pepper
- cooking spray

1.Take a pan and spray some cooking spray, then put over medium-high heat and melt butter.

2.Attach the veggies and fry until the veggies are tender-crisp for several minutes.

3.Add shrimp, water, and seasonings. Cover and simmer until desired doneness (usually it takes 4-5 minutes).

4.Sprinkle with parmesan cheese. Serve.

389.Naked salmon burgers with sriracha mayo

Total time: 20 min | **Serve:** 4

- 3 tbsp. mayonnaise (light, with olive oil)
- 1 tbsp. sriracha
- ¼ cup red bell pepper (diced)
- ¼ cup yellow bell pepper (diced)
- 6 tbsp. whole-wheat breadcrumbs
- 1 clove garlic (minced)
- 1 lb. salmon fillet
- 1 egg (lightly beaten)
- ½ tbsp. soy sauce
- 1 tsp. lemon juice
- ¼ tsp. salt
- cooking spray
- 4 cups baby arugula
- 4 oz. avocado (sliced)

1.Combine mayonnaise and sriracha and put it on the side.

2.Remove the skin-from the salmon and cut about a 4 oz. Piece off.

3.Place in a food-processor to finely chop. With a knife, finely chop the remaining salmon.

4.Take a bowl combine and the salmon with the bell peppers, whole-wheat breadcrumbs, and garlic.

5.In another bowl, combine egg, soy sauce, lemon juice, and salt, and then add to the salmon mixture, tossing gently to combine.

6.Form 4 patties and refrigerate at least one hour (in this way, burgers become firm and hold together during cooking).

7.Lightly coat a grill-pan with cooking spray. Place over medium-high heat until hot. Cook the patties until cooked through(about 4-5 minutes each side).

8.Place arugula on each plate, top each with a salmon burger, 1 tbsp, mayo, and avocado slices.

390.Salmon and Cream Cheese Bites

Prep Time: 10 min | **Cook Time:** 10 min | **Serve:** 2

- 3 medium eggs
- ¼ teaspoon salt or to taste
- ½ teaspoon dried dill
- 0.88 ounce fresh or smoked salmon, chopped ½ cup cream
- 0.88-ounce grated parmesan
- 0.88-ounce cream cheese, diced

1.Grease 18 wells of a mini muffin pan with some fat.

2.Make sure to preheat your oven to 130 C.

3.Add eggs into a bowl and whisk well. Add salt and cream and whisk well.

4.Add parmesan, cream cheese, and dill and stir.

5.Divide the egg mixture into the 18 wells of the mini muffin pan.

6.Drop at least 1 - 2 pieces of salmon in each well.

7.Place the mini muffin pan and bake for about 12 - 15 minutes or until set in the oven.

8.Cool the mini muffins on your countertop.

9.Remove them from the molds and serve.

391.Shrimp and Endives

Prep Time: 5 min | **Cook Time:** 12 min | **Serve:** 2

- 1 pound shrimp, peeled and deveined
- 2 tablespoons avocado oil
- 2 spring onions, chopped
- 2 endives, shredded
- 1 tablespoon balsamic vinegar
- 1 tablespoon chives, minced
- A pinch of salt and black-pepper from the sea

1.Over medium-high heat, heat a pan with the oil, add the spring onions, endives and chives, stir and cook for 4 minutes.

2.Add the shrimp and remaining ingredients, toss, cook for 8 more minutes over medium heat, divide into bowls.

Nutrition: Calories 378, Fat 2, Carbs 6, Protein 6, Sodium 290

392.Baked Fish Fillets

Prep Time: 5 min | **Cook Time:** 20 min | **Serve:** 2

- 2 tablespoons butter, melted
- A pinch of ground paprika
- 3 fish fillets (5 ounces)
- Pepper to taste
- 1 tablespoon lemon juice
- ½ teaspoon salt

1.Ensure that your oven is preheated to 350 ° F. By greasing it with some fat, prepare a pan for baking. Sprinkle the fillets with salt and pepper and put them in the pan. In a cup, add the butter, paprika and lemon juice and stir. Brush over the fillets with this mixture. In the oven, put the baking pan and cook the fillets.

Nutrition: Calories 245, Fat 12, Carbs 4, Protein 32, Sodium 455

393.Salmon Cakes

Prep Time: 10 min | **Cook Time:** 10 min | **Serving:** 2

- 2 cans salmon (14.75 ounces each), drained
- 8 tablespoons collagen
- 2 cups shredded mozzarella cheese
- 1 teaspoon onion powder
- 4 large pastured egg
- 4 teaspoons dried dill
- 1 pink sea salt teaspoon or to taste
- 4 tablespoons bacon grease

1.Add salmon, collagen, mozzarella, onion powder, eggs, dill, and salt into a bowl and mix well.

2.Make 8 patties from the mixture.

3.Place a large skillet with bacon grease over a medium-low flame.

4.Place the salmon cakes in the skillet once the fat is well heated and cook until it becomes golden brown on all sides.

5.Take off the pan from heat and let the patties remain in the cooked fat for 5 minutes. Serve.

Nutrition: Calories 204, Fat 10, Carbs 5, Protein 29, Sodium 643

394.Grilled Split Lobster

Prep Time: 10 min | **Cook Time:** 15 min | **Serve:** 2

- 4 tablespoons olive oil or melted butter Kosher salt to taste

- 4 live lobsters (1 ½ pound each)
- Freshly ground pepper to taste
- Melted butter to serve
- Hot sauce like Frank's hot sauce, to serve Lemon wedges to serve

1. For 15 minutes, put the live lobsters in the freezer.
2. Place them on your cutting board with the belly down on the cutting board. Hold the tail. Split the lobsters in half lengthwise. Start from the point where the tail joins the body and goes up to the head. Flip sides and cut it lengthwise via the tail.
3. Rub melted butter on the cut part immediately after cutting it. Sprinkle salt and pepper over it.
4. Set up your grill and preheat it to high heat for 5-10 minutes. Clean the grill grate and lower the heat to low heat.
5. Place the lobsters on the grill and press the claws on the grill until cooked— grill for 6-8 minutes.
6. Flip sides and cook until it is cooked through and lightly charred.
7. Transfer to a plate. Drizzle melted butter on top and serve.

Nutrition: Calories 433, Fat 4, Carbs 26, Protein 6, Sodium 455

395. Fish Bone Broth

Prep Time: 10 min
Cook Time: 4 hrs
Serve: 2

- 2 pounds of the fish head or carcass
- Salt to taste
- 7 – 8 quarts water + extra to blanch
- 2 inches ginger, sliced
- 2 tablespoons lemon juice

1. To blanch the fish: Add water and fish heads into a large pot. Place the pot over high heat.
2. Turn the heat off when it boils and discard the water.
3. Place the fish back in the pot. Pour 7-8 quarts of water.
4. Place the pot over high heat. Add ginger, salt, and lemon juice.
5. Reduce the heat as the mixture boils, and cover it with a lid.
6. Remove from heat. When it cools down, strain into a large jar with a wire mesh strainer.
7. Refrigerate for 5-6 days. Unused broth can be frozen.

Nutrition: Calories 254, Fat 4, Carbs 26, Protein 6, Sodium 455

396. Garlic Butter Shrimp

Prep Time: 10 min | **Cook Time:** 10 min | **Serve:** 2

- 1 cup unsalted butter, divided
- Kosher salt to taste
- ½ cup chicken stock
- Freshly ground pepper to taste
- ¼ cup chopped fresh parsley leaves
- 3 pounds medium shrimp, peeled, deveined garlic
- Juice of 2 lemons

1. Add 4 tablespoons butter into a large skillet and place the skillet over medium-high flame. Once butter melts, stir in salt, shrimp, and pepper and cook for 2 - 3 minutes. Stir every minute or so. Remove the shrimp with a spoon and place it on a tray.
2. Add garlic into the pot and cook until you get a nice aroma. Pour lemon juice and stock and stir.
3. Lower the heat and cook until the stock falls to half its initial volume until it comes to a boil.

4. Add the rest of the butter, a tablespoon each time, and stir until it melts each time.
5. Add shrimp and stir lightly until well coated.
6. Sprinkle parsley on top and serve.

Nutrition: Calories 484, Fat 21, Carbs 4, Protein 33, Sodium 370

397. Grilled Shrimp

Prep Time: 10 min | **Cook Time:** 5 min | **Serve:** 2
Shrimp Seasoning

- 2 teaspoons garlic powder
- 2 teaspoons Italian seasoning
- 2 teaspoons kosher salt
- ½ - 1 teaspoon cayenne pepper

Grilling

- 4 tablespoons extra-virgin olive oil
- 2 pounds shrimp, peeled, deveined
- 2 tablespoons fresh lemon juice
- Oil to grease the grill grated

1. You can grill the shrimp in a grill or boil it in an oven. Choose whatever method suits you and preheat the grill or oven to high heat.
2. In case you are broiling it in an oven, prepare a baking sheet by lining it with foil and greasing the foil as well, with some fat.
3. Add garlic powder, cayenne pepper, salt, and Italian seasoning into a large bowl and mix well.
4. Add lemon juice and oil and mix well.
5. Stir in the shrimp. Make sure that the shrimp are well coated with the mixture.
6. If using the grill, fix the shrimp on skewers; else, place them on the baking sheet.
7. Grease the grill grates with some oil. Grill the shrimp or broil them in an oven until they turn pink. It should take 180 seconds for each side.

Nutrition: Calories 309, Fat 12, Carbs 8, Protein 16, Sodium 340

398. Garlic Ghee Pan-Fried Cod

Prep Time: 5 min | **Cook Time:** 10 min | **Serve:** 2

- 2 cod fillets (4.8 ounces each)
- 3 cloves garlic, peeled, minced
- Salt to taste
- 1 ½ tablespoons ghee
- ½ tablespoon garlic powder (optional)

1. Place a pan over medium-high flame. Add ghee.
2. Once ghee melts, stir in half the garlic and cook for about 6 – 10 seconds.
3. Add fillets and season with garlic powder and salt.
4. Soon the color of the fish will turn white. This color should be visible for about half the height of the fish.
5. Turn the fish over and cook, adding remaining garlic.
6. When the entire fillet turns white, remove it from the pan.

Nutrition: Calories 193, Fat 16, Carbs 6, Protein 21, Sodium 521

399. Mussel And Potato Stew

Prep Time: 10 min | **Cook Time:** 20 min | **Serve:** 2

- potatoes
- broccoli
- olive oil
- filets
- garlic

1.Submerge potatoes in cold water in a medium saucepan. Put the salt, and boil. Allow cooling for 15 minutes till soft. Let drain.
2.Boil a saucepan of salted water. Put broccoli rabe, and allow to cook till just soft; it should turn bright green. Drain thoroughly, and slice into 2-inch lengths.
3.In a big, deep skillet, mix garlic, anchovies, and oil. Let cook over high heat for approximately a minute, crushing anchovies. In a skillet, scatter the mussels, put chopped parsley, broccoli rabe, and potatoes on top. Put half cup water, and add salt to season. Place the cover, and allow to cook till mussels are open.

Nutrition: Calories 254, Fat 9, Carbs 12, Protein 11, Sodium 326

400.Tuna and Tomatoes

Prep Time: 5 min | **Cook Time:** 20 min | **Serve:** 2
- 1 yellow onion, chopped
- 1 tablespoon olive oil
- 1 pound tuna fillets, boneless, skinless, and cubed
- 1 cup tomatoes, chopped
- 1 red pepper, chopped
- 1 teaspoon sweet paprika
- 1 tablespoon coriander, chopped

1.Over medium heat, heat a pan with the oil, add the onions and pepper and cook for 5 minutes.
2.Add the fish and the other ingredients, cook everything for 15 minutes, divide between plates and serve.

Nutrition: Calories 215, Fat 2, Carbs 34, Protein 16, Sodium 350

401.Mustard Salmon With Herbs

Prep Time: 10 min | **Cook Time:** 30 min | **Serve:** 2
- mustard
- mayonnaise
- dressing mix
- garlic powder, or to taste
- lemons
- salmon fillet
- 1 sprig fresh mint, stemmed, or to taste
- 1 sprig fresh rosemary, or to taste
- 2 spoons chopped fresh chives, or to taste
- 1 sprig fresh dill, or to taste
- 4 cloves garlic, crushed, or to taste

1.In a bowl, combine garlic powder, ranch dressing, Italian dressing, mayonnaise, and mustard. Squeeze over the mixture with 1/2 of the lemon. Cut the leftover lemon halves
2.Put the preheated oven in and cook for 30-45 minutes before the flesh can easily flake with a fork.

Nutrition: Calories 277, Fat 11, Carbs 26, Protein 18, Sodium 520

402.Nutty Coconut Fish

Prep Time: 10 min | **Cook Time:** 30 min | **Serve:** 2
- mayonnaise
- mustard
- bread crumbs
- shredded coconut
- mixed nuts
- granulated sugar
- 1 teaspoon salt

- 1/2 teaspoon cayenne pepper
- 1 pound whitefish fillets

1.The oven should be preheated to 190-195 degrees C.
2.Blend brown mustard and mayonnaise in a small bowl. Mix cayenne pepper, salt, sugar, chopped mixed nuts, shredded coconut, and dry breadcrumbs in a medium bowl.
3.Dip fish in mayonnaise mixture, then dip in breadcrumb mixture. In a baking dish, put coated fish fillets.
4.Bake for 20/3 minutes in a preheated oven until the fish flakes easily with a fork.

Nutrition: Calories 180, Fat 2, Carbs 12, Protein 6, Sodium 426

403.Olive Oil Poached Tuna

Prep Time: 10 min | **Cook Time:** 30 min | **Serve:** 2
- tuna steaks
- garlic
- thyme
- pepper flakes
- olive oil
- sea salt to taste

1.Set aside tuna for 10-15 minutes at room temperature.
2.In a heavy pan, mix red pepper flakes, garlic, and thyme. Pour in olive oil until an inch deep. On medium heat, heat for 5-10 minutes until the thyme and garlic sizzles.
3.Put the tuna lightly in the pan of hot oil, then turn heat to low. Cook steaks for 5-7 minutes while constantly spooning oil on top until the tuna is hot and white. Take off heat, move the steaks to a baking pan, and then pour hot oil and herbs on top. Let the fish cool down to temperature.
4.Use plastic wrap to tightly cover the baking dish and put the steaks in the refrigerator for 24 hours. Take the tuna out of the oil and top with sea salt.

Nutrition: Calories 208, Fat 21, Carbs 26, Protein 36, Sodium 543

404.One-Pot Tuna Casserole

Prep Time: 10 min | **Cook Time:** 20 min | **Serve:** 2
- 1 (16 ounces) package egg noodles
- 1 (10 ounces) package frozen green peas, thawed
- 1/4 cup butter
- 1 (10.75 ounces) can condense cream of mushroom soup
- 1 (5 ounces) can tuna, drained
- 1/4 cup milk
- 1 cup shredded Cheddar cheese

1.Boil a big pot with lightly salted water. Cook pasta in boiling water, till "al dente"; add peas at 3 final minutes of cooking and drain.
2.Melt butter overheats in the same pot. Add Cheddar cheese, milk, tuna, and mushroom soup; mix till mixture is smooth and cheese melts. Mix peas and pasta in till evenly coated.

Nutrition: Calories 398, Fat 16, Carbs 12, Protein 33, Sodium 455

405.Bacon-Wrapped Salmon

Prep Time: 10 min | **Cook Time:** 30 min | **Serve:** 2
- 4 (4 ounces) skin-on salmon fillets
- 1 teaspoon garlic powder
- 1 teaspoon dried dill weed
- salt and pepper to taste
- 1/2 pound bacon, cut in half

1.Preheat oven to 375°F. Generously brush olive oil on a cookie sheet.

2.Arrange salmon fillets skin down on the cookie sheet. Season fillets with dill, salt, pepper, and garlic powder. Cover the fillets completely with bacon strips. Arrange the bacon so they don't overlap each other.

3.Bake in the oven for 20-23 minutes, just until the fish's center is not translucent. To broil, change the oven setting and cook for another 1 to 2 minutes until the bacon becomes crispy.

Nutrition: Calories 307, Fat 23, Carbs 8, Protein 16, Sodium 590

406.Bagna Cauda

Prep Time: 10 min | **Cook Time:** 30 min | **Serve:** 2
- 1/2 cup butter
- 10 cloves garlic, minced
- fillets
- cream

1.Mix in garlic and cook until softened. Lower the heat to low. Mix in heavy cream and anchovy filets.

2.Bring the mixture back to medium heat, stirring from time to time, until bubbling.

Nutrition: Calories 670, Fat 34, Carbs 26, Protein 28, Sodium 430

407.Bermuda Fish Chowder

Prep Time: 10 min | **Cook Time:** 30 min | **Serve:** 2
- 2 tablespoons vegetable oil
- 3 stalks celery, chopped
- 2 carrots, chopped
- 1 onion, chopped
- 1 green bell pepper, chopped
- 3 cloves garlic, minced
- 3 tablespoons tomato paste
- 4 cups clam juice
- 2 potatoes, peeled and cubed
- 1 (14.5 ounces) can peeled tomatoes
- 2 spoons Worcestershire sauce
- 1 jalapeno pepper
- 1 little spoon ground black pepper
- 1 bay-leaf
- 1 pound red-snapper fillets, cut into 1 inch pieces

1.In a large soup pot, heat the oil over medium heat. Toss in the carrots, celery, green pepper, onion, and garlic and sauté them for about 8 minutes.

2.Pour in the tomato paste and cook and stir for 1 minute. Mix in the clam juice, canned tomatoes with juice, potatoes, Worcestershire sauce, bay leaf, jalapeno pepper, and ground black pepper. Let it simmer until the potatoes are already tender, stirring the soup for about every 30 minutes.

3.Put the fish in and let it simmer for about 10 minutes until the snapper easily flakes with a fork.

Nutrition: Calories 320, Fat 28, Carbs 21, Protein 36, Sodium 660

408.Salmon Tikka

Prep Time: 10 min | **Cook Time:** 30 min | **Serve:** 2
- red pepper
- turmeric
- salt
- salmon fillets
- cornstarch
- oil

1.In a bowl, combine salt, turmeric, and cayenne. Put salmon into the bowl; toss until evenly coated with seasoning mixture. Let fish rest for 15 minutes.

2.In a container, heat oil over medium heat. Meanwhile, sprinkle cornstarch all over salmon; toss to coat evenly.

3.Cook salmon in hot oil, about 1 minute on each side, until golden brown.

Nutrition: Calories 254, Fat 24, Carbs 12, Protein 26, Sodium 765

409.Almond And Parmesan Crusted Tilapia

Prep Time: 10 min | **Cook Time:** 30 min | **Serve:** 2
- 1 teaspoon olive oil, or as needed
- 3 cloves garlic, minced
- 1/2 cup grated Parmesan cheese
- almonds, crushed
- mayonnaise
- bread crumbs
- 2 tablespoons fresh lemon juice
- 1/4 teaspoon dried basil
- 1/4 teaspoon ground black pepper
- 1/8 teaspoon onion powder
- 1/8 teaspoon celery salt
- 1 pound tilapia fillets

1.Put the rack 6 inches away from the heat source and start preheating the oven's broiler. Use aluminum foil to line a broiling tray or use olive oil cooking spray to coat.

2.Heat olive oil in a frying container over medium heat, stir garlic while cooking for 3 to 5 minutes, or aromatic.

3.In a bowl, combine celery salt, onion powder, black pepper, basil, seafood seasoning, lemon juice, bread crumbs, mayonnaise, almonds, buttery spreads, garlic, and Parmesan cheese.

4.Set the tilapia fillets in a layer on top of the prepared pan, use aluminum foil to cover it.

5.Put the container in the preheated oven and start boiling for about 2 to 3 minutes. Flip the fillets, cover the pan with aluminum foil, and restart broiling for 2 to 3 more minutes. Remove aluminum foil and put the Parmesan cheese mixture on top to cover the fish. Broil in the oven for 2 more minutes until topping gets browned; fish can be shredded easily with a fork.

Nutrition: Calories 498, Fat 32, Carbs 26, Protein 8, Sodium 634

410.Crab And Shrimp Pasta Salad

Prep Time: 10 min | **Cook Time:** 30 min | **Serve:** 2
- 1 (16 ounces) package uncooked tri-colored spiral pasta
- 1/2 cup mayonnaise
- 1/4 cup apple cider vinegar
- 1/4 cup olive oil
- salt and pepper to taste
- 1 (8 ounces) package imitation crabmeat, flaked
- 1 (6.5 ounces) can tiny shrimp, drained
- 1-pint grape tomatoes halved
- 1 English cucumber, diced
- 1 (4 ounces) can slice black olives, drained
- 1 red bell pepper, seeded and chopped

1.Boil a big pot with lightly salted water. Add pasta. Cook for 10 minutes till tender, then drain. Cool by rinsing under cold water. Put into a big bowl, put aside.

2.Mix pepper, salt, olive oil, vinegar, and mayonnaise in a small bowl. Put on pasta; mix to coat. Add bell pepper, black olives, cucumber, tomatoes, shrimp, and crab. Gently mix to coat in dressing. Taste, then adjust seasoning if you want. Mix extra mayonnaise if the pasta is very dry.

Nutrition: Calories 480, Fat 24, Carbs 10, Protein 23, Sodium 680

411.Cream Of Salmon Soup

Prep Time: 10 min | **Cook Time:** 30 min | **Serve:** 2

Puff Pastry Triangles:
- 1 sheet frozen puff pastry, thawed
- 1 egg yolk, beaten
- 1 tablespoon sesame seeds

Salmon Soup:
- 1 1/2 tablespoons butter
- 1 onion, diced
- 18 ounces salmon fillets, diced
- 1 tablespoon tomato paste
- 2 1/2 cups fish stock
- 1/2 cup dry white wine
- 1 tablespoon cornstarch
- 1 1/4 cups heavy whipping cream
- A little saffron, salt and white pepper, freshly ground, to taste
- 3 little spoons chopped fresh dill

1.Set the oven at 400°F and start preheating.

2.On a lightly floured surface, place puff pastry; use a rolling pin to roll it out. Brush egg yolk over. Put sesame seeds on top; press in firmly. First, divide puff pastry into squares, then into triangles, put them on a baking sheet.

3.Start baking for about 15 minutes in the preheated oven till triangles are puffed up and golden brown.

4.In the meantime, place a pot on medium heat, melt in the butter and cook in onion till soft and translucent, about 5 minutes. 5.Include in salmon and cook for 5 minutes. Mix in tomato paste; cook for 1 minute. Add in white wine and fish stock. Boil everything; turn down the heat; simmer for 15 minutes. Let it boil.

6.Blend a little bit of water and cornstarch into a paste. Pour into the soup and let the mixture come to a boil. Cook till the soup is thickened, about 5 minutes. Make the soup into a smooth purée with an immersion blender. Mix in saffron and cream. Flavor with pepper and salt.

7.Dill for garnish and puff pastry triangles to serve with the soup.

Nutrition: Calories 436, Fat 32, Carbs 26, Protein 36, Sodium 663

412.Creamed Salmon On Toast

Prep Time: 10 min | **Cook Time:** 30 min | **Serve:** 2
- Butter
- flour
- milk
- green peas
- 1 (14.75 ounces) can salmon
- salt and pepper to taste

1.Set the heat to medium, then melt butter in a skillet or saucepan. Whisk the flour while stirring continuously to have a smooth paste. Carefully pour the milk while stirring continuously with the peas' leftover liquids to make a smooth thick gravy.

2.Break large pieces of the salmon into smaller pieces by flaking them into a bowl. Mix the peas and salmon carefully into the sauce using a wooden spoon to keep the peas from being mashed. Cook until thoroughly heated.

3.Use a toaster oven or a broiler pan to toast some bread. You can even add butter if you want and garnish it with some salmon mixture on top.

Nutrition: Calories 244, Fat 32, Carbs 26, Protein 6, Sodium 321

413.Coconut Salsa on Chipotle Fish Tacos

Prep Time: 10 min | **Cook Time:** 10 min | **Serve:** 4
- ¼ cup chopped fresh cilantro
- ½ cup seeded and finely chopped plum tomato
- 1 cup peeled and finely chopped mango
- 1 lime cut into wedges
- 1 tablespoon chipotle Chile powder
- 1 tablespoon safflower oil
- 1/3 cup finely chopped red onion
- 10 tablespoon fresh lime juice, divided
- 4 6-oz boneless, skinless cod fillets
- 5 tablespoon dried unsweetened shredded coconut
- 8 pcs of 6-inch tortillas, heated

1. Whisk well Chile powder, oil, and 4 tablespoon lime juice in a glass baking dish. Add cod and marinate for 12 – 15 minutes. Turning once halfway through the marinating time.

2. Make the salsa by mixing coconut, 6 tablespoon lime juice, cilantro, onions, tomatoes and mangoes in a medium bowl. Set aside.

3. On high, heat a grill pan. Place cod and grill for four minutes per side, turning only once.

4. Once cooked, slice cod into large flakes and evenly divide onto the tortilla.

5. Evenly divide salsa on top of cod and serve with a side of lime wedges.

Nutrition: Calories: 477 Protein: 35.0g Fat: 12.4g Carbs: 57.4g

414.Baked Cod Crusted with Herbs

Prep Time: 5 min | **Cook Time:** 10 min | **Serve:** 4
- ¼ cup honey
- ¼ teaspoon salt
- ½ cup panko
- ½ teaspoon pepper
- 1 tablespoon extra virgin olive oil
- 1 tablespoon lemon juice
- 1 teaspoon dried basil
- 1 teaspoon dried parsley
- 1 teaspoon rosemary
- 4 pieces of 4-oz cod fillets

1. With olive oil, grease a 9 x 13-inch baking pan and preheat oven to 375oF.

2. In a zip-top bag, mix panko, rosemary, salt, pepper, parsley and basil.

3. Evenly spread cod fillets in a prepped dish and drizzle with lemon juice.

4. Then brush the fillets with honey on all sides. Discard remaining honey, if any.

5. Then evenly divide the panko mixture on top of cod fillets.

6. Pop in the oven and bake for ten minutes or until fish is cooked.

Nutrition: Calories: 137 Protein: 5g Fat: 2g Carbs: 21g

415. Cajun Garlic Shrimp Noodle Bowl

Prep Time: 10 min | **Cook Time:** 15 min | **Serve:** 2

- ½ teaspoon salt
- 1 onion, sliced
- 1 red pepper, sliced
- 1 tablespoon butter
- 1 teaspoon garlic granules
- 1 teaspoon onion powder
- 1 teaspoon paprika
- 2 large zucchinis, cut into noodle strips
- 20 jumbo shrimps, shells removed and deveined
- 3 cloves garlic, minced
- 3 tablespoon ghee
- A dash of cayenne pepper
- A dash of red pepper flakes

1. Prepare the Cajun seasoning by mixing the onion powder, garlic granules, pepper flakes, cayenne pepper, paprika and salt. Toss in the shrimp to coat in the seasoning.
2. In a skillet, heat the ghee and sauté the garlic. Add in the red pepper and onions and continue sautéing for 4 minutes.
3. Add the Cajun shrimp and cook until opaque. Set aside.
4. In another pan, heat the butter and sauté the zucchini noodles for three minutes.
5. Assemble by placing the Cajun shrimps on top of the zucchini noodles.

Nutrition: Calories: 712 Fat: 30.0g Protein: 97.8g Carbs: 20.2g

416. Crazy Saganaki Shrimp

Prep Time: 10 min | **Cook Time:** 10 min | **Serve:** 4

- ¼ teaspoon salt
- ½ cup Chardonnay
- ½ cup crumbled Greek feta cheese
- 1 medium bulb. fennel, cored and finely chopped
- 1 small Chile pepper, seeded and minced
- 1 tablespoon extra virgin olive oil
- 12 jumbo shrimps, deveined with tails left on
- 2 tablespoon lemon juice, divided
- 5 scallions sliced thinly
- Pepper to taste

1. In a medium bowl, mix salt, lemon juice and shrimp.
2. On medium fire, place a saganaki pan (or large nonstick saucepan) and heat oil.
3. Sauté Chile pepper, scallions, and fennel for 4 minutes or until starting to brown and is already soft.
4. Add wine and sauté for another minute.
5. Place shrimps on top of the fennel, cover and cook for 4 minutes or until shrimps are pink.
6. Remove just the shrimp and transfer to a plate.
7. Add pepper, feta and 1 tablespoon lemon juice to the pan and cook for a minute or until cheese begins to melt.
8. To serve, place cheese and fennel mixture on a serving plate and top with shrimps.

Nutrition: Calories: 310 Protein: 49.7g Fat: 6.8g Carbs: 8.4g

417. Creamy Bacon-Fish Chowder

Prep Time: 10 min | **Cook Time:** 30 min | **Serve:** 8

- 1 1/2 lbs. cod
- 1 1/2 teaspoon dried thyme

- 1 large onion, chopped
- 1 medium carrot, coarsely chopped
- 1 tablespoon butter, cut into small pieces
- 1 teaspoon salt, divided
- 3 1/2 cups baking potato, peeled and cubed
- 3 slices uncooked bacon
- 3/4 teaspoon ground black pepper, divided
- 4 1/2 cups water
- 4 bay leaves
- 4 cups 2% reduced-fat milk

1. In a large skillet, add the water and bay leaves and let it simmer. Add the fish. Cover and let it simmer some more until the flesh flakes easily with a fork. Remove the fish from the skillet and cut it into large pieces. Set aside the cooking liquid.
2. Place Dutch oven in medium heat and cook the bacon until crisp. Remove the bacon and reserve the bacon drippings. Crush the bacon and set aside.
3. Stir potato, onion and carrot in the pan with the bacon drippings, cook over medium heat for 10 minutes. Add the cooking liquid, bay leaves, 1/2 teaspoon salt, 1/4 teaspoon pepper and thyme, let it boil. Lower the heat and let simmer for 11 minutes. Add the milk and butter, simmer until the potatoes become tender, but do not boil. Add the fish, 1/2 teaspoon salt, 1/2 teaspoon pepper. Remove the bay leaves.
4. Serve sprinkled with the crushed bacon.

Nutrition: Calories: 400 Carbs: 34.5g Protein: 20.8g Fat: 19.7g

418. Crisped Coco-Shrimp with Mango Dip

Prep Time: 10 min | **Cook Time:** 20 min | **Serve:** 4

- 1 cup shredded coconut
- 1 lb. raw shrimp, peeled and deveined
- 2 egg whites
- 4 tablespoon tapioca starch
- Pepper and salt to tast
- Mango Dip Ingredients:
- 1 cup mango, chopped
- 1 jalapeño, thinly minced
- 1 teaspoon lime juice
- 1/3 cup coconut milk
- 3 teaspoon raw honey

1. preheat oven to 4000F.
2. Ready a pan with a wire rack on top.
3. In a medium bowl, add tapioca starch and season with pepper and salt.
4. In a second medium bowl, add egg whites and whisk.
5. In a third medium bowl, add coconut.
6. To ready shrimps, dip first in tapioca starch, then egg whites, and then coconut. Place dredged shrimp on wire rack. Repeat until all shrimps are covered.
7. Pop shrimps in the oven and roast for 10 minutes per side.
8. Meanwhile, make the dip by adding all ingredients in a blender. Puree until smooth and creamy. Transfer to a dipping bowl.
9. Once shrimps are golden brown, serve with mango dip.

Nutrition: Calories: 294.2 Protein: 26.6g Fat: 7g Carbs: 31.2g

419. Cucumber-Basil Salsa on Halibut Pouches

Prep Time: 10 min | **Cook Time:** 17 min | **Serve:** 4

- 1 lime, thinly sliced into eight pieces

- 2 cups mustard greens, stems removed
- 2 teaspoon olive oil
- 4 – 5 radishes trimmed and quartered
- 4 4-oz skinless halibut filets
- 4 large fresh basil leaves
- Cayenne pepper to taste – optional
- Pepper and salt to taste
- Salsa Ingredients:
- 1 ½ cups diced cucumber
- 1 ½ finely chopped fresh basil leaves
- 2 teaspoon fresh lime juice
- Pepper and salt to taste

1. preheat oven to 400°F.
2. Prepare parchment papers by making 4 pieces of 15 x 12-inch rectangles. Lengthwise, fold in half and unfold pieces on the table.
3. Season halibut fillets with pepper, salt and cayenne—if using cayenne.
4. Just to the right of the fold, place ½ cup of mustard greens. Add a basil leaf on the center of mustard greens and topped with 1 lime slice. Around the greens, layer ¼ of the radishes. Drizzle with ½ teaspoon of oil, season with pepper and salt. Top it with a slice of halibut fillet.
5. Just as you would make a calzone, fold the parchment paper over your filling and crimp the edges of the parchment paper beginning from one end to the other end. To seal the end of the crimped parchment paper, pinch it.
6. Repeat the remaining ingredients until you have 4 pieces of parchment papers filled with halibut and greens.
7. Place pouches in a pan and bake in the oven until halibut is flaky around 15 to 17 minutes.
8. While waiting for halibut pouches to cook, make your salsa by mixing all salsa ingredients in a medium bowl.
9. Once halibut is cooked, remove it from the oven and make a tear on top. Be careful of the steam as it is very hot. Equally, divide salsa and spoon ¼ of salsa on top of halibut through the slit you have created.
Nutrition: Calories: 335.4 Protein: 20.2g Fat: 16.3g Carbs: 22.1g

420.Salmon with Mustard

Prep Time: 10 min | **Cook Time:** 8 min | **Serve:** 4
- ¼ teaspoon ground red pepper or chili powder
- ¼ teaspoon ground turmeric
- ¼ teaspoon salt
- 1 teaspoon honey
- 1/8 teaspoon garlic powder or a minced clove garlic 2 teaspoon. whole grain mustard 4 pcs 6-oz salmon fillets

1. In a small bowl, mix well salt, garlic powder, red pepper, turmeric, honey and mustard.
2. Preheat the oven to broil and grease a baking dish with cooking spray.
3. Place salmon on a baking dish with skin side down and spread evenly mustard mixture on top of salmon.
4. Pop in the oven and broil until flaky, around 8 minutes.
Nutrition: Calories: 324 Fat: 18.9 g Protein: 34 g Carbs: 2.9g

421.Dijon Mustard and Lime Marinated Shrimp

Prep Time: 10 min | **Cook Time:** 10 min | **Serve:** 8
- ½ cup fresh lime juice and lime zest as garnish

- ½ cup of rice vinegar
- ½ teaspoon hot sauce
- 1 bay leaf
- 1 cup of water
- 1 lb. uncooked shrimp, peeled and deveined
- 1 medium red onion, chopped
- 2 tablespoon capers
- 2 tablespoon Dijon mustard
- 3 whole cloves

1. Mix hot sauce, mustard, capers, lime juice and onion in a shallow baking dish and set aside.
2. Put the bay leaf, cloves, vinegar, and water to a boil in a large saucepan.
3. Once boiling, add shrimps and cook for a minute while stirring continuously.
4. Drain shrimps and pour shrimps into onion mixture.
5. For an hour, refrigerate while covered the shrimps.
6. Then serve shrimps cold and garnished with lime zest.
Nutrition: Calories: 232.2 Protein: 17.8g Fat: 3g Carbs: 15g

422.Dill Relish on White Sea Bass

Prep Time: 10 min | **Cook Time:** 12 min | **Serve:** 4
- 1 ½ tablespoon chopped white onion
- 1 ½ teaspoon chopped fresh dill
- 1 lemon, quartered
- 1 teaspoon Dijon mustard
- 1 teaspoon lemon juice
- 1 teaspoon pickled baby capers, drained
- 4 pieces of 4-oz white sea bass fillets

1. Preheat oven to 375°F.
2. Mix lemon juice, mustard, dill, capers and onions in a small bowl.
3. Prepare four aluminum foil squares and place 1 fillet per foil.
4. Squeeze a lemon wedge per fish.
5. Evenly divide into 4 the dill spread and drizzle over the fillet.
6. Close the foil over the fish securely and pop in the oven.
7. Bake for 12 minutes or until fish is cooked through.
8. Remove from foil and transfer to a serving platter.
Nutrition: Calories: 115 Protein: 7g Fat: 1g Carbs: 12g

423.Salmon & Arugula Omelet

Prep Time: 10 min | **Cook Time:** 7 min | **Serve:** 4
- 6 eggs
- 2 tablespoons unsweetened almond milk Salt and ground black pepper, as required 2 tablespoons olive oil
- 4 ounces smoked salmon, cut into bite-sized chunks
- 2 cups fresh arugula, chopped finely
- 4 scallions, chopped finely

1.In a bowl, place the eggs, coconut milk, salt and black pepper and beat well. Set aside.
2. Over medium pressure, heat the oil in a non-stick skillet.
3.Place the egg mixture evenly and cook for about 30 seconds without stirring.
4.Place the salmon kale and scallions on top of egg mixture evenly.
5. Lower the heat to a low level and cook covered for about 4-5 minutes or until omelet is done completely.
6.Uncover the skillet and cook for about 1 minute.
7.Carefully transfer the omelet onto a serving plate.

424. Tuna Omelet
Prep Time: 10 min | **Cook Time:** 5 min | **Serve:** 2
- 4 eggs
- ¼ cup unsweetened almond milk
- 1 tablespoon scallions, chopped
- 1 garlic clove, minced
- ½ of jalapeño pepper, minced
- Salt and ground black pepper, to taste
- 1 (5-ounce) can water-packed tuna, drained and flaked
- 1 tablespoon olive oil
- 3 normal spoons green bell pepper, seeded and chopped
- 3 tablespoons tomato, chopped
- ¼ cup low-fat cheddar cheese, shredded

1. In a bowl, add the eggs, almond milk, scallions, garlic, jalapeño pepper, salt, and black pepper, and beat well.
2. Add the tuna and stir to combine.
3. In a big-non-stick frying pan, heat oil over medium heat.
4. Place the egg mixture in an even layer and cook for about 1–2 minutes, without stirring.
5. Carefully lift the edges to run the uncooked portion flow underneath.
6. Spread the veggies over the egg mixture and sprinkle with the cheese.
7. Cover the frying pan and cook for about 30–60 seconds.
8. Remove the lid and fold the omelet in half.
9. Remove from the heat and cut the omelet into 2 portions.

425. Fish Stew
Prep Time: 15 min | **Cook Time:** 50 min | **Serve:** 10
- ¼ cup coconut oil
- ½ cup yellow onion, chopped
- 1 cup celery stalk, chopped
- ½ cup green bell pepper, seeded and chopped
- 1 garlic clove, minced
- 4 cups water
- 4 beef bouillon cubes
- 20 ounces okra, trimmed and chopped
- 2 (14-ounce) cans sugar-free diced tomatoes with liquid
- 2 bay leaves
- 1 teaspoon dried thyme, crushed
- 2 teaspoons red pepper flakes, crushed
- ¼ teaspoon hot pepper sauce
- Salt and ground black pepper, as required
- 32 ounces catfish fillets
- ½ cup fresh cilantro, chopped

1. In a big skillet, melt the coconut oil over medium heat and sauté the onion, celery and bell pepper for about 4-5 minutes.
2. Meanwhile, in a large soup pan, mix together bouillon cubes and water and bring to a boil over medium heat.
3. Transfer the onion mixture and remaining ingredients except catfish into the pan of boiling water and bring to a boil.
4. Decrease the heat to low, cook for about 30 minutes, protected.
5. Stir in catfish fillets and cook for about 10-15 minutes.
6. Stir in the cilantro and remove from the heat.

426. Salmon & Veggie Salad
Prep Time: 15 min | **Serve:** 2
- 6 ounces cooked wild salmon, chopped
- 1 cup cucumber, sliced
- 1 cup red bell-pepper, seeded and sliced ½ cup grape tomatoes, quartered
- 1 tablespoon scallion green, chopped
- 1 cup lettuce, torn
- 1 cup fresh spinach, torn
- 2 tablespoons olive oil
- 2 tablespoons fresh lemon juice

1. In a salad bowl, place all ingredients and gently toss to coat well.

427. Tuna Salad
Prep Time: 15 min | **Serve:** 4
For Dressing:
- 2 tablespoons fresh dill, minced
- 2 tablespoons olive oil
- 1 tablespoon fresh lime juice
- Salt and ground black pepper, to taste

For Salad:
- 4 cups fresh spinach, torn
- 2 (6-ounce) cans water-packed tuna, drained and flaked
- 6 hard-boiled eggs, peeled and sliced
- 1 cup tomato, chopped
- 1 large cucumber, sliced

1. For Dressing: place dill, oil, lime juice, salt, and black pepper in a small bowl and beat until well combined.
2. Divide the spinach onto serving plates and top each with tuna, egg, cucumber, and tomato.
3. Drizzle with dressing.

428. Shrimp & Greens Salad
Prep Time: 15 min | **Cook Time:** 6 min | **Serve:** 6
- 3 tablespoons olive oil, divided
- 1 garlic clove, crushed and divided
- 2 tablespoons fresh rosemary, chopped
- 1-pound shrimp, peeled and deveined
- Salt and ground black pepper, as required
- 4 cups fresh arugula
- 2 cups lettuce, torn
- 2 tablespoons fresh lime juice

1. In a large wok, heat 1 normal spoon of oil over medium heat and sauté 1 garlic clove for about 1 minute.
2. Add the shrimp with salt and black pepper and cook for about 4-5 minutes.
3. Remove from the heat and place to cool aside.
4. Ina large bowl, add the shrimp, arugula, remaining oil, lime juice, salt and black pepper and gently, toss to coat.

429. Shrimp, Apple & Carrot Salad
Prep Time: 20 min | **Cook Time:** 3 min | **Serve:** 4
- 12 medium shrimp
- 1½ cups Granny Smith apple, cored and sliced thinly 1½ cups carrot, peeled and cut into matchsticks
- ½ cup fresh mint leaves, chopped
- 2 tablespoons balsamic vinegar
- ¼ cup extra-virgin olive oil
- 1 teaspoon lemongrass, chopped
- 1 teaspoon garlic, minced

- 2 sprigs fresh cilantro, leaves separated and chopped

1. In a large pan of the salted boiling water, add the shrimp and lemon and cook for about 3 minutes.
2. Remove from the heat and drain the shrimp well.
3. Set aside to cool.
4. After cooling, peel and devein the shrimps.
5. Transfer the shrimp into a large bowl.
6. Add the remaining all ingredients except cilantro and gently, stir to combine.
7. Cover the bowl and refrigerate for about 1 hour.
8. Top with cilantro just before serving.

430. Shrimp & Green Beans Salad
Prep Time: 20 min | **Cook Time:** 8 min | **Serve:** 5
For Shrimp:
- 2 tablespoons olive oil
- 2 tablespoons fresh key lime juice
- 4 large garlic cloves, peeled
- 2 sprigs fresh rosemary leaves
- ½ teaspoon garlic salt
- 20 large shrimp, peeled and deveined

For Salad:
- 1-pound fresh green beans, trimmed
- ¼ cup olive oil
- 1 onion, sliced
- Salt and ground black pepper, as required ½ cup garlic and herb feta cheese, crumbled

1. For shrimp marinade: in a blender, add all the ingredients except shrimp and pulse until smooth.
2. Transfer the marinade in a large bowl.
3. Add the shrimp and coat with marinade generously.
4. Cover the bowl and refrigerate for a minimum of 31 minutes to marinate.
5. Preheat the broiler of oven. Arrange the rack in top position of the oven. Line a large baking sheet with a piece of foil.
6. Place the shrimp with marinade onto the prepared baking sheet.
7. Broil for about 3-4 minutes per side.
8. Transfer the shrimp mixture into a bowl and refrigerate until using.
9. Meanwhile, For Salad: in a pan of the salted boiling water, add the green beans and cook for about 3-4 minutes.
10. Drain the green beans well and rinse under cold running water.
11. Transfer the green beans into a large bowl.
12. Add the onion, shrimp, salt and black pepper and stir to combine.
13. Cover and refrigerate to chill for about 1 hour.
14. Stir in cheese just before serving.

431. Shrimp & Olives Salad
Prep Time: 15 min | **Cook Time:** 3 min | **Serve:** 4
- 1-pound shrimp, peeled and deveined
- 1 lemon, quartered
- 2 tablespoons olive oil
- 2 teaspoons fresh lemon juice
- Salt and freshly ground-black-pepper, to taste
- 2 tomatoe, sliced
- ¼ cup onion, sliced
- ¼ cup green olives
- ¼ cup fresh cilantro, chopped finely

1. In a tub of boiling water that is finely salted, add the quartered lemon.
2. Then, add the shrimp and cook for about 2-3 minutes or until pink and opaque.
3. With a slotted spoon, transfer the shrimp into a bowl of ice water to stop the cooking process.
4. Drain the shrimp completely and then pat dry with paper towels.
5. In a small bowl, add the oil, lemon juice, salt, and black pepper, and beat until well combined.
6. Divide the shrimp, tomato, onion, olives, and cilantro onto serving plates.
7. Drizzle with oil mixture.

432. Shrimp & Arugula Salad
Prep Time: 15 min | **Cook Time:** 5 min | **Serve:** 4
For Shrimp:
- 1-pound large shrimp, peeled and deveined ½ tablespoon fresh lemon juice

For Salad:
- 6 cups fresh arugula
- 2 tablespoons extra-virgin olive oil
- 1 tablespoons fresh lemon juice
- Salt and ground black pepper, as required

1. In a large pan of salted boiling water, add the shrimp and lemon juice and cook for about 2 minutes.
2. Withdraw the shrimp from the pan with a slotted-spoon and put it in an ice bath.
3. Drain the shrimp well.
4. In a large bowl, add the shrimp, arugula, oil, lemon juice, salt and black pepper and gently, toss to coat.

433. Shrimp & Veggies Salad
Prep Time: 20 min | **Cook Time:** 5 min | **Serve:** 6
For Dressing:
- 2 tablespoons natural almond butter
- 1 garlic clove, crushed
- 1 tablespoon fresh cilantro, chopped
- 2 tablespoons fresh lime juice
- 1 tablespoon maple syrup
- ½ teaspoon cayenne pepper
- ¼ teaspoon salt
- 1 tablespoon water
- 1/3 cup olive oil

For Salad:
- 1-pound shrimp, peeled and deveined Salt and ground black pepper, as required
- 1 teaspoon olive oil
- 1 cup carrot, peeled and julienned
- 1 cup red cabbage, shredded
- 1 cup green cabbage, shredded
- 1 cup cucumber, julienned
- 4 cups fresh baby arugula
- ¼ cup fresh basil, chopped
- ¼ cup fresh cilantro, chopped
- 4 cups lettuce, torn
- ¼ cup almonds, chopped

1. For Dressing: in a bowl, add all ingredients except oil and beat until well combined.
2. Slowly, add oil, beating continuously until smooth.
3. For Salad: in a bowl, add shrimp, salt, black pepper and oil and toss to coat well.

4. Heat a skillet over medium-high heat and cook the shrimp on each side for about two minutes.

5.Detach from the heat to cool and set aside.

6.In a large serving bowl, add all the cooked shrimp, remaining salad ingredients and dressing and toss to coat well.

434.Salmon Lettuce Wraps

Prep Time: 10 min | **Serve:** 2

- ¼ cup low-fat mozzarella cheese, cubed ¼ cup tomato, chopped
- 2 tablespoons fresh dill, chopped
- 1 teaspoon fresh lemon juice
- Salt, as required
- 4 lettuce leaves
- 1/3 pound cooked salmon, chopped

1.In a small bowl, combine mozzarella, tomato, dill, lemon juice, and salt until well combined.

2.Arrange the lettuce leaves onto serving plates.

3.Divide the salmon and tomato mixture over each lettuce leaf

435.Tuna Burgers

Prep Time: 15 min | **Cook Time:** 6 min | **Serve:** 2

- 1 (15-ounce) can water-packed tuna, drained
- ½ celery stalk, chopped
- 2 tablespoon fresh parsley, chopped
- 1 teaspoon fresh dill, chopped
- 2 tablespoon walnuts, chopped
- 2 tablespoon mayonnaise
- 1 egg, beaten
- 1 tablespoon butter
- 3 cups lettuce

1.For Burgers: add all ingredients except the butter and lettuce in a bowl and mix until well combined.

2.Make 2 equal-sized patties from mixture.

3.In a frying pan, melt butter over medium heat and cook the patties for about 2-3 minutes.

4.Carefully flip the side and cook for about 2-3 minutes.

5.Divide the lettuce onto serving plates.

6.Top each plate with 1 burger and serve.

436.Spicy Salmon

Prep Time: 105 min | **Cook Time:** 8 min | **Serve:** 4

- 4 tablespoons extra-virgin olive oil, divided
- 2 tablespoons fresh lemon juice
- 1 teaspoon ground turmeric
- 1 teaspoon ground cumin
- Salt and ground black pepper, as required
- 4 (4-ounce) boneless, skinless salmon fillets
- 6 cups fresh arugula

1.In a bowl, mix together 2 normal spoons of oil, lemon juice, turmeric, cumin, salt and black pepper.

2.Add the salmon fillets and coat with the oil mixture generously. Set aside.

3.In a non-stick wok, heat remaining oil over medium heat.

4.Place salmon fillets, skin-side down and cook for about 3-5 minutes.

5.Change the side and cook for about 2-3 minutes more.

6.Divide the salmon onto serving plates and serve immediately alongside the arugula.

437.Lemony Salmon

Prep Time: 10 min | **Cook Time:** 14 min | **Serve:** 4

- 2 garlic cloves, minced
- 1 tablespoon fresh lemon zest, grated
- 2 tablespoons olive oil
- 2 tablespoons fresh lemon juice
- Salt and ground black pepper, to taste
- 4 (6-ounce) boneless, skinless salmon fillets
- 6 cups fresh spinach

1. Preheat the grill to medium-high heat.

2.Grease the grill grate.

3.In a bowl, place all-ingredients except for salmon and spinach and mix well.

4.Add the salmon fillets and coat with garlic mixture generously.

5.Grill the salmon fillets for about 6-7 minutes per side.

6.Serve immediately alongside the spinach.

438.Zesty Salmon

Prep Time: 10 min | **Cook Time:** 10 min | **Serve:** 4

- 1 tablespoon butter, melted
- 1 tablespoon fresh lemon juice
- 1 teaspoon Worcestershire sauce
- 1 teaspoon lemon zest, grated finely.
- 4 (6-ounce) salmon fillets
- Salt and ground black pepper, to taste

1.In a baking dish, place butter, lemon juice, Worcestershire sauce, and lemon zest, and mix well.

2.Coat the fillets with mixture and then arrange skin side-up in the baking dish.

3.Set aside for about 15 minutes.

4.Preheat the broiler of oven.

5.Arrange the oven rack about 6-inch from heating element.

6.Line a broiler pan with a piece of foil.

7.Remove the salmon fillets from baking dish and season with salt and black pepper.

8.Arrange the salmon fillets onto the prepared broiler pan, skin side down.

9.Broil for about 8-10 minutes.

439.Stuffed Salmon

Prep Time: 15 min | **Cook Time:** 16 min | **Serve:** 4

For Salmon:

- 4 (6-ounce) skinless salmon fillets
- Salt and ground black pepper, as required
- 2 tablespoons fresh lemon juice
- 2 tablespoons olive oil, divided
- 1 tablespoon unsalted butter

For Filling:

- 4 ounces low-fat cream cheese, softened
- ¼ cup low-fat Parmesan cheese, grated finely
- 4 ounces frozen spinach, thawed and squeezed
- 2 teaspoons garlic, minced
- Salt and ground black pepper, as required

1.Season each salmon-fillet with salt and black-pepper and then, drizzle with lemon juice and 1 tablespoon of oil.

2.Arrange the salmon fillets onto a smooth surface.

3.With a sharp knife, cut a pocket into each salmon fillet about ¾ of the way through, take care not to cut the whole way.

4.For filling: in a bowl, add the cream cheese, Parmesan cheese, spinach, garlic, salt and black pepper and mix well.

5.Place about 1-2 tablespoons of spinach mixture into each salmon pocket and spread evenly.

6.In a skillet, heat the remaining oil and butter over medium-high heat and cook the salmon fillets for about 6-8 minutes per side.

7.Remove the salmon fillets from heat and transfer onto the serving plates.

440.Salmon with Asparagus

Prep Time: 10 min | **Cook Time:** 20 min | **Serve:** 6
- 6 (4-ounce) salmon fillets
- 2 tablespoons extra-virgin olive oil
- 3 tablespoons fresh parsley, minced
- ¼ teaspoon ginger powder
- Salt and freshly ground black-pepper, to taste
- 1½ pounds fresh asparagus

1.Preheat your oven to 400 degrees.
2.Grease a large baking dish.
3.In a bowl, place all-ingredients and mix well.
4.Arrange the salmon fillets into prepared baking dish in a single layer.
5.Bake for approximately 16-21 minutes or until desired doneness of salmon.
6.Meanwhile, in a pan of the boiling water, add asparagus and cook for about 4-5 minutes.
7.Drain the asparagus well.
8.Divide the asparagus onto serving plates evenly and top each with 1 salmon fillet and serve.

441.Salmon Parcel

Prep Time: 15 min | **Cook Time:** 20 min | **Serve:** 6
- 6 (4-ounce) salmon-fillets
- Salt and freshly ground-black-pepper, to taste 1 yellow bell pepper, seeded and cubed
- 1 red bell pepper, seeded and cubed
- 4 plum tomatoes, cubed
- 1 small onion, sliced thinly
- ½ cup fresh parsley, chopped
- ¼ cup extra-virgin olive oil
- 2 tablespoons fresh lemon juice

1.Preheat your oven to 400 degrees F.
2.Arrange 6 pieces of foil onto a smooth surface.
3.Place one salmon-fillet on each piece of foil and sprinkle with salt and black pepper.
4.In a bowl, mix together bell peppers, tomato and onion.
5.Place veggie mixture over each fillet evenly and top with parsley and capers evenly.
6.Drizzle with oil and lemon juice.
7.Fold the each piece of foil around salmon mixture to seal it.
8.Arrange the foil packets onto a large baking sheet in a single layer.
9.Bake for approximately 25 minutes.
10.Remove from the oven and place the foil packets onto serving plates.
11.Carefully unwrap each foil packet and serve.

442.Salmon with Cauliflower Mash

Prep Time: 15 min | **Cook Time:** 20 min | **Serve:** 4
For Cauliflower Mash:
- 1-pound cauliflower, cut into florets
- 1 tablespoon extra-virgin olive oil
- 3 garlic cloves, minced
- 1 teaspoon fresh thyme leaves
- Salt and freshly ground black-pepper, to taste

For Salmon:
- 1 (1-inch) piece fresh ginger, grated finely
- 1 tablespoon honey
- 1 tablespoon fresh lemon juice
- 1 tablespoon Dijon mustard
- 2 tablespoons olive oil
- 4 (6-ounce) salmon fillets
- 2 tablespoons fresh parsley, chopped

1.For mash: in a large saucepan of water, arrange a steamer basket and bring to a boil.
2.Place the cauliflower florets in steamer basket and steam covered for about 10 minutes.
3.Drain the cauliflower and set aside.
4.In a small-frying pan, heat the oil over-medium heat and sauté the garlic for about 2 minutes.
5.Remove the frying pan from heat and transfer the garlic oil in a large food processor.
6.Add the cauliflower, thyme, salt and black-pepper and pulse until smooth.
7.Transfer the cauliflower mash into a bowl and set aside.
8.Meanwhile, in a bowl, mix together ginger, honey, lemon juice and Dijon mustard. Set aside.
9.In a large non-stick skillet, heat olive-oil over medium-high heat and cook the salmon fillets for about 3-4 minutes per side.
10.Stir in honey mixture and immediately remove from heat.
11.Divide warm cauliflower mash onto serving plates.
12. Top each plate with one salmon fillet and serve.

443.Salmon with Salsa

Prep Time: 15 min | **Cook Time:** 8 min | **Serve:** 4
For Salsa:
- 2 large ripe avocados, peeled, pitted and cut into small chunks
- 1 small tomato, chopped
- 2 tablespoons red onion, chopped finely ¼ cup fresh cilantro, chopped finely
- 1 tablespoon jalapeño pepper, seeded and minced finely
- 1 garlic clove, minced finely
- 3 tablespoon fresh lime juice
- Salt and ground black pepper, as required

For Salmon:
- 4 (5-ounce) (1-inch thick) salmon fillets
- Sea salt and ground black-pepper, as required
- 3 tablespoons olive oil
- 1 tablespoon fresh rosemary leaves, chopped
- 1 tablespoon fresh lemon juice

1.For salsa: add all ingredients in a bowl and gently, stir to combine.
2.With a plastic-wrap, cover the bowl and refrigerate before serving.
3.For salmon: season each salmon fillet with salt and black pepper generously.
4.In a big-skillet, heat the oil over medium-high heat.
5.Place the salmon fillets, skins side up and cook for about 4 minutes.
6.Carefully change the side of each salmon fillet and cook for about 4 minutes more.
7.Stir in the rosemary and lemon juice and remove from the heat.
8.Divide the salsa onto serving plates evenly.
9.To each plate with 1 salmon fillet and serve.

444. Walnut Crusted Salmon

Prep Time: 15 min | **Cook Time:** 20 min | **Serve:** 2

- ½ cup walnuts
- 1 tablespoon fresh dill, chopped
- 2 tablespoons fresh lemon rind, grated
- Salt and ground black pepper, as required
- 1 tablespoon coconut oil, melted
- 3-4 tablespoons Dijon mustard
- 4 (3-ounce) salmon fillets
- 4 teaspoons fresh lemon juice
- 3 cups fresh baby spinach

1. Preheat your oven to 350 degrees F.
2. Line the parchment paper with a large baking sheet.
3. Place the walnuts in a food processor and pulse until chopped roughly.
4. Add the dill, lemon rind, garlic salt, black pepper, and butter, and pulse until a crumbly mixture forms.
5. Place the salmon fillets onto prepared baking sheet in a single layer, skin-side down.
6. Coat the top of each salmon-fillet with Dijon mustard.
7. Place the walnut mixture over each fillet and gently, press into the surface of salmon.
8. Bake for approximately 15–20 minutes.
9. Remove the salmon fillets from oven and transfer onto the serving plates.
10. Drizzle with the lemon juice and serve alongside the spinach.

445. Garlicky Tilapia

Prep Time: 10 min | **Cook Time:** 5 min | **Serve:** 4

- 2 tablespoons olive oil
- 4 (5-ounce) tilapia fillets
- 3 garlic cloves, minced
- 1 tablespoon fresh ginger, minced
- 2-3 tablespoons low-sodium chicken broth Salt and ground black pepper, to taste
- 6 cups fresh baby spinach

1. In a big sauté-pan, heat the oil over medium heat and cook the tilapia fillets for about 3 minutes.
2. Flip the side and stir in the garlic and ginger.
3. Cook for about 1-2 minutes.
4. Add the broth and cook for about 2-3 more minutes.
5. Stir in salt and black pepper and remove from heat.
6. Serve hot alongside the spinach.

446. Tilapia Piccata

Prep Time: 15 min | **Cook Time:** 8 min | **Serve:** 4

- 3 tablespoons fresh lemon juice
- 2 tablespoons olive oil
- 2 garlic cloves, minced
- ½ teaspoon lemon zest, grated
- 2 teaspoons capers, drained
- 2 tablespoons fresh basil, minced
- 4 (6-ounce) tilapia fillets
- Salt and ground black pepper, as required 6 cups fresh baby kale

1. Preheat the broiler of the oven.
2. Arrange an oven rack about 4-inch from the heating element.
3. Grease a broiler pan.
4. In a little-bowl, add the lemon juice, oil, garlic and lemon zest and beat until well combined.
5. Add the capers and basil and stir to combine.

6. Reserve 2 tablespoons of mixture in a small bowl.
7. Coat the fish fillets with remaining capers mixture and sprinkle with salt and black pepper.
8. Place the tilapia fillets onto the broiler pan and broil for about 3-4 minutes side.
9. Remove from the oven and place the fish fillets onto serving plates.
10. Drizzle with reserved capers mixture and serve alongside the kale.

447. Cod in Dill Sauce

Prep Time: 10 min | **Cook Time:** 13 min | **Serve:** 2

- 2 (6-ounce) cod fillets
- 1 teaspoon onion powder
- Salt and ground black pepper, as required 3 tablespoons butter, divided
- 2 garlic cloves, minced
- 1-2 lemon slices
- 2 teaspoons fresh dill weed
- 3 cups fresh spinach, torn

1. Season each cod fillet evenly with the onion powder, salt and black pepper.
2. In a medium skillet, heat 1 normal spoon of oil over high heat and cook the cod fillets for about 4-5 minutes per side.
3. Transfer the cod fillets onto a plate.
4. Meanwhile, in a frying-pan, heat the remaining oil over low heat and sauté the garlic and lemon slices for about 40-60 seconds.
5. Stir in the cooked cod fillets and dill and cook, covered for about 1-2 minutes.
6. Remove the cod fillets from heat and transfer onto the serving plates.
7. Top with the pan sauce and serve immediately alongside the spinach.

448. Cod & Veggies Bake

Prep Time: 15 min | **Cook Time:** 20 min | **Serve:** 4

- 1 teaspoon olive oil
- ½ cup onion, minced
- 1 cup zucchini, chopped
- 1 garlic clove, minced
- 2 tablespoons fresh basil, chopped
- 2 cups fresh tomatoes, chopped
- Salt and ground black pepper, as required
- 4 (6-ounce) cod steaks
- 1/3 cup feta cheese, crumbled

1. Preheat your oven to 450 degrees F.
2. Grease a large shallow baking dish.
3. In a skillet, heat oil over-medium heat and sauté the onion, zucchini and garlic for about 4-5 minutes.
4. Stir in the basil, tomatoes, salt and black pepper and immediately remove from heat.
5. Place the cod steaks into prepared baking dish in a single layer and top with tomato mixture evenly.
6. Sprinkle with the cheese evenly.
7. Bake for approximately 16 minutes or until desired doneness.

449. Cod & Veggie Pizza

Prep Time: 20 min | **Cook Time:** 1 h | **Serve:** 3

For Base:
- Olive oil cooking spray
- ¼ cup oat flour
- 2 teaspoons dried rosemary, crushed
- Freshly ground black pepper, to taste
- 4 egg whites
- 2½ teaspoons olive oil
- ½ cup low-fat Parmesan cheese, grated freshly 2 cups zucchini, grated and squeezed

For Topping:
- 1 cup tomato paste
- 1 teaspoon fresh rosemary, minced
- 1 teaspoon fresh basil, minced
- Freshly ground black pepper, to taste
- 4 cups fresh mushrooms, chopped
- 1 tomato, chopped
- 3 ounces boneless cod fillet, chopped
- 1½ cups onion, sliced into rings
- 1 red bell pepper, seeded and chopped
- 1 green bell-pepper, seeded and chopped 1/3 cup low-fat mozzarella, shredded

1.Preheat your oven to 400 degrees F.
2.Grease a pie dish with cooking spray.
3.For base: in a large bowl, add all the ingredients and mix until well combined.
4.Transfer the mixture into prepared pie dish and press to smooth the surface.
5.Bake for approximately 40 minutes.
6. Remove from the oven to cool and set aside for at least 15 minutes.
7.Carefully turn out the crust onto a baking sheet.
8.For topping: in s bowl, add tomato paste, herbs and black pepper.
9.Spread tomato sauce mixture over crust evenly.
10.Arrange the vegetables over tomato sauce, followed by the cheese.
11.Bake for about 21 minutes or until cheese is melted.

450.Garlicky Haddock
Prep Time: 10 min | **Cook Time:** 11 min | **Serve:** 2
- 2 tablespoons olive oil, divided
- 4 garlic cloves, minced and divided
- 1 teaspoon fresh ginger, grated finely
- 2 (4-ounce) haddock fillets
- Salt and freshly ground black-pepper, to taste 3 C. fresh baby spinach

1.In a skillet, heat one normal spoon of oil over medium heat and sauté 2 garlic cloves and ginger for about 1 minute.
2.Add the haddock fillets, salt and black pepper and cook for about 3-5 minutes per side or until desired doneness.
3. Meanwhile, heat the remaining oil over medium heat in another skillet, and heat and sauté the remaining garlic for about 1 minute.
4.Ad the spinach, salt and black pepper and cook for about 4-5 minutes.
5.Divide the spinach onto serving plates and top each with 1 haddock fillet.

DESSERT AND SALAD

451.Chocolate Bars
Prep Time: 10 min | **Cook Time:** 20 min | **Serve:** 16
- 15 oz cream cheese, softened
- 15 oz unsweetened dark chocolate
- 1 tsp vanilla
- 10 drops liquid stevia

1.Grease 8-inch square dish and set aside.
2.In a saucepan, dissolve chocolate over low heat.
3.Add stevia and vanilla and stir well.
4.Remove pan from heat and set aside.
5.Add cream cheese into the blender and blend until smooth.
6.Add melted chocolate mixture into the cream cheese and blend until just combined.
7.Transfer mixture into the prepared dish and spread evenly, and place in the refrigerator until firm.
Nutrition: Calories: 230 Fat: 24 g Carbs: 7.5 g Sugar: 0.1 g Protein: 6 g Cholesterol: 29 mg

452.Blueberry Muffins
Prep Time: 15 min | **Cook Time:** 35 min | **Serve:** 12
- 2 eggs
- 1/2 cup fresh blueberries
- 1 cup heavy cream
- 2 cups almond flour
- 1/4 tsp lemon zest
- 1/2 tsp lemon extract
- 1 tsp baking powder
- 5 drops stevia
- 1/4 cup butter, melted

1.heat the cooker to 350 F. Line muffin tin with cupcake liners and set aside.
2.Add eggs into the bowl and whisk until mix.
3.Add remaining ingredients and mix to combine.
4.Pour mixture into the prepared muffin tin and bake for 25 minutes.
Nutrition: Calories: 190 Fat: 17 g Carbs: 5 g Sugar: 1 g Protein: 5 g Cholesterol: 55 mg

453.Chia Pudding
Prep Time: 20 min | **Cook Time:** 0 min | **Serve:** 2
- 4 tbsp chia seeds
- 1 cup unsweetened coconut milk
- 1/2 cup raspberries

1.Add raspberry and coconut milk into a blender and blend until smooth.
2.Pour mixture into the glass jar.
3.Add chia seeds in a jar and stir well.
4.Seal the jar with a lid and shake well and place in the refrigerator for 3 hours.
5.Serve chilled and enjoy.
Nutrition: Calories: 360 Fat: 33 g Carbs: 13 g Sugar: 5 g Protein: 6 g Cholesterol: 0 mg

454.Avocado Pudding
Prep Time: 20 min | **Cook Time:** 0 min | **Serve:** 8
- 2 ripe avocados, pitted and cut into pieces
- 1 tbsp fresh lime juice
- 14 oz can coconut milk
- 2 tsp liquid stevia
- 2 tsp vanilla

1.Inside the blender, Add all ingredients and blend until smooth.
Nutrition: Calories: 317 Fat: 30 g Carbs: 9 g Sugar: 0.5 g Protein: 3 g Cholesterol: 0 mg

455. Delicious Brownie Bites

Prep Time: 20 min | **Cook Time:** 0 min | **Serve:** 13

- 1/4 cup unsweetened chocolate chips
- 1/4 cup unsweetened cocoa powder
- 1 cup pecans, chopped
- 1/2 cup almond butter
- 1/2 tsp vanilla
- 1/4 cup monk fruit sweetener
- 1/8 tsp pink salt

1. Add pecans, sweetener, vanilla, almond butter, cocoa powder, and salt into the food processor and process until well combined.
2. Transfer the brownie mixture into the large bowl. Add chocolate chips and fold well.
3. Make small round shape balls from brownie mixture and place them onto a baking tray.
4. Place in the freezer for 20 minutes.

Nutrition: Calories: 108 Fat: 9 g Carbs: 4 g Sugar: 1 g Protein: 2 g Cholesterol: 0 mg

456. Wasabi Tuna Asian Salad

Prep Time: 30 min | **Cook Time:** 10 min | **Serve:** 1

- Lime juice (1 teaspoon)
- Non-stick cooking spray
- Pepper/dash of salt
- Wasabi paste (1 teaspoon)
- Olive oil (2 teaspoons)
- Chopped or shredded cucumbers (1/2 cup)
- Bok Choy stalks (1 cup)
- Raw tuna steak (8 oz.)

1. Fish: preheat your skillet to medium heat. Mix your wasabi and lime juice; coat the tuna steaks.
2. Use a non-stick cooking spray on your skillet for 10 seconds.
3. Put your tuna steaks on the skillet and cook over medium heat until you get the desired doneness.
4. Salad: Slice the cucumber into match-stick tiny sizes. Cut the bok Choy into minute pieces. Toss gently with pepper, salt, and olive oil if you want.

Nutrition: Protein: 61g, Fiber: 1g, Cholesterol: 115mg, Saturated fats: 2g, Calories: 380

457. Lemon Greek Salad

Prep Time: 25 min | **Cook Time:** 25 min | **Serve:** 1

- Chicken breast (140 oz)
- Chopped cucumber (1 cup)
- Chopped orange/red bell pepper (1 cup)
- Wedged/sliced/chopped tomatoes (1 cup)
- Chopped olives (1/4 cup)
- Fresh parsley (2 tablespoons), finely chopped.
- Finely chopped red onion (2 tablespoons)
- Lemon juice (5 teaspoons)
- Olive oil (1 teaspoon)
- Minced garlic (1 clove)

1. Preheat your grill to medium heat.
2. Grill the chicken and cook on each side until it is no longer pink or for 5 minutes.
3. Cut the chicken into tiny pieces. In your serving bowl, mix garlic, olives, and parsley. Whisk in olive oil (1 teaspoon) and lemon juice (4 teaspoons). Add onion, tomatoes, bell pepper, and cucumber.

4. Toss gently. Coat the ingredients with dressing. Add another teaspoon of lemon juice to taste. Divide the salad into two servings and put 6oz chicken on top of each salad.

Nutrition: Protein: 56g, Fiber: 4g, Total carbs: 14g, Sodium: 280mg, Cholesterol: 145mg, Saturated fat: 2.5g, Total fat: 12g, Calories: 380

458. Broccoli Salad

Prep Time: 5 min | **Cook Time:** 25 min | **Serve:** 1

- 1/3 tablespoons sherry vinegar
- 1/24 cup olive oil
- 1/3 teaspoons fresh thyme, chopped
- 1/6 teaspoon Dijon mustard
- 1/6 teaspoon honey
- Salt to taste
- 1 1/3 cups broccoli florets
- 1/3 red onions
- 1/12 cup parmesan cheese shaved
- 1/24 cup pecans

1. Mix the sherry vinegar, olive oil, thyme, mustard, honey, and salt in a bowl.
2. In a serving bowl, blend the broccoli florets and onions.
3. Drizzle the dressing on top.
4. Sprinkle with the pecans and parmesan cheese before serving.

Nutrition: Calories: 199, Fat: 17.4g, Saturated fat: 2.9g, Carbohydrates: 7.5g, Fiber: 2.8g, Protein: 5.2g

459. Potato Carrot Salad

Prep Time: 15 min | **Cook Time:** 10 min | **Serve:** 1

Water

- 1 potato, sliced into cubes
- 1/2 carrots, cut into cubes
- 1/6 tablespoon milk
- 1/6 tablespoon Dijon mustard
- 1/24 cup mayonnaise

Pepper to taste

- 1/3 teaspoons fresh thyme, chopped
- 1/6 stalk celery, chopped
- 1/6 scallions, chopped
- 1/6 slice turkey bacon, cooked crispy and crumbled

1. Fill your pot with water.
2. Place it over medium-high heat.
3. Boil the potatoes and carrots for 10 to 12 minutes or until tender.
4. Drain and let cool.
5. In a bowl, mix the milk, mustard, mayonnaise, pepper, and thyme.
6. Stir in the potatoes, carrots, and celery.
7. Coat evenly with the sauce.
8. Cover and refrigerate for 4 hours.
9. Top with the scallions and turkey bacon bits before serving

Nutrition: Calories: 106, Fat: 5.3g, Saturated fat: 1g, Carbohydrates: 12.6g, Fiber: 1.8g, Protein: 2g

460. Marinated Veggie Salad

Prep Time: 4 h and 30 m | **Cook Time:** 3 m | **Serve:** 1

- 1 zucchini, sliced
- 4 tomatoes, sliced into wedges
- ¼ cup red onion, sliced thinly
- 1 green bell pepper, sliced
- 2 tablespoons fresh parsley, chopped

- 2 tablespoons red-wine vinegar
- 2 tablespoons olive oil
- 1 clove garlic, minced
- 1 teaspoon dried basil
- 2 tablespoons water
- Pine nuts, toasted and chopped

1. In a bowl, combine the zucchini, tomatoes, red onion, green bell pepper, and parsley.
2. Pour the vinegar and oil into a glass jar with a lid.
3. Add the garlic, basil, and water.
4. Seal the jar and stir well to combine.
5. Pour the dressing into the vegetable mixture.
6. Cover the bowl.
7. Marinate in the refrigerator for 4 hours.
8. Garnish with the pine nuts before serving.

Nutrition: Calories: 65, Fat: 4.7g, Saturated fat: 0.7g, Carbohydrates: 5.3g, Fiber: 1.2g, Protein: 0.9g

461. Mediterranean Salad
Prep Time: 20 min | **Cook Time:** 5 min | **Serve:** 1
- 1 teaspoon balsamic vinegar
- 1/2 tablespoon basil pesto
- 1/2 cup lettuce
- 1/8 cup broccoli florets, chopped
- 1/8 cup zucchini, chopped
- 1/8 cup tomato, chopped
- 1/8 cup yellow bell pepper, chopped
- 1/2 tablespoons feta cheese, crumbled

1. Arrange the lettuce on a serving platter.
2. Top with the broccoli, zucchini, tomato, and bell pepper.
3. In a bowl, mix the vinegar and pesto.
4. Drizzle the dressing on top.
5. Sprinkle the feta cheese.

Nutrition: Calories: 100, Fat: 6g, Saturated fat: 1g, Carbohydrates: 7g, Protein: 4g

462. Potato Tuna Salad
Prep Time: 4 h 20 m | **Cook Time:** 10 m | **Serve:** 1
- 1 potato, peeled and sliced into cubes
- 1/12 cup plain yogurt
- 1/12 cup mayonnaise
- 1/6 clove garlic, crushed and minced
- 1/6 tablespoon almond milk
- 1/6 tablespoon fresh dill, chopped
- ½ teaspoon lemon zest
- Salt to taste
- 1 cup cucumber, chopped
- ¼ cup scallions, chopped
- ¼ cup radishes, chopped
- (9 oz) canned tuna flakes
- 1/2 hard-boiled eggs, chopped
- 1 cups lettuce, chopped

1. Fill your pot with water.
2. Add the potatoes and boil.
3. Cook for 15 minutes or till slightly tender.
4. Drain and let cool.
5. In a bowl, mix the yogurt, mayo, garlic, almond milk, fresh dill, lemon zest, and salt.
6. Stir in the potatoes, tuna flakes, and eggs.
7. Mix well.
8. Chill in the refrigerator for 4 hours.
9. Stir in the shredded lettuce before serving.

Nutrition: Calories: 243, Fat: 9.9g, Saturated fat: 2g, Carbohydrates: 22.2g, Fiber: 4.6g, Protein: 17.5g

463. High Protein Salad
Prep Time: 5 min | **Cook Time:** 5 min | **Serve:** 1
Salad:
- 1 (15 oz) can green kidney beans
- 1/4 tablespoon capers
- 1/4 handfuls arugula
- 1 (15 oz) can lentils

Dressing:
- 1/1 tablespoon caper brine
- 1/1 tablespoon tamari
- 1/1 tablespoon balsamic vinegar
- 2/2 tablespoon peanut butter
- 2/2 tablespoon hot sauce
- 2/1 tablespoon tahini

For the dressing:
1. In a bowl, stir all the ingredients until they come together to form a smooth dressing.
For the salad:
2. Mix the beans, arugula, capers, and lentils. Top with the dressing and serve.

Nutrition: Calories: 205, Fat: 2g, Protein: 13g, Carbs: 31g, Fiber: 17g

464. Rice and Veggie Bowl
Prep Time: 5 min | **Cook Time:** 15 min | **Serve:** 1
- 1/3 tablespoon coconut oil
- 1/2 teaspoon ground cumin
- 1/2 teaspoon ground turmeric
- 1/3 teaspoon chili powder
- 1 red bell pepper, chopped
- 1/2 tablespoon tomato paste
- 1 bunch of broccoli, cut into bite-sized-florets with short stems 1/2 teaspoon salt, to taste
- 1 large red onion, sliced
- 1/2 garlic cloves, minced
- 1/2 head of cauliflower, sliced into bite-sized florets 1/2 cups cooked rice
- Newly ground black pepper to taste

1. Start with warming up the coconut oil over medium-high heat.
2. Stir in the turmeric, cumin, chili powder, salt, and tomato paste.
3. Cook the content for 1 minute. Stir repeatedly until the spices are fragrant.
4. Add the garlic and onion. Fry for 2,5 to 3,3 minutes until the onions are softened.
5. Add the broccoli, cauliflower, and bell pepper. Cover, then cook for 3 to 4 minutes and stir occasionally.
6. Add the cooked rice. Stir so it will combine well with the vegetables. Cook for 2 to 3 minutes. Stir until the rice is warm.
7. Check the seasoning and change to taste if desired.
8. Lessen the heat and cook on low for 2 to 3 more minutes so the flavors will meld.
9. Serve with freshly ground black pepper.

Nutrition: Calories: 260, Fat: 9g, Protein: 9g, Carbs: 36g, Fiber: 5g

465. Squash Black Bean Bowl
Prep Time: 5 min | **Cook Time:** 30 min | **Serve:** 1

- 1 large spaghetti squash, halved,
- 1/3 cup water (or 2 tablespoon olive oil, rubbed on the inside of squash)

Black bean filling:
- 1/2 (15 oz) can of black beans, emptied and rinsed 1/2 cup fire-roasted corn (or frozen sweet corn) 1/2 cup thinly sliced red cabbage
- 1/2 tablespoon chopped green onion, green and white parts ¼ cup chopped fresh coriander
- ½ lime, juiced or to taste
- Pepper and salt, to taste

Avocado mash:
- One ripe avocado, mashed
- ½ lime, juiced or to taste
- ¼ teaspoon cumin
- Pepper and pinch of sea salt

1. Preheat the oven to 400°F.
2. Chop the squash in part and scoop out the seeds with a spoon, like a pumpkin.
3. Fill the roasting pan with 1/3 cup of water. Lay the squash, cut side down, in the pan. Bake for 30 minutes until soft and tender.
4. While this is baking, mix all the ingredients for the black bean filling in a medium-sized bowl.
5. In a small dish, crush the avocado and blend in the avocado mash ingredients.
6. Eliminate the squash from the oven and let it cool for 5 minutes. Scrape the squash with a fork so that it looks like spaghetti noodles. Then, fill it with black bean filling and top with avocado mash.

Nutrition: Calories: 85, Fat: 0.5g, Protein: 4g, Carbs: 6g, Fiber: 4g

466. Pea Salad

Prep Time: 40 min | **Cook Time:** 0 min | **Serve:** 1
- 1/2 cup chickpeas, rinsed and drained
- 1/2 cups peas, divided
- Salt to taste
- 1 tablespoon olive oil
- ½ cup buttermilk
- Pepper to taste
- 2 cups pea greens
- 1/2 carrots shaved
- 1/4 cup snow peas, trimmed

1. Add the chickpeas and half of the peas to your food processor.
2. Season with salt.
3. Pulse until smooth. Set aside.
4. In a bowl, toss the remaining peas in oil, milk, salt, and pepper.
5. Transfer the mixture to your food processor.
6. Process until pureed.
7. Transfer this mixture to a bowl.
8. Arrange the pea greens on a serving plate.
9. Top with the shaved carrots and snow peas.
10. Stir in the pea and milk dressing.
11. Serve with the reserved chickpea hummus.

Nutrition: Calories: 214, Fat: 8.6g, Saturated fat: 1.5g, Carbohydrates: 27.3g, Fiber: 8.4g, Protein: 8g

467. Snap Pea Salad

Prep Time: 1 h | **Cook Time:** 0 min | **Serve:** 1
- 1/2 tablespoons mayonnaise
- ¾ teaspoon celery seed
- ¼ cup cider vinegar
- 1/2 teaspoon yellow mustard
- 1/2 tablespoon sugar
- Salt and pepper to taste
- 1 oz. radishes, sliced thinly
- 2 oz. sugar snap peas, sliced thinly

1. In a bowl, combine the mayonnaise, celery seeds, vinegar, mustard, sugar, salt, and pepper.
2. Stir in the radishes and snap peas.
3. Refrigerate for 30 minutes.

Nutrition: Calories: 69, Fat: 3.7g, Saturated fat: 0.6g, Carbohydrates: 7.1g, Fiber: 1.8g, Protein: 2g

468. Cucumber Tomato Chopped Salad

Prep Time: 15 min | **Cook Time:** 0 min | **Serve:** 1
- 1/4 cup light mayonnaise
- 1/2 tablespoon lemon juice
- 1/2 tablespoon fresh dill, chopped
- 1/2 tablespoon chive, chopped
- 1/4 cup feta cheese, crumbled
- Salt and pepper to taste
- 1/2 red onion, chopped
- 1/2 cucumber, diced
- 1/2 radish, diced
- 1 tomato, diced
- Chives, chopped

1. Combine the mayonnaise, lemon juice, fresh dill, chives, feta cheese, salt, and pepper in a bowl.
2. Mix well.
3. Stir in the onion, cucumber, radish, and tomatoes.
4. Coat evenly.
5. Garnish with the chopped chives.

Nutrition: Calories: 187, Fat: 16.7g, Saturated fat: 4.1g, Carbohydrates: 6.7g, Fiber: 2g, Protein: 3.3g

469. Zucchini Pasta Salad

Prep Time: 4 min | **Cook Time:** 0 min | **Serve:** 1
- 1 tablespoon olive oil
- 1/2 teaspoons dijon mustard
- 1/3 tablespoons red-wine vinegar
- 1/2 clove garlic, grated
- 2 tablespoons fresh oregano, chopped
- 1/2 shallot, chopped
- ¼ teaspoon red pepper flakes
- 4 oz. zucchini noodles
- ¼ cup Kalamata olives pitted
- 1 cups cherry tomato, sliced in half
- ¾ cup parmesan cheese shaved

1. Mix the olive oil, Dijon mustard, red wine vinegar, garlic, oregano, shallot, and red pepper flakes in a bowl.
2. Stir in the zucchini noodles.
3. Sprinkle on top the olives, tomatoes, and parmesan cheese.

Nutrition: Calories: 299, Fat: 24.7g, Saturated fat: 5.1g, Carbohydrates: 11.6g, Fiber: 2.8g, Protein: 7g

470. Egg Avocado Salad

Prep Time: 10 min | **Cook Time:** 0 min | **Serve:** 1
- 1/2 avocado
- 1 hard-boiled egg, peeled and chopped
- 1/4 tablespoon mayonnaise

- 1/4 tablespoons freshly squeezed lemon juice ¼ cup celery, chopped
- 1/2 tablespoons chives, chopped
- Salt and pepper to taste

1. Add the avocado to a large bowl.
2. Mash the avocado using a fork.
3. Stir in the egg and mash the eggs.
4. Add the mayonnaise, lemon juice, celery, chives, salt, and pepper.
5. Chill in the refrigerator for at least 20 to 30 minutes before serving.

Nutrition: Calories: 224, Fat: 18g, Saturated fat: 3.9g, Carbohydrates: 6.1g, Fiber: 3.6g, Protein: 10.6g

471. Sweet Potato Muffins Fueling Hack

Prep Time: 15 min | **Cook Time:** 15 min | **Serve:** 4
- 1 packet Honey Sweet potatoes
- 2 Tablespoon liquid egg (like Eggbeaters) 1/2 C water
- 1/4 tsp baking powder
- 2 pinches Sinful Cinnamon Seasoning

1. Preheat oven to 400 degrees.
2. Sift the baking powder into the liquid egg.
3. Puree the sweet potatoes and add to the egg/baking powder mix.
4. Go on a light run and bring the water to a boil; add to the potato mix.
5. Bring in the cinnamon and the seasoning.
6. Whisk until well-combined.
7. Fill about ¾ of the way with the muffin cups with this mix.
8. Place into the oven for 15 minutes.

Nutrition: Energy (calories): 189 kcal Protein: 39.52 g Fat: 10.02 g Carbohydrates: 1.98 g Calcium, Ca44 mg Magnesium, Mg48 mg Phosphorus, P200 mg

472. Asian Cabbage Salad

Prep Time: 10-15 min | **Cook Time:** 2 m | **Serve:** 4-8
- 4 C green-cabbage, shredded
- 1/4 C rice wine-vinegar (no sugar added) 1 Tablespoon low sodium soy-sauce
- 4 little spoon Stacey Hawkins Valencia Orange Oil (optional- can be made fat free simply by leaving out)
- 1 normal spoon Asian style seasoning 2 teaspoons lime juice
- 1/4 C cilantro, chopped to taste with salt and pepper

1. Combine shredded cabbage with shredded cabbage in a large bowl, green onions, cilantro, citrus dressing, and Asian seasoning (seeds removed, ground In a coffee grinder, or in a pestle and mortar, with a pestle); mix well. Chill in the refrigerator.

Nutrition: Energy (calories): 99 kcal Protein: 4.13 g Fat: 4.53 g Carbohydrates: 12.47 g Calcium, Ca92 mg Magnesium, Mg35 mg Phosphorus, P95 mg

473. Tangy Kale Salad

Prep Time: 20 min | **Cook Time:** 6 min | **Serve:** 6
- One-half cup olive oil
- One-fourth cup lemon juice 2 tablespoons Dijon mustard 1 tablespoon minced shallot
- 1 small garlic clove, finely minced
- One-fourth teaspoon salt, or more to taste ground black pepper to taste

Salad:
- 1 teaspoon olive oil
- One-third cup sliced almonds
- 1 bunch kale, center stems discarded and leaves thinly sliced 8 ounces Brussels sprouts, shredded
- 1 cup grated Pecorino Romano cheese

1. Whisk together the lemon Juice to create the dressing, olive oil, shallot, garlic, mustard, ¼ teaspoon salt and pepper. Set aside.
2. To make the salad, heat the oil over medium-high heat in a large skillet. Add the almonds and cook, sometimes stirring, until the almonds are cooked. Almonds are ready. They are fragrant, and the oil is very aromatic about 2 minutes. Transfer to a plate. Attach the skillet to the kale and cook until it begins to wilt and become colorful for about 4 minutes.
3. Add the Brussels sprouts, reduce the heat to medium-low. Season with salt and pepper. Stuff the leaves with the cheese. Drizzle with the dressing.
4. Top with the almonds.

Nutrition: Energy (calories): 193 kcal Protein: 1.74 g Fat: 19.11 g Carbohydrates: 5.56 g Calcium, Ca23 mg Magnesium, Mg14 mg

474. Crunchy Cauliflower Salad

Prep Time: 10 min | **Cook Time:** 10 min | **Serve:** 8
- 4 cups cauliflower florets
- 1 Tablespoon (one capful) Stacey Hawkins Tuscan Fantasy Seasoning
- 1/4 cup apple cider vinegar

In a wide bowl,
1. Position the cauliflower florets and coat them with a vinegar solution. Add Stacey Hawkins Tuscan Fantasy Seasoning and stir well. Let sit to allow cauliflower to marinate for 10 minutes.
2. Preheat the oven to 450 degrees and Put a baking sheet on top of it—heavy-duty foil. On a baking sheet, put the marinated cauliflower and bake in the 450-degree oven for 10-12 minutes. Remove and allow to cool.

Nutrition: Energy (calories): 29 kcal Protein: 1.72 g Fat: 0.24 g Carbohydrates: 5.36 g Calcium, Ca20 mg Magnesium, Mg13 mg Phosphorus, P39 mg

475. Crisp Summer Cucumber Salad

Prep Time: 15 min | **Cook Time:** 0 min | **Serve:** 4
- 4 C sliced cucumbers (peels on or off- your choice) 2 T apple cider vinegar
- 1/4 C sliced white onion
- 2 tsp Stacey Hawkins Dash of Desperation Seasoning

1. Reserve some cucumber slices for garnish.
2. In a tub, mix up the rest of the ingredients.
3. Pour over remaining cucumber slices and place in a pretty bowl.
4. Enable 15 minutes to sit down to absorb the flavor and serve.

Nutrition: Energy (calories): 20 kcal Protein: 0.29 g Fat: 0.53 g Carbohydrates: 3.08 g Calcium, Ca3 mg Magnesium, Mg3 mg Phosphorus, P6 mg

476. Decadently Dark Chocolate Mousse

Prep Time: 10 min | **Cook Time:** 0 min | **Serve:** 2

- 2 ripe avocados
- One-half cup unsweetened, dark cocoa powder 1 T vanilla
- One-fourth cup stevia powder
- One-fourth cup Unsweetened pinch of almond milk salt

1. Combine all ingredients into a high-speed blender and blend until smooth. (This can be done in a food processor as well. I would skip the blending and just mash the ingredients with a mortar and pestle.)
2. Preserve this mousse in a closed container in the fridge for up to 5 days.

Nutrition: Energy (calories): 466 kcal Protein: 9.27 g Fat: 38.35 g Carbohydrates: 31.21 g Calcium, Ca132 mg Magnesium, Mg154 mg Phosphorus, P259 mg

477. Fresh Strawberry Salad Dressing

Prep Time: 10 min | **Cook Time:** 0 min | **Serve:** 2

- 1 C – Fresh Ripe Strawberries
- 1 T – Balsamic Vinegar Mosto Cotto 2 T – Lemon Oil
- 1/4 tsp Peppercorns 1 Pinch Sea Salt

1. Put all the ingredients into a food-processor or blender and blend until creamy, then transfer to a serving bowl or pitcher for serving.

Nutrition: Energy (calories): 339 kcal Protein: 0.57 g Fat: 1.83 g Carbohydrates: 82.37 g Calcium, Ca12 mg Magnesium, Mg13 mg Phosphorus, P21 mg

478. Pumpkin Balls

Prep Time: 15 min | **Cook Time:** 0 min | **Serve:** 18

- 1 cup almond butter
- 5 drops liquid stevia
- 2 tbsp coconut flour
- 2 tbsp pumpkin puree
- 1 tsp pumpkin pie spice

1. Mix pumpkin puree in a large bowl and almond butter until well combined.
2. Add liquid stevia, pumpkin pie spice, and coconut flour and mix well.
3. Make little balls from the mixture and place them on a baking tray.
4. Place in the freezer for 1 hour.

Nutrition: Calories: 96 Fat: 8 g Carbs: 4 g Sugar: 1 g Protein: 2 g Cholesterol: 0 mg

479. Smooth Peanut Butter Cream

Prep Time: 10 min | **Cook Time:** 0 min | **Serve:** 8

- 1/4 cup peanut butter
- 4 overripe bananas, chopped
- 1/3 cup cocoa powder
- 1/4 tsp vanilla extract
- 1/8 tsp salt

1. In the blender, add all the listed ingredients and blend until smooth.

Nutrition: Calories: 101 Fat: 5 g Carbs: 14 g Sugar: 7 g Protein: 3 g Cholesterol: 0 mg

480. Vanilla Avocado Popsicles

Prep Time: 20 min | **Cook Time:** 0 min | **Serve:** 6

- 2 avocadoes
- 1 tsp vanilla
- 1 cup almond milk
- 1 tsp liquid stevia
- 1/2 cup unsweetened cocoa powder

1. In the blender, add all the listed ingredients and blend smoothly.
2. Pour blended mixture into the Popsicle molds and place in the freezer until set.

Nutrition: Calories: 130 Fat: 12 g Carbs: 7 g Sugar: 1 g Protein: 3 g Cholesterol: 0 mg

481. Chocolate Popsicle

Prep Time: 20 min | **Cook Time:** 10 min | **Serve:** 6

- 4 oz unsweetened chocolate, chopped
- 6 drops liquid stevia
- 1 1/2 cups heavy cream

1. Add heavy cream into the microwave-safe bowl and microwave until it just begins the boiling.
2. Add chocolate into the heavy cream and set aside for 5 minutes.
3. Add liquid stevia into the heavy cream mixture and stir until chocolate is melted.
4. Pour mixture into the Popsicle molds and place in freezer for 4 hours or until set.

Nutrition: Calories: 198 Fat: 21 g Carbs: 6 g Sugar: 0.2 g Protein: 3 g Cholesterol: 41 mg

482. Raspberry Ice Cream

Prep Time: 10 min | **Cook Time:** 0 min | **Serve:** 2

- 1 cup frozen raspberries
- 1/2 cup heavy cream
- 1/8 tsp stevia powder

1. Blend all the specified ingredients in a blender until smooth.

Nutrition: Calories: 144 Fat: 11 g Carbs: 10 g Sugar: 4 g Protein: 2 g Cholesterol: 41 mg

483. Chocolate Almond Butter Brownie

Prep Time: 10 min | **Cook Time:** 16 min | **Serve:** 4

- 1 cup bananas, overripe
- 1/2 cup almond butter, melted
- 1 scoop protein powder
- 2 tbsp unsweetened cocoa powder

1. Preheat to 325 F the air fryer. Air fryer baking pan and set aside.
2. Preheat to 325 F the air fryer.
3. In the prepared pan, pour the batter, put it in the air fryer's basket, and cook for 16 minutes.

Nutrition: Calories: 82 Fat: 2 g Carbs: 11 g Sugar: 5 g Protein: 7 g Cholesterol: 16 mg

484. Peanut Butter Fudge

Prep Time: 10 min | **Cook Time:** 10 min | **Serve:** 20

- 1/4 cup almonds, toasted and chopped
- 12 oz smooth peanut butter
- 15 drops liquid stevia
- 3 tbsp coconut oil
- 4 tbsp coconut cream
- Pinch of salt

1. Line baking tray with parchment paper.
2. In a pan, melt the coconut-oil over low heat. Add peanut butter, coconut cream, stevia, and salt in a saucepan. Stir well.
3. Pour fudge mixture into the prepared baking tray and sprinkle chopped almonds on top.
4. Place the tray in the refrigerator for 1 hour or until set.
Nutrition: Calories: 131 Fat: 12 g Carbs: 4 g Sugar: 2 g Protein: 5 g Cholesterol: 0 mg

485. Almond Butter Fudge
Prep Time: 10 min | **Cook Time:** 10 min | **Serve:** 18
- 3/4 cup creamy almond butter
- 1 1/2 cups unsweetened chocolate chips

1. Line 8*4-inch pan with parchment paper and set aside.
2. Add chocolate chips and almond butter into the double boiler and cook over medium heat until the chocolate-butter mixture is melted. Stir well.
3. place the mixture into the prepared pan and place it in the freezer until set.
Nutrition: Calories: 197 Fat: 16 g Carbs: 7 g Sugar: 1 g Protein: 4 g Cholesterol: 0 mg

486. Homemade Coconut Ice Cream
Prep Time: 10 min | **Cook Time:** 95 min | **Serve:** 4
- 2 cups evaporated low-fat milk
- ⅓ cup low-fat condensed milk
- 1 cup low-fat coconut milk
- 1 cup stevia/xylitol/bacon syrup
- 2 scoops whey protein concentrate
- 2 tsp. sugar-free coconut extract
- 1 tsp. dried coconut

1. Mix all the ingredients together in a bowl.
2. Heat the mixture over medium heat until it starts to bubble.
3. Remove from the heat and then leave the mixture to cool.
4. Chill mixture for about an hour, then freeze in ice cream maker as outlined by the manufacturer's directions.
Nutrition: Calories: 182, Fat: 2 g, Carbohydrates: 20 g, Protein: 22 g

487. Coconut Panna Cotta
Prep Time: 5 min | **Cook Time:** 20 min | **Serve:** 2
- 2 cups skimmed milk
- 1/2 cup water
- 1 tsp. sugar-free coconut extract
- 1 envelope powdered grass-fed – organic gelatin – sugar-free
- 2 scoops whey protein isolate
- 4 tbsp. stevia/xylitol/yacon syrup
- ⅓ cup fresh raspberries
- 2 tbsp. fresh mint

1. In a non-stick pan, pour the milk, stevia, water, and coconut Extract.
2. Bring to a boil.
3. Slowly add the gelatin and stir well until the mixtures start to thicken.
4. When ready, divide the mix among the small silicon cups.
5. Refrigerate overnight to relax and hang up.
6. Remove through the fridge and thoroughly turn each cup over ahead of a serving plate.
7. Garnish with raspberries and fresh mint, serve and revel in.

Nutrition: Calories: 130, Fat: 3 g, Carbohydrates: 14 g, Protein: 29 g

488. Blueberry Lemon Cake
Prep Time: 10 min | **Cook Time:** 40 min | **Serve:** 4
For the cake:
- 2/3 cup almond flour
- 5 eggs
- ⅓ cup almond milk, unsweetened
- ¼ cup erythritol
- 2 tsp. vanilla extract
- Juice of 2 lemons
- 1 tsp. lemon zest
- ½ tsp. baking soda
- Pinch of salt
- ½ cup fresh blueberries
- 2 tbsp. butter, melted

For the frosting:
- ½ cup heavy cream
- Juice of 1 lemon
- 1/8 cup erythritol

1. Preheat the oven to 35˚F
2. In a bowl, add the almond flour, eggs, and almond milk and mix well until smooth.
3. Add the erythritol, a pinch of salt, baking soda, lemon zest, lemon juice, and vanilla extract. Mix and combine well.
4. Fold in the blueberries.
5. Use the butter to grease the pans.
6. Pour the batter into the greased pans.
7. Put on a baking sheet for even baking.
8. Put in the oven to bake until cooked through in the middle and slightly brown on the top, about 35 to 40 minutes.
9. Let cool before removing from the pan.
10. Mix the erythritol, lemon juice, and heavy cream. Mix well.
11. Pour frosting on top.
Nutrition: Calories:274, Fat: 23 g, Carbohydrates: 8 g, Protein: 9 g

489. Rich Chocolate Mousse
Prep Time: 10 min | **Cook Time:** 15 min | **Serve:** 3
- ¼ cup low-fat coconut cream
- 2 cups fat-free Greek-style yogurt, strained
- 4 tsp. powered cocoa, no added sugar
- 2 tbsp. stevia/xylitol/bacon syrup
- 1 tsp. natural vanilla extract

1. Combine all the ingredientsin a medium bowl and mix well.
2. Put individual serving bowls or glasses and refrigerate.
Nutrition: Calories: 269, Fat: 3 g, Carbohydrates: 20 g, Protein: 43 g

490. Raspberry Cheesecake
Prep Time: 10 min | **Cook Time:** 25 min | **Serve:** 6
- 2/3 cup coconut oil, melted
- ½ cup cream cheese
- 6 eggs
- 3 tbsp. granulated sweetener
- 1 tsp. vanilla extract
- ½ tsp. baking powder
- ¾ cup raspberries

1. In a bowl, beat together the coconut oil and cream cheese until smooth.
2. Beat in eggs, then beat in the sweetener, vanilla, and baking powder until smooth.
3. Pour the batter into a pan and finally smooth the top. Scatter the raspberries on top.
4. Bake for 25/30 minutes or until the center is firm.
Nutrition: Calories: 176, Fat: 18 g, Carbohydrates: 3 g, Protein: 6 g

491. Peanut Butter Brownie Ice Cream Sandwiches

Prep Time: 2 min | **Cook Time:** 2 min | **Serve:** 2
- 1 packet Medifast Brownie Mix
- 3 tablespoons water
- 1 Peanut Butter Crunch Bar or any bar of your choice
- 2 tablespoons Peanut Butter Powder
- 1 tablespoon water
- 2 tablespoons cool whip

1. Melt the Brownie Mix with water.
2. Add in the Peanut Butter Crunch until a dough is formed.
3. Spoon 4 dough balls on a plate and flatten using the palm of your hands.
4. Make sure that the dough is 1/4 inch thick.
5. Place in a microwave oven and cook for 2 minutes.
6. Meanwhile, mix the Peanut Butter Powder and water to form a paste.
7. Add cool whip. Leave to cool in the fridge for minimun 1 hour.
8. Take the cookies out from the microwave oven and allow it to cool.
9. Once cooled, spoon the peanut butter ice cream in between two cookies.
Nutrition: Calories per serving: 410 Cal, Protein: 8.3 g, Carbohydrates: 57.6 g, Fat: 13.2 g, Sugar: 5.3g

492. Chocolate Frosty

Prep Time: 20 min | **Cook Time:** 0 min | **Serve:** 4
- 2 tbsp unsweetened cocoa powder
- 1 cup heavy whipping cream
- 1 tbsp almond butter
- 5 drops liquid stevia
- 1 tsp vanilla

1. Add cream into the medium bowl and beat using the hand mixer for 5 minutes.
2. Add remaining ingredients and blend until thick cream forms.
3. Pour in serving bowls and place them in the freezer for 30 minutes.
Nutrition: Calories: 137 Fat: 13 g Carbs: 3 g Sugar: 0.5 g Protein: 2 g, Cholesterol: 41 mg

493. Tiramisu Milkshake

Cook Time: 5 min | **Serve:** 1
- 1 sachet Frosty Coffee Soft Serve Treat ½ cup ice
- 6 ounces plain low-fat Greek yogurt
- ½ cup almond milk
- 2 tablespoons sugar-free chocolate
- 2 tablespoons whipped topping

1.Place all ingredients, except the whipped, in a blender.
2.Pulse until smooth.
3.Pour in glass and top with whipped topping.

Nutrition: Calories per serving: 239; Protein: 23.7g; Carbs: 64.2g; Fat: 22.8g Sugar: 15.2g

494. Weight Watchers Macaroni Salad Recipe with Tuna

Prep Time: 15 min | **Cook Time:** 10 min
- 1/2 Cup of Mayonnaise Medium
- 1 tbsp of Red Vinegar
- 1 Tbsp Dijon Mustard
- 1/2 Tbsps Ground Garlic
- 1 Cup of Chopped Celery
- 1/3 Red Onion Cup, Chopped
- 2 Tbsps of Chopped Fresh Parsley
- Salt & Pepper
- 3 Tuna Ounces, In Water
- Macaroni Whole Wheat Elbow (8 Ounces)

1. We must cook the macaroni in salted water first. In order to get the exact times and water measurements, use the kit. Drain the pasta and, after it is cooked, set it aside in a wide tub.
2. When the pasta cooks, the mayonnaise, vinegar, mustard, and garlic powder blend together.
3. Add the mixture of mayonnaise to the cooked pasta, and stir until well mixed.
4. The salmon, celery, cabbage, and parsley are rolled in. Season with salt and pepper to taste.
5. Depending on your tastes, you can serve the dish warm or cold.

495. Big Mac Salad

Prep Time: 10 min | **Cook Time:** 10 min
Salad Ingredients
- 1 pound lean ground beef
- 1 tsp of Worcestershire sauce
- 1/2 tsp of onion salt
- 1 tsp of minced garlic
- 1 large head romaine, chopped
- 1 large diced tomato
- 1/2 diced small red or white onion
- 1 cup of light cheddar cheese
- 12 diced dill pickles

Dressing Ingredients
- 2 Tbsp of Light Mayo Best Foods or Light Kraft Mayo
- 2 tbsp of nonfat Greek
- 2 tbsp of Ketchup Heinz
- 1/2 tbsp of water
- 1 tbsp of minced white onion
- 1 tsp of sugar
- 1 tsp of sweet pickle relish
- 1 tsp of white vinegar
- dash of salt

1. Spray with non-stick cooking spray on a large skillet. Add the lean ground beef and onion salt and cook, occasionally stirring, for around 5-7 minutes. Using a fork to make the meat crumble.
2. Add sauce from Worcestershire and garlic mined. Stir before the garlic is added. Cook meat until it isn't pink anymore. Take off the heat to cool it down.
3. Measure out 4 ounces of ground beef using a food scale and split equally between the salads. Divide the romaine into four servings, the tomatoes equally.

4. Place 4 ounces of meat on top of lettuce, 1/4 cup cheese, add tomatoes, 2 cups of dressing, and top with diced pickles

Dressing Ingredients:

1.Whisk or mix light mayonnaise, white vinegar, plain fat or Greek yogurt, sugar ketchup, salt, water, sweet pickle relish, minced white onion, and sugar in a small bowl or in a food processor. Pour into an airtight jar. Place dressing in the refrigerator for a minimum of 30 minutes.

496.Loaded Caesar Salad with Crunchy Chickpeas

Prep Time: 5 min | **Cook Time:** 20 min | **Serve:** 6

For the chickpeas
- 2 (15-ounce) cans chickpeas, drained and rinsed
- 2 tablespoons extra-virgin olive oil
- 1 teaspoon kosher salt
- 1 teaspoon garlic powder
- 1 teaspoon onion powder
- 1 teaspoon dried oregano

For the dressing
- ½ cup mayonnaise
- 2 tablespoons grated Parmesan cheese
- 2 tablespoons freshly squeezed lemon juice
- 1 clove garlic, peeled and smashed
- 1 teaspoon Dijon mustard
- ½ tablespoon Worcestershire sauce
- ½ tablespoon anchovy paste

For the salad
- 3 heads romaine lettuce, cut into bite-size pieces

To make the chickpeas:

1. Preheat the oven to 450°F. Line a baking sheet with parchment paper.
2. Add the chickpeas, oil, salt, garlic powder, onion powder, and oregano in a small container. Scatter the coated chickpeas on the prepared baking sheet.
3. Roast for about 20 minutes, tossing occasionally, until the chickpeas are golden and have a bit of crunch.

To make the dressing:

1. In a small bowl, whisk the mayonnaise, Parmesan, lemon juice, garlic, mustard, Worcestershire sauce, and anchovy paste until combined.

To make the salad:

1. In a large container combine the lettuce and dressing. Toss to coat. Top with the roasted chickpeas and serve.

Cooking Tip: Don't wash out that bowl you used for the chickpeas — the remaining oil adds a great punch of flavor to blanched green beans or another simply cooked vegetable.

Nutrition: Calories: 367, Total fat: 22 g, Total carbs: 35 g, Cholesterol: 9 mg, Fiber: 13 g, Protein: 12 g, Sodium: 407 mg

497.Shrimp Cobb Salad

Prep Time: 25 min | **Cook Time:** 10 min | **Serve:** 2

- 4 slices center-cut bacon
- 1 lb. large shrimp, peeled and deveined
- 1/2 teaspoon ground paprika
- 1/4 teaspoon ground black pepper
- 1/4 teaspoon salt, divided
- 2 1/2 tablespoons fresh lemon juice
- 1 1/2 tablespoons extra-virgin olive oil
- 1/2 teaspoon whole grain Dijon mustard
- 1 (10 oz.) package romaine lettuce hearts, chopped
- 2 cups cherry tomatoes, quartered
- 1 ripe avocado, cut into wedges
- 1 cup shredded carrots

1. Cook the bacon for 4 minutes on each side in a large skillet over medium heat till crispy.
2. Take away from the skillet and place on paper towels; let cool for 5 minutes. Break the bacon into bits. Throw out most of the bacon fat, leaving behind only 1 tablespoon in the skillet.
3. Bring the skillet back to medium-high heat. Add black pepper and paprika to the shrimp for seasoning.
4. Cook the shrimp around 2 minutes each side until it is opaque.
5. Sprinkle with 1/8 teaspoon of salt for seasoning.
6. Combine the remaining 1/8 teaspoon of salt, mustard, olive oil and lemon juice together in a small bowl. Stir in the romaine hearts.
7. On each serving plate, place on 1 and 1/2 cups of romaine lettuce. Add on top the same amounts of avocado, carrots, tomatoes, shrimp and bacon.

Nutrition: Calories: 528, Total Carbohydrate: 22.7 g, Cholesterol: 365 mg, Total Fat: 28.7 g, Protein: 48.9 g, Sodium: 1166 mg

499.Strawberry, Orange & Rocket Salad

Prep Time: 15 min | **Serve:** 4

For Salad:
- 6 cups fresh rocket
- 1½ cups fresh strawberries, hulled and sliced 2 oranges, peeled and segmented

For Dressing:
- 2 tablespoons fresh lemon juice
- 1 tablespoon raw honey
- 2 teaspoons extra-virgin olive oil
- 1 teaspoon Dijon mustard
- Salt and ground black pepper, as required

1.For Salad: in a salad bowl, place all ingredients and mix.
2.For Dressing: place all ingredients in another bowl and beat until well combined.
3.Place dressing on top of salad and toss to coat well.

500.Strawberry & Asparagus Salad

Prep Time: 15 min | **Cook Time:** 5 min | **Serve:** 8

- 2 pounds fresh asparagus, trimmed and sliced
- 3 cups fresh strawberries, hulled and sliced
- ¼ cup extra-virgin olive oil
- ¼ cup balsamic vinegar
- 2 tablespoons maple syrup
- Salt and ground black pepper, as required

1.In a pan of water, add the asparagus over medium-high heat and bring to a boil.
2.Boil the asparagus for about 2-3 minutes or until al dente.
3.Drain the asparagus and immediately transfer into a bowl of ice water to cool completely.
4.With paper towels, drain the asparagus and pat dry.
5.In a big bowl, add the asparagus and strawberries and mix.
6.In a little bowl, add the olive oil, vinegar, honey, salt and black pepper and beat until well blended.
7. Place the dressing over the asparagus strawberry mixture and gently toss to coat.
8. Refrigerate for about 1 hour before serving.

CPSIA information can be obtained
at www.ICGtesting.com
Printed in the USA
BVHW011750150321
602550BV00009B/771